Clinical Guide to Sports Injuries

Roald Bahr, MD, PhD

Sverre Mæhlum, MD, PhD

Editors

Tommy Bolic

Medical Illustrator

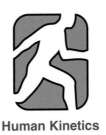

Human Kinetics

Library of Congress Cataloging-in-Publication Data

Idrettsskader. English.

Clinical guide to sports injuries / Roald Bahr, Sverre Mæhlum, editors; Tommy Bolic, medical illustrator.

p. ; cm.

Includes index.

ISBN 0-7360-4117-6

1. Sports injuries--Patients--Rehabilitation.

[DNLM: 1. Athletic Injuries--rehabilitation. 2. Sports Medicine--methods. QT 261 I21 2003a] I. Bahr, Roald, 1957- II. Mæhlum, Sverre, 1944- III. Title.

RD97.I3713 2003

617.1'027--dc21   2003051124

ISBN: 0-7360-4117-6

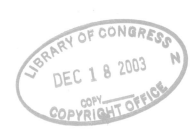

Figure 1.1 is adapted from *Clinical Sports Medicine,* vol. 11, "Cell-matrix response in tendon injury," pp. 533-578, Copyright 1992, with permission from Elsevier. Figure 1.4 is adapted, by permission, from S.L. Woo et al., 1987, "The biomechanical and morphological changes in the medial collateral ligament of the rabbit after immobilization and remobilization," *Journal of Bone and Joint Surgery American* 69:1200-1211. Figure 3.1 is adapted, by permission, from W.H. Meeuwisse, 1994, "Assessing causation in sport injury: A multifactorial model," *Clinical Journal of Sport Medicine* 4: 166-170.

This book is an English translation of *Idrettsskader,* published in 2002 by Gazette bok.

Managing Editors: Petter Thorsrud, Maggie Schwarzentraub, and Anne Cole; **Translator:** Edith Matteson; **Medical Reader for the English Translation:** Jonathan Reeser, MD, PhD; **Copyeditor:** Felice Bassuk; **Proofreader:** Red Inc.; **Indexer:** Marie Rizzo; **Permission Manager:** Dalene Reeder; **Graphic Designer:** Børre Gammelsrud and Nancy Rasmus; **Graphic Artist:** Yvonne Griffith; **Art/Photo Manager:** Kelly Hendren; **Cover Designer:** Keith Blomberg; **Illustrators:** Tommy Bolic (medical art) and Lill-Ann Prøis (rehabilitation exercises); **Printer:** Maracle; **Financial Support for Translation:** Marketing Unit for Norwegian International Non-fiction (MUNIN)

Printed in Canada   10 9 8 7 6 5 4 3 2 1

Human Kinetics
Web site: www.HumanKinetics.com

United States: Human Kinetics, P.O. Box 5076, Champaign, IL 61825-5076
800-747-4457
e-mail: humank@hkusa.com

Canada: Human Kinetics, 475 Devonshire Road Unit 100, Windsor, ON N8Y 2L5
800-465-7301 (in Canada only)
e-mail: orders@hkcanada.com

Europe: Human Kinetics, 107 Bradford Road, Stanningley, Leeds LS28 6AT, United Kingdom
+44 (0) 113 255 5665
e-mail: hk@hkeurope.com

Australia: Human Kinetics, 57A Price Avenue, Lower Mitcham, South Australia 5062
08 8277 1555
e-mail: liahka@senet.com.au

New Zealand: Human Kinetics, P.O. Box 105-231, Auckland Central
09-523-3462
e-mail: hkp@ihug.co.nz

Contents

Types and Causes of Injuries

Roald Bahr and Sverre Mæhlum

Regular physical activity is probably the most important thing a person can do to stay healthy. Today we know that physical activity reduces the risk of premature death in addition to the risk of cardiovascular disease, high blood pressure, type 2 diabetes, and even some types of cancer. Indeed, physical inactivity can present as great a health risk as smoking, obesity, hypercholesterolemia, or hypertension. In fact, intense exercise is not required to accrue significant health benefits, which can be achieved through moderate physical activity even at an advanced age. Furthermore, individuals who are the least fit are the ones who stand to derive the greatest health benefits from regular physical activity.

Unfortunately, physical activity–whether in the form of work, sport, outdoor activity, play, or physical education–is not without potential side effects. Injuries are a particular risk. Nevertheless, the net health effect of exercise is positive–the benefits of physical activity far outweigh the physical problems caused by injuries.

Acute Injuries and Overuse Injuries

A sports injury may be defined as tissue damage that occurs as a result of participation in sport or exercise. However, in this book the term applies to any damage that results from any form of physical activity. Physical activity can be defined as moving or using one's body, and it may include numerous forms of exertion such as work, fitness exercise, outdoor pursuits, recreational play, training, general conditioning, "working out," and structured physical education activities.

Sports injuries can be divided into *acute injuries* and *overuse injuries*, depending on the mechanism of injury and the onset of symptoms. Acute injuries occur suddenly and have a clearly defined cause or onset. In contrast, overuse injuries occur gradually. In most cases, it is easy to classify an injury as either acute or due to overuse. In some cases, however, it can be difficult to distinguish between the two, particularly when the symptoms have a sudden onset even though the injury may actually represent the end result of a chronic process. For example, an athlete with a stress fracture of the second metatarsal will often state that their symptoms originated during a specific run and perhaps even from a specific step. By the previous definition, then, the injury could be classified as an acute injury. In actuality the stress fracture occurred because the involved bone had become fatigued and weakened from overuse over time. Consequently, such injuries should be classified as overuse injuries.

As shown in figure 1.1, the tissue injury process has often been under way for a period of time before the athlete becomes symptomatic. Repetitive low-grade forces that lead to tissue microtrauma may result in overuse injuries. In most cases, the tissue will undergo repair without demonstrable clinical symptoms. However, if the process of tissue overload continues, over time the ability of the tissue to repair itself can be exceeded, resulting in a symptomatic clinical overuse injury.

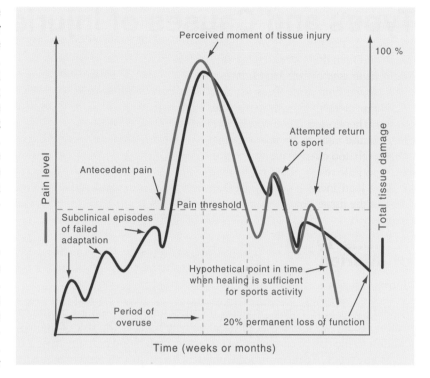

Figure 1.1 Hypothetical overview of pain and tissue injury in a typical overuse injury.

The difference between acute injuries and overuse injuries can also be described in biomechanical terms. Dynamic or static muscle action creates internal resistance in the loaded structures (stress) that counteracts tissue deformation (strain). All tissue has a characteristic ability to tolerate deformation and stress, and injuries occur when this tolerance level is exceeded. Acute injuries occur when tissue loading is sufficient to cause sudden irreversible deformation of the tissue. By contrast, overuse injuries occur as a result of repeated overloading, each incidence of which, alone, is not enough to cause irreversible deformation, but which when accumulated over time exceeds the tissue injury threshold.

Acute injuries occur most commonly in sports featuring high speeds, a high risk of falling (e.g., downhill skiing), and in team sports characterized by frequent, high energy contact between players (e.g., ice hockey and soccer). Overuse injuries make up the large portion of injuries in aerobic sports that require lengthy training sessions with a monotonous routine (e.g., long-distance running, bicycling, or cross-country skiing). In addition, overuse injuries may also occur in technical sports, in which the same movement is repeated numerous times (e.g., tennis, javelin throwing, weightlifting, and high jumping).

Why Do Injuries Occur?

The basic principle of training is that the body reacts predictably to a specific physical training load with tissue-specific adaptation. Loading that exceeds what an athlete is accustomed to will cause the tissue being trained to attempt to adapt to the new demands being placed on it. For example, resistance training provides a stimulus that causes the muscles to increase production of contractile proteins. The muscle fibers subsequently become larger (hypertrophy) and more numerous (hyperplasia). In addition, the trained muscle specifically adapts to training that is primarily aerobic (endurance oriented) or anaerobic (strength oriented). This principle of specific adaptation to imposed demands applies to all types of tissue, including bone, tendon, ligament, muscle, and cartilage, all of which adapt accordingly by becoming stronger and more resilient (figure 1.2).

If the training load exceeds the tissue's ability to adapt, injuries will eventually occur. The risk of overuse injuries increases when training load increases, such as an increase in the duration of individual training sessions or an increase in training intensity or the frequency of training sessions. Often the duration, intensity, and frequency of training increase at the same time, such as at a training camp or at the beginning of the season. Therefore, it is common to say that overuse injuries are due to doing "too much, too often, too quickly, and with too little rest," which means that training load increases at a rate that exceeds the tissue's ability to adapt.

Various Types of Injuries

Sports injuries can be divided into *soft-tissue injuries* (cartilage injuries, muscle injuries, tendon injuries, and ligament injuries) and *skeletal injuries* (fractures). The various types of tissue have distinctly different biomechanical properties and their ability to adapt to training also varies. This chapter examines the characteristics of the various types of tissue and the ways in which the skeleton, cartilage, muscles, tendons, and ligaments can be injured.

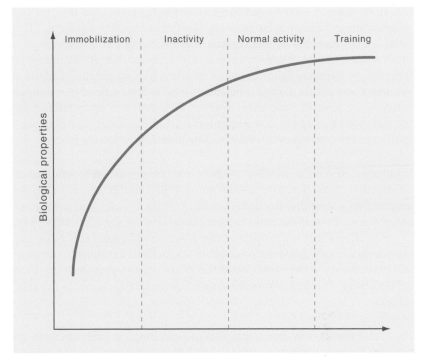

Figure 1.2 Adaptation to training. Inactivity significantly weakens the tissue's biological properties, whereas exercise improves function.

Ligaments

Structure and Function

Ligaments consist of collagen tissue that connects one bone to another. Ligaments function primarily to passively stabilize the joints. In addition, ligaments serve an important proprioceptive function.

Ligaments primarily consist of cells, collagen fibers, and proteoglycans. Fibroblasts are the most abundant cell type, and they function to produce collagen (primarily type I, in addition to several other types as well). The amount of proteoglycan is much lower than the amount found in cartilage. Although the collagen fibers in tendons are organized in a parallel manner (in the longitudinal direction of the muscles), the orientation of the collagen fibers in ligaments can be parallel, oblique, or even spiral (e.g., the anterior cruciate ligament). The organization of fiber direction is specific to the function of each ligament. In addition, ligaments contain slightly more elastic fibers than do tendons.

Ligaments may insert directly or indirectly into the bone. Direct insertion occurs with a transition zone consisting of fibrocartilage and mineralized fibrocartilage (including specialized collagen fibers that go down into the bone vertically). Indirect insertion occurs when the ligament grows into the surrounding periosteum.

Ligaments may be intra-articular (i.e., localized within a joint or inside the joint capsule), capsular (where the ligament projects as a thickening of the joint capsule), or extracapsular (localized outside the joint capsule). The cruciate ligaments are intra-articular ligaments. The anterior talofibular ligament is a capsular ligament, where it may be difficult to distinguish between the ligament and the rest of the capsule, whereas the calcaneofibular ligament is an extracapsular ligament. The type of ligament is important for its healing potential following a total rupture. A total rupture of an intra-articular ligament, such as the anterior cruciate ligament, will not heal, whereas the capsular ligaments have excellent healing potential. Blood supply to the ligaments also differs. Capsular ligaments tend to have a good blood supply, just as the surrounding joint capsule does, whereas intra-articular ligaments are supplied from the ends with a marginal vascularization zone in the midzone. Adequate blood supply is an important component of the healing potential following injury.

Ligaments contain a number of different peripheral nerve endings that transmit information about position, movement, and pain to the central nervous system. This information is essential to effective control of the muscles that surround a joint (such as the knee). Even if the main function is passive stabilization of the joint, much evidence indicates that the proprioceptive function of ligaments is more important than previously thought. Ligamentous injuries may reduce the ability to register the position and movements of the joint, even if the injury does not result in significant mechanical instability. This loss of proprioceptive awareness may increase the risk of recurrent injuries.

Figure 1.3 shows how ligaments react to stretching. At first, the wavy pattern of the collagen fibers straightens out and very little force is required to cause a significant change in length. If force increases further, the collagen fibers will be stretched, and the relationship between load and deformation becomes linear. This means that the ligament serves as an ideal spring in the elastic zone, as long as the change in length does not exceed about 4%. If a force causes a change in length in excess of this, the collagen fibers will rupture—individual fibers initially and then all fibers will fail (a total rupture). The strength and stiffness of a ligament depend on its length and cross-sectional area. The greater the cross-sectional area, the stronger and stiffer the ligament. A longer ligament is less stiff, but the maximum tensile strength does not change if the cross-sectional area is the same.

Adaptation to Training

Connective tissue adapts slowly to repetitive loading but weakens rapidly as a result of immobilization (figure 1.4). Ligaments adapt to training by increasing the cross-sectional area, as well as by changing the material properties so that they become stronger per area unit. Normal everyday activity (without specific training) is apparently sufficient to maintain 80% to 90% of a ligament's mechanical potential. Systematic training increases ligament strength by 10% to 20%. The negative effect of immobilization sets in quickly, however. After a few weeks, strength is reduced to about one-half of the pre-immobilization baseline value. Systematic training over several weeks can restore the tensile strength of the ligament

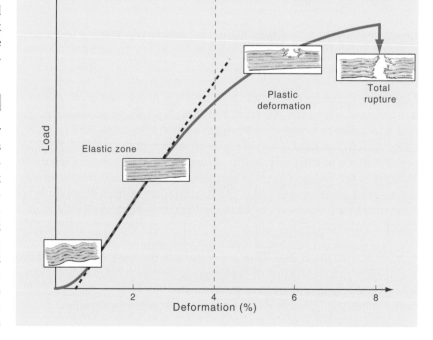

Figure 1.3 Stress deformation curve for ligaments.

substance, although the ligament-bone junction will remain weaker for several months despite regular loading.

Ligament Injuries

Unlike tendons, which are subject to both acute and overuse injuries, ligaments are usually injured as the result of acute trauma. The typical injury mechanism involves sudden overloading, stretching the ligament while the joint is in an extreme position. For example, traumatic ankle inversion may cause the lateral ligaments—primarily the anterior talo-fibular ligament—to rupture.

Ruptures may occur in the mid-substance of the ligament or at the ligament-bone junction (figure 1.5). Sometimes avulsion fractures also occur, when the ligament pulls a piece of the bone off with it. This fragment is usually shaped like the top of a hard boiled egg. Several factors (including the athlete's age) determine the location of the rupture. For example, children are more susceptible to avulsion fractures, midsubstance ruptures occur more commonly in adolescents and young adults, while the ligament-bone junction is typically the point of tissue failure in middle-aged patients, and avulsion fractures are more common in the elderly, particularly if the skeleton is osteoporotic.

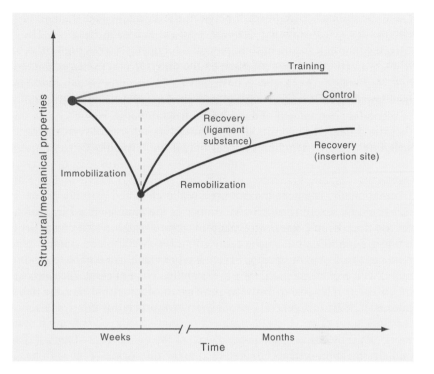

Figure 1.4 Relationship between training, immobilization, and remobilization of the ligaments.

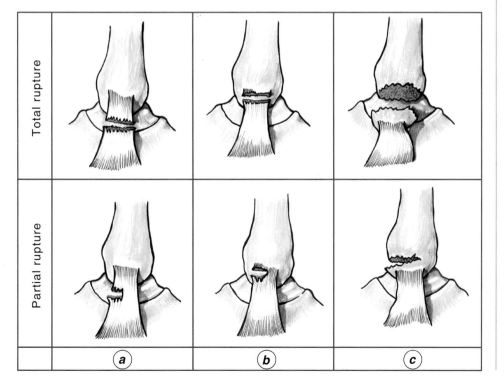

Figure 1.5 Ligament injuries. Total and partial ruptures may occur *(a)* in the midsubstance and *(b)* at the site of ligament insertion and *(c)* as avulsion fractures.

Overuse injuries of ligaments are rare, and symptomatic inflammatory conditions seldom occur. Nevertheless, overuse injuries may occur if a ligament is gradually stretched out due to repetitive microtrauma. One such example is the shoulder joint, where throwers and other overhead athletes (e.g., javelin throwers and baseball, hand-ball, and volleyball players) may stretch out their anterior capsular ligaments. This may impair glenohumeral stability and predispose the athlete to shoulder pain due to secondary entrapment of the subacromial structures. However, one must be aware that the primary ligament injury (overstretching) does not typically result in clinical symptoms. Rather, symptoms appear only if the instability causes muscular dysfunction and/or results in injury to other associated structures (e.g., the rotator cuff).

Internationally, ligament injuries are usually classified as mild (grade 1), moderate (grade 2), or severe (grade 3). Mild injuries are characterized by structural damage on the microscopic level, with slight local tenderness. Partial tears are classified as moderate injuries, and usually result in visible swelling and notable tenderness, but tend not to affect joint stability. Severe injuries result in a complete rupture of the ligament, with significant swelling and instability. Nevertheless, because of the variable, inconsistent relationship between the degree of structural damage, tenderness, and joint instability, this general classification of ligamentous injuries is almost worthless for clinical purposes. Instead, ligament or joint-specific classification systems may be more clinically useful to grade the degree of the injury. These types of diagnostic tests and classification systems are described in the discussion of the various relevant body regions in chapters 4-15.

An acute ligament rupture sets off a series of events–termed the inflammatory cascade–which can be divided into three stages: the inflammatory phase (phase 1), the proliferative phase (phase 2), and the maturation phase (phase 3).

The Inflammatory Process

Inflammation is a local response that occurs in vascularized tissue in response to loading of sufficient magnitude that it results in cell damage. Inflammation consists of a characteristic chain of vascular, biochemical, and cellular events that may result in repair, regeneration, or formation of scar tissue. The five cardinal signs of inflammation are rubor (redness), tumor (swelling), calor (heat, increased temperature), dolor (pain), and *functio laesa* (loss of function). Of the cardinal signs, pain is generally the most prominent in sports injuries, both as a symptom that the patient experiences subjectively and as a finding on physical exam (tenderness to palpation). However, it should be noted that painful conditions are by no means always related to inflammation, as will be described later in the section on tendon injuries. Under normal conditions, the cellular elements of the blood are (for the most part) isolated intravascularly. However, an injury to the vascular endothelium may result in leakage of plasma components, as well as erythrocytes and leukocytes, into the extravascular space. The acute inflammatory process is activated by a series of different mediators that primarily result in increased vascular permeability, activation of leukocytes, blood platelets, and the coagulation system (figure 1.6). Vasoactive mediators bind to specific receptors on endothelial cells and smooth muscle cells, resulting in either vasoconstriction or dilatation. Neutrophilic granulocytes, monocytes, and lymphocytes are attracted to the injury site by chemotactic factors released from the injured tissue. These "white blood cells" in turn release a series of inflammatory mediators, including prostaglandins and leukotrienes.

The Inflammatory Phase (Phase 1)

The inflammatory phase begins with bleeding and plasma exudation. Activation of the coagulation cascade initiates clotting, which eventually forms a meshwork of fibrin, fibronectin, and collagen.

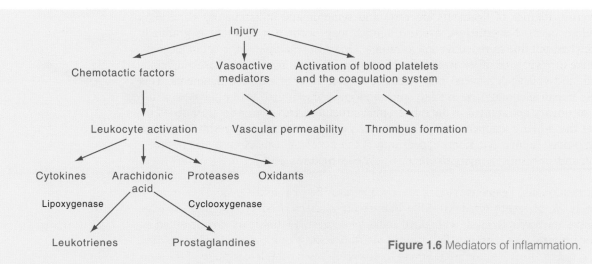

Figure 1.6 Mediators of inflammation.

This meshwork provides some initial strength to the clot. Neutrophilic granulocytes release a series of proteolytic enzymes that dissolve the damaged extracellular matrix. Platelets and macrophages release growth factors that not only attract pericytes, endothelial cells, and fibroblasts but also stimulate cell division. The inflammatory phase lasts a few days.

The Proliferative Phase (Phase 2)

The proliferative phase is characterized by the accumulation of large numbers of endothelial cells, myofibroblasts, and fibroblasts at the site of the injury. Ingrowth of new capillaries begins at the edge of the injury site, and within a few days a rich capillary network is established. The myofibroblasts and fibroblasts organize themselves perpendicularly to the capillaries resulting in the formation of an immature granulation tissue. These cells produce an extracellular network that initially consists of fibronectin and proteoglycans. After a week, the production of collagen increases greatly. At the same time, there is continuous breakdown of the initial clot, the injured extracellular matrix, and the newly formed matrix. The macrophages accomplish this by phagocytosing the superfluous cellular components. Through the continuous deposition and removal of extracellular matrix and cellular debris, the injured tissue is gradually repaired and remodeled, demonstrating an increased tensile strength. The proliferation stage lasts a few weeks.

The Maturation Phase (Phase 3)

The maturation stage establishes the final tissue structure through continuous remodeling of the scar tissue. During this phase, the number of macrophages is significantly reduced and the mature blood supply is finally established by selective removal of capillaries with low blood flow. Thicker collagen fibers are formed in the direction of tissue tension, and a network of cross bridges is established between them. Therefore, the form and function of the scar tissue depends on the degree to which the tissue is subjected to loading during this stage, which may last several months.

Tendons

Structure and Function

Tendons consist of connective tissue that attaches muscle to bone. Their essential function is to transfer force from the muscles to the skeleton, thereby producing motion and contributing to joint stabilization. Tendons are comprised primarily of type I collagen, which makes up 80% to 90% of the tendon. Structurally, tendons closely resemble ligaments. The collagen in tendon is arranged in parallel arrays of tropocollagen, which are in turn organized into successively larger structures, termed microfibrils, subfibrils, fibrils,

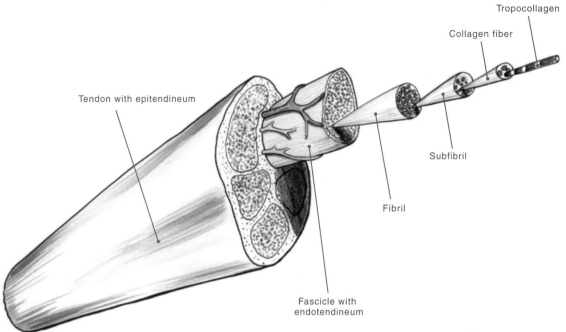

Tropocollagen

Collagen fiber

Tendon with epitendineum

Subfibril

Fibril

Fascicle with
endotendineum

Figure 1.7 The structure
of tendons.

and fascicles (figure 1.7). The strict organization into parallel bundles of various sizes is the principle structural difference between tendons and ligaments. The organization of collagen in ligaments is more variable and dependent on function.

Fascicles are surrounded by a loose connective tissue (endotenon), which makes the fascicles mobile in relation to each other. The endotenon also contains veins, nerve fibers, and lymphatics. The surface of the tendon is surrounded by epitenon, a white synovial-like membrane made of loose connective tissue that also supports blood vessels, lymphatics, and nerves. Some tendons are covered by a loose areolar connective tissue (paratenon), which envelopes the entire tendon.

The muscle cell ends in a number of microscopic membranous infoldings that protrude like small fingers into the myotendinous junction. The collagen fibers creep into the folds that form between the fingers and attach to the basal membrane of the muscle. At the other end, the tendons attach to bone via fibrocartilage and mineralized fibrocartilage. A few collagen fibers (Sharpey's fibers) penetrate the mineralized fibrocartilage into the subchondral bone, contributing to better attachment.

The relationship between stress and deformation of tendons is similar to that of ligaments (figure 1.3). Initially, the collagen fibers are easily stretched from their normal wavy appearance. In the elastic zone the tendon behaves like an ideal spring, whereas ruptures occur in the deformation zones: single fibers first, then total tendon ruptures.

Adaptation to Training

Tendons adapt to training in the same manner as do ligaments—by increasing in cross-sectional area and improving the material properties of the connective tissues of which they are composed.

Tendon Injuries

Tendons are subject to both acute and overuse injuries. Because tendons are usually superficial, they can be severed by a penetrating trauma (such as a stab wound) or a deep laceration (such as one caused by the edge of a skate). Acute tendon ruptures occur if force is applied that exceeds the tendon's tolerance. Tendon ruptures usually occur in connection with eccentric force generation, such as in the Achilles tendon when pushing off at the start of a sprint run. Tendon ruptures, which may be partial or total, usually occur in the mid-tendon substance but may also occur at the bone-tendon junction or as avulsion fractures. Acute tendon injuries occur most commonly in athletes between 30 and 50 years of age who participate in "explosive" sports. Tendon ruptures may occur without previous symptoms or warning. However, more detailed study reveals that degenerative changes are often present in the tendon, thereby apparently predisposing the athlete to more serious injury.

Tendons are the tissue most susceptible to overuse injury. Several different terms are used to describe these overuse injuries: tendinitis (tendon inflammation), tenosynovitis (tendon sheath inflammation), tenoperiostitis (inflammation of tendon insertions and origins), periostitis (periosteal inflammation), and bursitis/hemobursitis (bursal inflammation, possibly with associated hemorrhage). Each of these terms describes a part of the tendon or the surrounding tissue that appears to be affected. Note that all of the descriptors end in "itis," suggesting that the underlying pathophysiology is inflammatory.

Although tendon injuries have traditionally been characterized as inflammatory, the actual pathogenesis of overuse tendon injuries remains uncertain. While tendon loading does not normally cause more than a 4% change in length (i.e., within the physiological elastic zone), some sports require repetitive loading in excess of this (4% to 8% change in length), potentially causing collagen fibrils to rupture. Therefore, one possible explanation for what has been called tendinitis is repetitive microtrauma that exceeds the instrinsic ability of the tendon to repair itself, resulting in inflammation. It is also possible that cumulative microtrauma might affect collagen cross-bridges, other matrix proteins, or microvascular elements of the tendon.

However, one problem with this explanation is that the histological findings are not consistent with inflammation. Surgical specimens are typically devoid of inflammatory cells. However, degenerative changes including the loss of collagen, altered fiber organization, reduced cell count, vascular ingrowth, and, occasionally, local necrosis with or without calcification are seen. The concept of tendinosis was introduced to describe these types of focal degenerative changes. Because the relationship between the microscopic degenerative changes and the athlete's clinical symptoms is unclear, the term "tendinopathy" is often used to describe chronic tendon pain. Table 1.1 provides an overview of old and new terminology for tendon disorders and injuries. The new terminology has been developed in an effort to reflect current thinking with regard to the underlying cellular mechanisms. Thus, the term "tendinitis" should be reserved to describe tendon pathology that includes a posttraumatic inflammatory response.

Skeleton

Structure and Function

The skeleton consists of bone, which may be thought of as a special type of connective tissue that remodels continuously in a response to the complex interplay between mechanical loading, systemic hormones, and calcium homeostasis. Bone may be classified as either cortical (compact) or trabecular (spongious), and the two types of bone have different functions and properties. The long bones consist primarily of cortical bone, whereas the vertebrae in the spinal column consist of trabecular bone. Bone serves many important functions, including providing protection for underlying organs, providing the body's most important calcium store, and, through hematopoiesis that occurs in the marrow of long bones, producing blood

New	Old	Definition	Histological Findings
Paratenonitis	Tenosynovitis Tenovaginitis Peritendinitis	An inflammation of only the paratenon, either lined by synovium or not	Inflammatory cells in paratenon or peritendinous areolar tissue
Paratenonitis with tendinosis	Tendinitis	Paratenon inflammation associated with intratendinous degeneration	Same as above, with loss of tendon collagen, fiber disorientation, scattered vascular ingrowth, but no prominent intratendinous inflammation
Tendinosis	Tendinitis	Intratendinous degeneration due to atrophy (aging, microtrauma, vascular compromise, etc.)	Noninflammatory intratendinous collagen degeneration with fiber disorientation, hypocellularity, scattered vascular ingrowth, occasional local necrosis, and/or calcification
Tendinitis	Tendon strain or tear - acute (less than 2 weeks) - subacute (4–6 weeks) - chronic (over 6 weeks)	Symptomatic degeneration of the tendon with vascular disruption and inflammatory repair response	Three recognized subgroups: Each displays variable histology from pure inflammation with hemorrhage and tear, to inflammation superimposed upon preexisting degeneration, to calcification and tendinosis changes in chronic conditions. In chronic stage there may be interstial microinjury, central tendon necrosis, frank partial rupture, or acute complete rupture.

Table 1.1 Terminology for tendon disorders and tendon injuries.

cells. However, in regard to musculoskeletal function, the skeleton's most important function is that of a lever in the locomotor apparatus.

Like other connective tissue, bone consists of cells, collagen fibers, and an extracellular matrix. The bone cells, which include osteocytes, osteoblasts, and osteoclasts, develop from stem cells in the bone marrow. The osteoblasts and osteoclasts are responsible for remodeling bone. Located on the bone surface, osteoblasts are the most important bone-forming cells. When an osteoblast has formed enough bone to be completely surrounded by a mineralized matrix, it is called an osteocyte. Osteoclasts are also found on the bone surface, and their job is to absorb bone. Osteocytes communicate with each other and with osteoblasts and osteoclasts through channels in the extracellular matrix, and it is assumed that this represents an important signal pathway by which mechanical loading leads to bone remodeling. Optimum remodeling of bone depends on an adequate supply of vitamins and minerals. Recommended daily allowances for calcium, magnesium, and vitamin D have been established.

The extracellular bone matrix consists of both organic and inorganic components. The inorganic component constitutes more than half the bone mass and consists primarily of calcium and phosphate (in the form of hydroxyapatite crystals). The inorganic components contribute greatly to the hardness and strength that are characteristic of bone. Strength increases with increasing bone mineral density, but skeletal architecture is also important. The main organic component is collagen, which contributes to bone's elastic properties.

The skeletal surface is covered by a thick layer of fibrous connective tissue, called "periosteum." Periosteum is richly supplied by nerves and blood. For this reason, direct trauma that results in bleeding in or underneath the periosteum can be very painful. The periosteum is particularly well attached to bone in areas where muscles, tendons, and ligaments attach to the skeleton. In these areas, collagen bundles (Sharpey's fibers) extend down from the periosteum into the underlying osseous tissue.

The longitudinal growth of the skeleton takes place in "growth zones" (termed physeal plates) (figure 1.8). The growth zones are subject to injuries: 15% of all acute fractures in children involve the physes. In addition, the apophyses are subject to overuse injuries during growth spurts. During developmental periods marked by rapid increases of muscular strength, the apophyses are vulnerable to injury if subjected to high training loads (e.g., the tibial tubercle is affected in Osgood-Schlatter disease, and the calcaneal apophysis is affected in Sever's disease). Bone mass also increases during the growth period and peaks when the athlete is in her thirties (figure 1.9). After that, bone mineral density decreases gradually, particularly in some postmenopausal women.

Bone has characteristic stress-deformation curves (figure 1.10). Initially, in the elastic zone, there is a linear relationship between load and deformation. If the load increases into the plastic deformation zone, even small changes in force will cause greater and greater deformation. Bone that is loaded beyond the elastic zone will change shape permanently (e.g., it may remain deformed even after loading ends). Greater loading in the deformation zone results in a complete fracture.

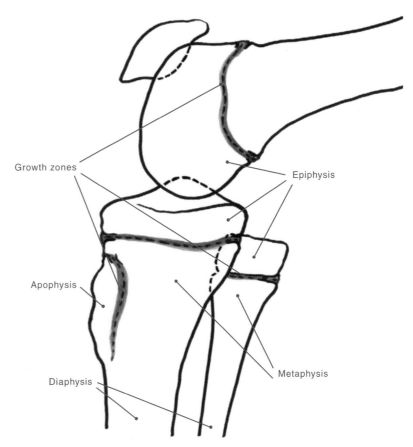

Figure 1.8 Growth zones in the long bones, such as the femur, fibula and tibia. The physeal plates are vulnerable to injury during growth spurts.

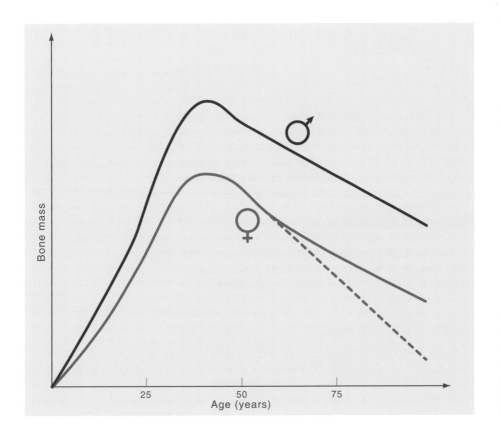

Figure 1.9 The development of bone mass as a function of age and sex. The dotted line shows the potential development in osteoporotic postmenopausal women.

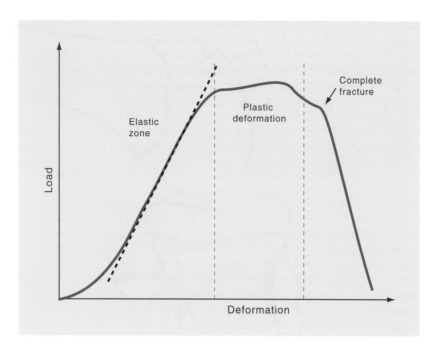

Figure 1.10 Load-deformation curve for bone.

Adaptation to Training

Physical training results in increased bone mineral density, but this increase is specific to each bone and not all types of activity increase bone mass. When a bone is loaded beyond the normal load to which it is typically subjected, the deformation will result in a signal to increase bone formation. It is likely that activities that involve more deformation, such as jumps and landings, result in increased bone formation. Athletes in power and jumping sports, like weight lifters, gymnasts, volleyball players, and squash players, tend to have the greatest bone mineral density. Runners may also have increased bone mineral density, whereas cyclists and swimmers have no higher bone mineral density than nonathletic control groups. That the response is specific to the bones being loaded is evident by the unilateral increases in bone mineral density demonstrated in the dominant arms of tennis and squash players. The response to physical activity is greatest during the growth stage, but even in postmenopausal women intense strength training has been found to stop and even reverse the expected decrease in bone mineral density.

Fractures

Fractures can be classified in various ways, but perhaps the most important differences exist between acute fractures and stress fractures. Acute fractures are caused by acute trauma that exceeds the tissues' tolerance, either from direct trauma (e.g., a kick to the leg), or indirect trauma (e.g., twisting of the lower leg).

Acute fractures can be broadly classified as transverse fractures, comminuted fractures, oblique (or spiral) fractures, and compression fractures. The type and magnitude of force that caused the fracture usually contributes to their characteristic appearance. Transverse fractures are generally caused by direct trauma to a small area, while comminuted fractures are caused by high energy trauma to a larger area. Oblique or spiral fractures are caused by indirect trauma in which rotational or torsional forces are applied to the bone, and compression fractures are caused by vertical forces on the bone (e.g., the femoral condyle being pressed down into the tibial plateau). Avulsion fractures can occur at the site of tendon or ligament insertion. In addition, two special types of fractures occur in children: (1) "greenstick fractures" (in which the bone is "bent" like a soft twig) and (2) physeal plate fractures (i.e., loosening of and possibly fracture through the growth plate).

Diagnostic signs of fractures include structural malalignment, unnatural movement, or shortening of an extremity. Pain, swelling, and reduced range of motion are also usually present but are less specific signs of fracture.

Unlike acute fractures, stress fractures do not necessarily result from any specific triggering trauma. Instead, there is a continuum of clinical reactions to repetitive loading of bone. As mentioned, bone remodels continuously throughout life. Increased loading results in microtrauma, circulatory compromise, and accelerated remodeling, with increased osteoclast and osteoblast activity. No symptoms are typically present during the phase of accelerated remodeling, and routine X rays will not demonstrate any changes. Magnetic Resonance Imaging (MRI) may demonstrate bone marrow edema, however, and scintigraphy will demonstrate increased uptake of technetium. If excessive loading continues, mild pain will occur some time after the training session begins. As trauma accumulates, symptoms generally occur earlier and earlier into the training session. This pattern is distinctly different from the pain associated with soft tissue injuries (e.g., tendinopathy), which usually occurs at the beginning of a training session then decreases after a thorough warm-up. Continued training will increase the intensity of the stress-reaction pain, and eventually the pain will linger after training sessions and during other activities such as regular walking. Radiographically, both MRI and scintigraphy will usually be positive during the stress reaction phase, whereas plain X rays frequently are unremarkable except for a subtle periosteal reaction. Once bone fatigue results in a completed fracture, plain radiography should be diagnostic. The development of stress fractures represents a physiological and clinical continuum from normal remodeling to accelerated remodeling, stress reaction, and completed stress fractures. Early diagnosis reduces treatment time.

As with other injuries due to progressive overload, a combination of factors contributes to bone stress. Most important among these potential contributing factors are training errors ("too much, too often, and too quickly, and with too little rest"); muscle fatigue (which presumably affects the shock-absorbing ability of the foot when running); malalignment of the lower extremities; the training surface; and the athlete's equipment (particularly footwear). If training is accurately documented, it will usually be seen that the athlete has made significant changes in her training regimen in the weeks preceding the onset of symptoms. Menstrual and eating disorders can also cause reduced bone mineral density and increase the risk of stress fractures.

Cartilage

Structure and Function

Cartilage consists of the basic elements of connective tissue, including cells and an extracellular matrix. There are three types of cartilage–elastic, hyaline, and fibrocartilage–of which hyaline is the most important. Hyaline cartilage consists of several layers characterized by a horizontal cellular organization in the extracellular matrix of the surface layer, and a vertical cellular organization in the deeper layers (figure 1.11).

The articular surface of most joints is covered by hyaline cartilage that is 1 to 5 mm thick. Cells constitute less than 10% of the volume of the hyaline cartilage, with the remainder consisting of macromolecules (20%) and water (70%). The macromolecules are primarily collagen fibers and proteoglycans. Cartilage strength is mainly a function of collagen content–primarily type II–and structural organization. The collagen is organized into a network of long fibrils, with proteoglycans woven into this network. Proteoglycans have two important properties: (1) they bind water, and (2) they are negatively charged, so that they repel each other. Consequently, hyaline cartilage naturally absorbs water and swells. The amount of proteoglycan and water is greatest in younger athletes and declines with age.

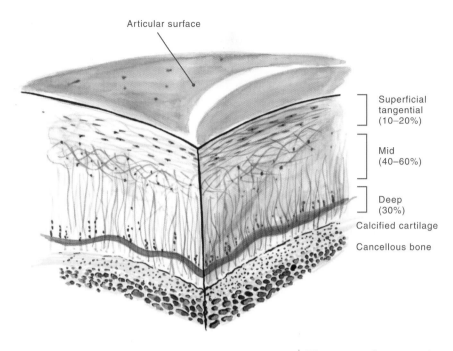

Figure 1.11 Structure of cartilage.

Hyaline cartilage is not supplied with nerves, blood vessels, or lymphatics. The cellular elements in cartilage obtain oxygen and nutrients from the surrounding tissue and articular fluid and dispose of waste matter through diffusion. Joint loading compresses the cartilage on the articular surfaces, pumping fluid out of the cartilage. When unloaded, water and dissolved substances are resorbed. Hylaine cartilage receives its nutrients and exchanges its waste products through this process of cyclic loading and unloading. Another key element of joint function is that the film of synovial fluid between the two hyaline cartilaginous surfaces makes friction extremely low, as low as wet ice on glass.

To understand the relationship between loading and deformation of hyaline cartilage, it is important to remember that the collagen fibers are organized as a meshwork–horizontally on the surface, multidirectionally in the middle section, and more vertically in the deep layer. When loading begins, the fibers have a wavy appearance histologically (figure 1.12). Deformation increases linearly with increasing load, and the collagen fibers straighten out until tearing occurs–initially among individual fibers and later among larger groups of fibers.

Fibrocartilage is strong and flexible; it is located near joints, tendons, ligaments, and in the intervertebral disks, where it forms a protective surface between the tendons, ligaments,

Figure 1.12 Stress deformation curve for hyaline cartilage showing the relationship between load and deformation.

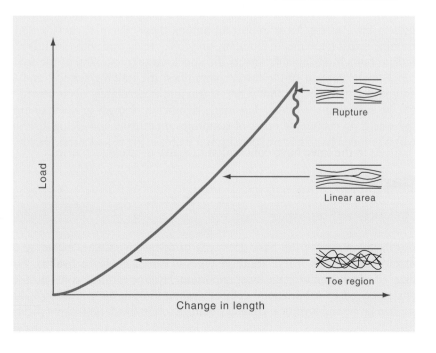

and bone. Therefore, fibrocartilage is primarily found in larger joints, such as the hip, shoulder (glenoid labrum), knee (menisci), and wrist (triangular fibrocartilage complex). In the knee, the fibrocartilagenous menisci help to improve the articular congruence between the hyaline cartilaginous surfaces of the femoral condyle and the tibial plateau and to absorb shock. In the hip, shoulder, and wrist fibrocartilage contributes to expanding the articular surface, as well, thereby increasing joint stability. Unlike hyaline cartilage, fibrocartilage generally has a blood and/or a nerve supply. For example, the nucleus fibrosis of the intervertebral discs has a nerve supply in the outer superficial portion, whereas the menisci in the knees have a blood supply in the outer portion, which has thus been referred to as the "red zone".

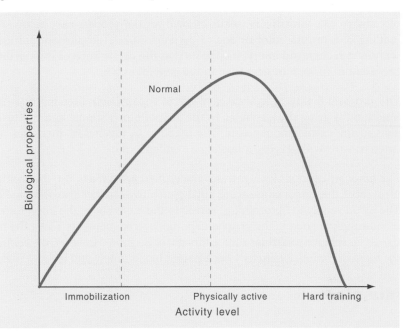

Adaptation to Training

Active loading of the articular cartilage causes the nutrients to cycle in and around the cartilage. Consequently, regular loading is necessary to maintain normal cartilage health and function. Cartilage adapts to activity like most other tissues (figure 1.13). Immobilization, such as when a joint is casted, therefore impairs cartilage homeostasis and function. It is also assumed that too much loading reduces biological properties. With time, overloading may contribute to the development of osteoarthritis of the affected joint.

Figure 1.13 Hypothetical relationship between activity level and the development of biological properties of hyaline cartilage.

Cartilage Injury

Hyaline cartilage can be injured through acute contusion, which may cause cracking, or by shear forces applied to the joint, causing vertical and horizontal rifts. Cartilage injuries frequently occur in connection with acute joint trauma. Two out of three patients with acutely sprained ankles that result in lateral ligament injuries have macroscopic cartilage injuries. Of those patients who have an arthroscopic examination after having sustained an acute knee ligament injury, 5% to 7% have a full-thickness cartilage injury of more than 2 cm^2. Some patients may have an isolated cartilage injury; others have osteochondral injuries in which the underlying bone is also injured. About one of five patients with anterior cruciate ligament injuries in the knee have concomitant localized cartilage injuries.

Articular cartilage injuries are classified on the basis of the size and depth of the lesion and the cause and accompanying pathology of the injury. The most important step is to distinguish between degenerative cartilaginous injuries (osteoarthritis), where changes are found in several places in the joint, and focal articular cartilage injuries (where localized changes are found in one or two places in the joint). In most of these patients, the injury does not produce symptoms during the acute stage; the danger is the degenerative changes that occur in the long term. For example, in osteoarthritis, the hyaline cartilage degenerates, the underlying bone becomes sclerotic, and the cartilage at the outer edges of the joints becomes ossified, leading to osteophyte formation. Acute ligament injuries, such as anterior cruciate ligament injuries, increase the risk of developing secondary osteoarthritis in the future. However, it is not known whether arthritis develops in the injured joint because the acute injury starts the degenerative processes or because the loading pattern in the involved knee is changed as a result of increased laxity. The cause of primary osteoarthritis is still unknown, yet the process may be due to increased loading of a normal joint or due to cartilage failure despite normal loading. Even without a recognized injury, it appears that the occurrence of osteoarthritis is more prevalent in former athletes than in the general public.

The intrinsic ability of hyaline cartilage to repair itself after injury is limited. This limitation is generally attributed to the lack of blood supply and the relative lack of cells in the cartilaginous tissue. The inability to regenerate increases the risk that osteoarthritis will develop following a cartilage injury.

The fibrocartilagenous knee menisci and glenoid labrum are also frequently injured. In most cases, these injuries are acute, but degenerative changes also occur in fibrocartilage. The blood supply to fibrocartilage varies. In the meniscus of the knee, for example, the blood supply is good in the peripheral portions ("red meniscus"), and the repair potential of this relatively vascular zone is thought to be good. However, the central portion of the menisci ("white meniscus") has a poorer blood supply and is thus difficult to repair.

Muscle

Structure and Function

Muscles make up 40% to 45% of body mass. The structure of the musculature (figure 1.14) reflects its central function–to generate power. The muscle fiber, which

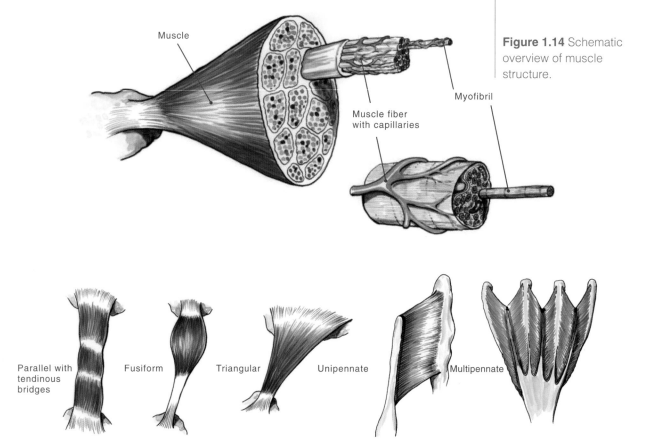

Muscle

Muscle fiber with capillaries

Myofibril

Figure 1.14 Schematic overview of muscle structure.

Parallel with tendinous bridges

Fusiform

Triangular

Unipennate

Multipennate

constitutes the basic macroscopic functional unit of muscle, can be organized in several ways, including unipennate, multipennate, or fusiform patterns. Pennate muscles are generally stronger than fusiform muscles, because several muscle fibers work in parallel to each other. However, because they contain shorter fibers, the maximum contraction speed of pennate muscles is slower than fusiform muscles. The primary subcellular element of muscle is the myofibril, which is composed of protein filaments (mainly actin and myosin). Capillaries surround the fibers, so that the ability to supply muscle with oxygen and nutrients is very good.

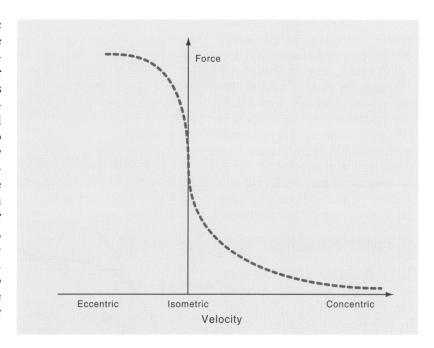

Figure 1.15 Relationship between force and velocity for different types of muscular action.

The ability of muscles to generate force depends on the working conditions, as shown in figure 1.15. The generation of force without changing the joint angle is called an "isometric" or "static" muscle action. The generation of power while the muscle is shortening is called a "concentric" muscle action, whereas the term "eccentric" action is used to describe muscle which lengthens while producing force. For concentric muscle action, maximal force production is reduced as the speed of contraction increases, whereas in eccentric muscle activity, muscle force increases with increasing speed. As a result, the risk of muscle injuries is greater during eccentric activation than during concentric muscle action.

That working conditions play a decisive role in the generation of force can be illustrated by comparing various types of jumps. Figure 1.16 shows a notable difference between the generation of ground reactive force from a squat jump (a strict concentric

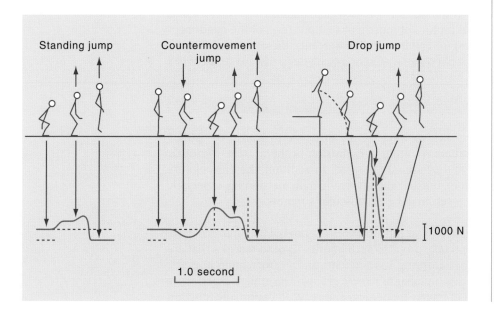

Figure 1.16 Force generation in various types of jumps.

jump from a 90° knee bend), a countermovement jump (a continuous eccentric-concentric movement), and a drop jump (jumping immediately after dropping from a height). The greater force generated from a drop jump significantly increases the risk of acute strains, and the risk of overuse injuries is high in sports characterized by this type of muscle action. This is true not only of the muscles but also of other musculoskeletal structures, such as tendons, cartilage, and bone.

Adaptation to Training

Muscle shows the greatest and most rapid response to training of all the soft tissues. Muscle volume and strength increase significantly after a short period of specific strength training (figure 1.17). Two factors contribute to increasing strength: (1) the ability to recruit several muscle fibers at the same time (neural factors) and (2) muscle volume (muscular factors). Muscle volume primarily increases as a result of individual muscle fibers increasing their cross-sectional area (hypertrophy), but also increases by the formation of new muscle cells (hyperplasia) derived from stem cells called "satellite cells" located in the periphery of the myofiber. Neural factors contribute most to the initial strength increase that occurs in response to training, whereas hypertrophy is primarily responsible for subsequent strength gains.

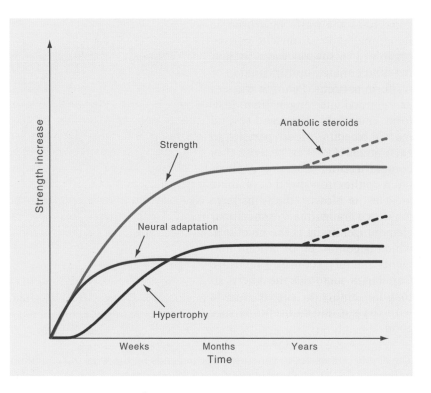

Figure 1.17 Increase in strength as a result of systematic strength training.

While muscular strength increases after just a few weeks of training, tendons, cartilage, and bone require months to adapt, and there is therefore a risk of developing overuse injuries following the introduction of systematic strength and jump training. The patellar and the Achilles tendons are particularly vulnerable to such overuse pathology in adult athletes. Notably, when the athlete has used anabolic steroids, there seems to be an increased risk for total rupture of muscle or tendons (e.g., of the quadriceps or the pectoralis major muscles). In children and adolescents, these types of overuse problems usually affect the apophyses (e.g., Osgood-Schlatter's disease and Sever's disease).

Muscle Injuries

Muscle injuries generally occur in two ways: (1) by distension (strains, or "pulled muscles") and (2) by direct trauma resulting in contusion of the muscle. Muscular lacerations also occur, although they are rare in sport. In addition, the musculature is sometimes injured as a result of unusual and atypically difficult training, especially eccentric training, which may result in delayed muscular soreness.

Strains usually occur at the myotendinous junction during a bout of maximal eccentric muscle action. Sprinters are especially prone to such injuries. Typical muscles that are prone to strain injury include the hamstring, hip adductor, and gastrocnemius muscles. Strains may, however, affect a large number of muscle groups. The athlete experiences immediate pain at the moment of injury. Tenderness and reduced contractile function ensue, and the athlete may occasionally feel a bump in the muscle immediately after the injury, if a significant tissue rupture has occurred. Swelling, due to bleeding or subsequent edema, is also a characteristic finding.

Contusions occur most commonly in the quadriceps muscles, which are exposed frontally and laterally on the thigh and therefore can easily be traumatized (e.g., by an opponent's kneecap). All types of muscle injuries, regardless of cause, result in internal bleeding in the musculature. This occurs because the musculature is well vascularized and because the regional blood flow is usually high at the moment of injury. Therefore, hematomas are quite common with this type of injury. Bleeding may be either intramuscular, if there is no injury to the muscle fascia, or intermuscular, if the blood can escape from the involved muscle compartments through associated trauma to the fascia (figure 11.3). In general, healing time is significantly longer in the presence of intramuscular bleeding than it is for intermuscular hemorrhage.

Tissue injury and bleeding result in an inflammatory reaction which forms the basis of the healing response leading to the formation of scar tissue. After a significant muscle injury, there is little muscle tissue regeneration. Instead, the injured muscle tissue is replaced by fibrous scar tissue without contractile properties, thereby contributing to an increased risk of recurrent injuries (e.g., hamstrings strains).

Occasionally, muscle hematomas can lead to an unfortunate complication known as myositis ossificans, which may be defined as calcification or ossification of the injured tissue. The most common location for myositis ossificans to develop is the thigh. As many as 20% of athletes who sustain a quadriceps contusion will develop myositis ossificans. Not all these patients will develop symptoms, even though calcification of the hematoma may be visible in X rays. The pathophysiology of heterotopic bone formation is not completely understood. Two to four weeks post-injury, new bone formation usually becomes visible on X ray, and is normally attached to the underlying bone. Bone mass can increase in size for several months, but it does not always do so. It is important to be aware that the early radiographic appearance of the heterotopic bone mass can easily be confused with osteogenic sarcoma. The two conditions can be difficult to distinguish on histologic examination as well. Heterotopic bone often will be resorbed over time, but this does not always happen. Nevertheless, normal function of the affected muscle is seldom regained.

Compartment syndrome can further complicate management of muscle contusions that result in intramuscular hemorrhage. Bleeding and soft tissue edema can cause such an increase in tissue hydrostatic pressure that circulation to the involved muscle compartment becomes compromised. This affects the muscle primarily on the capillary level and only rarely involves the large vessels passing though the compartment. Thus, the finding of a good pulse distal to the hematoma does not necessarily exclude the possibility of compartment syndrome. The primary symptom of compartment syndrome is pain (often described as extreme if the diagnosis is not made and the condition progresses), and the muscle compartment may be hard on palpation. Nerve function may be affected so that the patient feels paresthesias distally. If left untreated, compartment syndrome may result in necrosis of the muscles of the involved compartment, with major functional sequelae in the long term.

Muscle lacerations are rare in sport but may occur as a result of cuts from the edge of a skate or a downhill ski. Transverse lacerations cut across the muscle fibers. The wound is repaired with a fibrous scar tissue that lacks contractile properties, potentially affecting the function of the affected muscle.

Muscle stiffness (delayed-onset muscle soreness [DOMS]) is a troublesome but generally harmless symptom that occurs after muscular exertion to which the athlete is unaccustomed. Soreness is experienced primarily after demanding eccentric exercise. Symptoms generally increase gradually during the hours after training, peak after about 48 hours, and disappear in the next 2 to 3 days. DOMS is caused by the destruction of skeletal muscle architecture and is accompanied by a temporary, slight (10-15%) reduction in muscle strength. This type of muscle soreness is generally experienced only after the first few times a new eccentric exercise is performed. Stretching does not appear to prevent DOMS.

Treating Sports Injuries

Sverre Mæhlum and Roald Bahr

Treating Acute Injuries—The PRICE Principle

Most acute injuries, whether they affect the muscles, ligaments, tendons, or bone, are characterized by bleeding immediately after the injury. A muscular hematoma can occur as early as 30 seconds after a muscle injury. If the patient sustains an acute ligament rupture and remains untreated, a significant hematoma will be visible within a few minutes.

Therefore, the goal of acute treatment for acute injuries is to limit internal bleeding as much as possible and prevent or relieve pain, in order to improve conditions for subsequent treatment and healing of the injury. Measures to limit bleeding after an acute injury have traditionally been called ICE therapy, an acronym for Ice (cooling), Compression (with a pressure bandage), and Elevation (of the injured part of the body). Recently this acronym has been expanded to PRICE, with "P" standing for Protection and "R" for Rest. The PRICE principle has become well established.

It is essential that effective PRICE treatment begins as soon as possible after an injury (figure 2.1, a through h). Even if, in principle, it is always desirable to know exactly which injury the patient has, during the acute stage starting treatment right away has priority. It takes a few minutes to accurately examine a knee or ankle joint, but during this time significant bleeding may occur. Therefore, it is recommended that treatment be started as soon as possible after a quick preliminary examination to rule out major dislocations or fractures and to determine which area requires treatment. Later, a more detailed examination can be made.

The PRICE treatment continues after the patient has been transported home or to the hospital for further testing. If treatment continues at home, the patient must be given detailed instructions. Bleeding and plasma exudation will continue for 48 hours after an acute soft-tissue injury occurs. Therefore, to be effective, PRICE treatment must continue for 2 days.

Protection and Rest

The goals of protection and rest are to avoid further injury and to reduce the blood supply to the injured area (which can be more than ten times higher during sports activity than at rest). This is particularly true of tissue with a high blood flow during activity–for example, in the case of muscle injury. Rest alone is not enough to stop

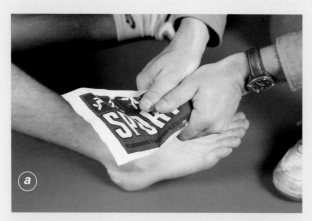
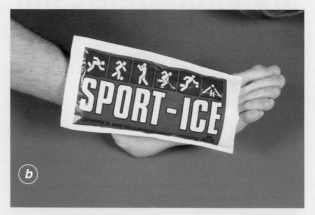

Figure 2.1 Example of PRICE therapy for an acute sprained ankle after inversion trauma, with a suspected lateral ligament injury. The patient must not bear weight, and stay off his ankle. The contents of the inner bag should be released by squeezing (*a*), and the cold pack should be placed over the lateral malleolus (*b*).

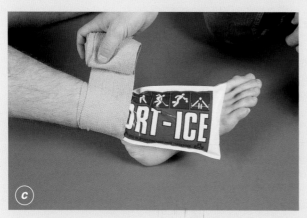
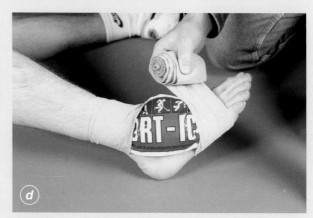

To attach the cold pack, the elastic bandage should be wrapped around the proximal (*c*) and distal (*d*) ends of the foot, and then the compression bandage should be applied tightly around the cold pack. When placed properly, the cold pack will augment the compression effect.

a hematoma from developing after a muscle or ligament injury, but further activity will cause the volume of bleeding to increase. Therefore, it is crucial to interrupt activity immediately. After sustaining an acute soft-tissue injury with bleeding in a lower extremity, the patient should not bear weight on the injured area for 2 days (48 hours). The patient would benefit from walking on crutches during this period.

Cold Treatment (Ice)

There is a long tradition of treating sports injuries with cold. In all likelihood, the main effect is pain relief. Cooling has a good analgesic effect, although the term "anesthesia dolorosa" (painful anesthesia) is used to indicate the discomfort the patient experiences initially before the analgesic effect sets in. However, cold treatment alone is not very effective in reducing bleeding. When a regular ice bag is

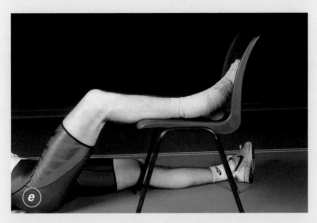

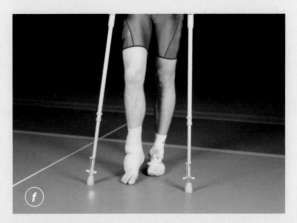

The patient must keep his leg as high above heart level as possible for at least half an hour *(e)*. Periodically shaking the cold pack (or the foot to which it is bandaged) will mix the chemicals and prolong the cold effect produced. If the patient needs to move, he should use crutches so that he bears absolutely no weight on the injured leg. The cold pack is used to provide maximum compression during transport, even if the effect of the cold treatment has subsided *(f)*.

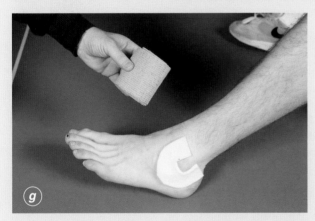

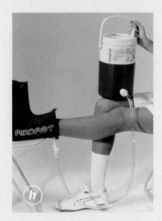

The comprehensive clinical examination should be deferred until a minimum of 30 minutes of PRICE therapy has been administered. At home, the patient continues compression treatment, wearing an elastic bandage continuously for the first 2 days, preferably with a horseshoe-shaped, foam-rubber pad placed around the malleolus *(g)*. Cooling has a good analgesic effect and may be provided without compression by using running cold water from the tap with the plug in. Special equipment for cold treatment *(h)*, available for most joints, can also be used for this purpose. If an ice pack is used, a thin cloth should be placed under the ice to avoid frostbite.

applied, the blood flow 2 cm below the surface of the skin is reduced by only 5% to 10% during the first 10 minutes but by more than 50% within a half hour. Consequently, the blood flow is significantly reduced, but this takes a while, and cold treatment alone is insufficient to stop bleeding during the first critical minutes after an injury occurs.

There are several ways of administering cold treatment: using disposable ice bags, cold water, ice cubes, or even snow. Disposable bags have the advantage of being easy to use in combination with a compression bandage, which provides maximum compression over the injury site. An inner bag separates the two components in the bag. When the inner bag is broken, the two components mix in an endothermic reaction that produces a cooling effect. The peak cooling effect occurs during the first 5 to 10 minutes, but it can be extended by shaking the bag periodically so that the contents are mixed up even more.

If ice cubes are used, they should be wrapped in a wet cloth; a pressure bandage may also be applied over the ice pack. The same is true of snow. Cold running water can also be used, but it is difficult to effectively combine it with compression during the acute stage. Later in the course, cold water is an excellent alternative. If pain makes it necessary, cooling can be repeated for 20-minute intervals every 3 to 4 hours for the first 48 hours.

Compression Treatment

Compression treatment using an elastic bandage is probably the most essential measure in limiting the development of hematoma. Diastolic pressure in an extremity at rest is about 40 to 70 mmHg. An elastic bandage that is pulled tight increases diastolic blood pressure under the bandage to about 85 mmHg, effectively reducing the blood supply by about 95% within a few seconds. After warm-up an athlete has a blood pressure of about 80 mmHg in the vastus lateralis muscle, but with a tight, elastic bandage blood flow under the bandage is 0% to 10% of the normal flow. Reduced blood flow increases linearly with pressure underneath the bandage, so that if the elastic bandage is loosely fit, the blood flow is reduced only by about 60%. Applying a firm pad underneath the compression bandage can increase local pressure over the injury site. An ice bag works in the same manner.

Elevation

Elevation of the injured body part is one of the five recommended PRICE measures, but of course it is suited primarily to distal extremity injuries. Because of effective autoregulation of blood flow, no reduction in blood flow occurs until the injured area is raised more than 30 cm above the level of the heart. At 50 cm elevation, blood flow is reduced to 80%; at 70 cm elevation, blood flow is still about 65% of the normal blood flow. Combining elevation with compression treatment may contribute to even more effective reduction of blood flow.

Elevation is recommended for the first 2 days whenever the patient is lying down or sitting still. The practitioner must remember that when the patient sits with his legs on a bench, the ankle is still the lowest point in the body. The injured area must be kept as far above heart level as possible and needs to be well propped up in bed at night.

Treating Overuse Injuries— Changing the Loading Pattern

Overuse injuries represent a significant proportion of injuries in a variety of sports. Athletes in endurance sports that require large amounts of training (with respect to frequency, duration, and intensity), and where the training may be monotonous (as in long-distance running, bicycling, and cross-country skiing), are particularly vulnerable. However, athletes in technical sports, where the same movement is repeated numerous times (e.g., tennis, golf, and throwing sports), also sustain overuse injuries.

Unlike acute injuries, overuse injuries generally do not have a well-defined triggering trauma. As the term suggests, overuse injuries are the result of too much loading over time. Therapy needs to be based on a determination of which factors contributed to the injury. Risk factors can be divided into intrinsic and extrinsic factors (also see chapter 3). A precise understanding of the process that resulted in the injury makes causal treatment possible, by wholly or partially eliminating the causal factors (figure 2.2). Because the injury is the result of overuse, the loading pattern must be changed for the therapy to succeed.

The basis of an overuse injury is often removed once the internal and external factors are successfully corrected. Many athletes are able to recover by taking this measure alone (figure 2.2). In other cases, however, it is necessary to include other measures to counteract inactivity, suppress inflammation, and stimulate healing of the injured tissue to enable the athlete to return to the desired activity level.

External Risk Factors

External risk factors may include a number of factors, e.g., improper training, new equipment, cold weather, and a slippery or hard surface. A thorough training history usually reveals that the injury is the result of changes in training load: "too much, too often, too soon, or with too little rest." The goal of taking the training history is to document how the athlete trained—how much, how often, how hard, and how long—and particularly focus on any changes in the training routine, if the athlete increased the amount of training during the period before the injury occurred. Usually the practitioner finds that the athlete increased the amount or intensity of training too quickly. This is true both of top-level athletes and of people who are exercising for fitness purposes. People involved in fitness training are particularly vulnerable during the first stage when they begin training without an established fitness base: they start at a level that is too high and proceed too quickly. Many athletes train extremely hard and thus are constantly on the verge of sustaining an overuse injury. Occasionally, overuse injuries occur when an athlete is resuming training after a vacation, an illness, an injury, or simply a pause in training. However, the practitioner should also be aware that the injury is not always caused by increasing the total amount of training but can also result when the loading pattern has changed, such as when new training exercises were started or the athlete changed her technique. This is particularly true when the season changes— for example, when a cross-country skier switches from training on snow to running.

Changes in training load that may result in injuries may also be caused by external factors other than the training itself. Some athletes use equipment that is not adjusted for them or the amount of training they are doing. A change of equipment, even to better equipment, is also a risk factor. New equipment may cause a change in the loading pattern, which by itself or in combination with other factors may trigger an overuse injury. Practitioners should check the footwear of patients with injuries to the lower extremities. However, other sports equipment, such as rackets, skis, bicycles, and oars, may contribute to the development of injuries. For example, the load on a tennis player's elbow depends on the size of the racket and handle and how tight the strings are.

Climate and surface are other factors that may trigger injuries. For example, runners, whether they are sprinters or long-distance runners, experience more muscle and tendon problems in cold climates than in warm climates. Volleyball and basketball players sustain overuse injuries to their knees more easily when they jump on a hard surface than on soft sand. Runners who train on a slippery or uneven surface may need to change their running technique to avoid acute injuries. Because most roads are highest in the middle and slope down toward the sides to ensure the drainage of water, running on only one side of the road increases loading. One foot will be subjected to increased pronation, the other to increased supination.

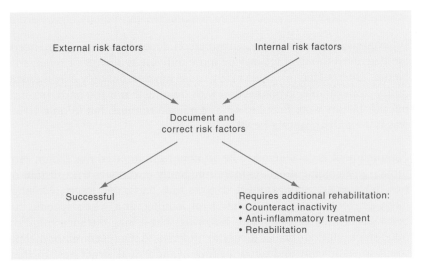

Figure 2.2 Treatment strategy for overuse injuries.

Internal Risk Factors

Internal risk factors (also known as person-dependent factors) also need to be documented, even though they may be more difficult to correct or remove than external factors. Internal factors alone rarely cause injuries, but they may increase the risk of injury—for example, in connection with training that is too hard. In one study, internal risk factors were found in 40% of injured runners, but in only 10% of the cases was it the only triggering factor.

Malalignment is considered to be an important internal risk factor. However, even though malalignment occurs more frequently in runners who sustain overuse injuries, no specific malalignment triggers any particular injury. Malalignment very likely prevents optimal distribution of loading, and when specific structures are overloaded, injuries can result. Knowing that a long-distance runner takes about 5000 steps per hour makes it easy to understand that even minor malalignment can result in significant undesired loading of individual structures. In theory, a varus position in the lower extremity (figure 13.11) will result in increased compression forces on the medial side and increased distension forces on the lateral side of the ankles and knees, whereas a valgus position (figure 13.10) should result in the opposite loading pattern. Alignment should be examined both at rest and during loading. To uncover alignment in some athletes, a high-speed video camera recording may be required to better analyze their mechanics while running on a treadmill. However, it is important to evaluate the deviation in relation to the loading they are subjected to. Malalignment that is insignificant to a person who runs only for fitness purposes may be crucial to a marathon runner who runs 150 to 200 km per week.

Poor muscle strength or poor balance in relative strength between muscles that have opposite effects on a joint can contribute to injuries. For example, some athletes have weak hamstring muscles relative to the strength of the quadriceps muscles. This may cause asymmetric loading of the knee or of the muscles close to the knee, a pattern that can make it easier for an injury to occur. This can easily happen to an athlete who was injured previously. If rehabilitation was not optimal, the patient may have an abnormal movement pattern and may develop an overuse injury.

Athletes with particularly good strength or flexibility, or who have rapidly increased their strength or flexibility, may be at risk for overuse injuries. For example, a talented javelin thrower could rapidly increase his throwing distance, or a high jumper her jumping height, over a short period, by using specific strength training. Although muscles rapidly adjust to strength training, cartilage, tendons, and ligaments take longer to adjust. Thus, increased strength or flexibility may cause an overuse injury in these structures.

Joint mobility very likely affects the risk of injuries. Poor mobility (hypomobility) may result in overuse injuries. For example, short, stiff hamstring muscles will cause the pelvis to tilt forward when the athlete lifts his knees high while running fast. This increases loading at the lowest part of the lumbar region, increasing the risk that the patient will have back pain. Stretching the hamstring muscles may improve the situation and may contribute to reducing back pain. Excessive mobility (hypermobility) may also result in injuries. Some patients have generalized joint laxity; others are hypermobile only in a single joint. In either case, the athlete should attempt to strengthen his muscles that act on the joint so that the muscles can take over some of the protective function that is not provided by the passive structures.

The list of internal factors that may result in overuse injuries is long. Some factors, such as age, are impossible to change. Other factors, such as poor muscle strength, poor mobility, and being overweight, can be changed. Correcting internal factors that trigger injuries is crucial to treating an overuse injury.

Preventing Inactivity

Patients who have an overuse injury often reduce their activity level, either on their own or because they have been told to do so by health care personnel. An important part of treating overuse injuries is preventing this type of inactivity, because inactivity leads to atrophy of all parts of the musculoskeletal system. In addition, inactivity is destructive to the general physical condition, which makes it even more difficult to return to the desired activity level. Atrophy often occurs very rapidly in connection with inactivity, and atrophy of musculature can be visible within a few weeks. Cartilage and ligaments also atrophy quickly. Therefore, inactivity, particularly complete immobilization, must be avoided to the greatest extent possible.

Atrophy of the muscles occurs even in situations in which the athlete is unaware that the musculature is being "rested." Reflex inhibition from pain can trigger atrophy. Among other things, joint swelling can cause atrophy through reflex inhibition. Aerobic muscle fibers (Type I fibers) atrophy the quickest, and a transition can also occur between fiber types. Isometric contractions can counteract the atrophy but cannot prevent it altogether. Electrostimulation of the musculature may also reduce atrophy, but it is primarily reserved for situations in which voluntary contractions are not possible.

Articular cartilage (hyaline cartilage) is particularly vulnerable to atrophy. Histologic changes are already visible after 6 days of immobilization, with reduced proteoglycan synthesis and aggregation. If this process takes place over time, it can lead to the development of osteoarthritis. However, the point at which this development becomes irreversible is unknown. The atrophy is counteracted by using the joint. Therefore, early mobilization is key, and in situations in which the patient cannot or is not permitted to move the joint on his own, such as after surgery, continuous passive motion should be used. The results seem to be particularly good for small non-weight-bearing joints. However, after immobilization, activity that is too intense may further damage the cartilage. Thus, when activity is resumed after a period of non-weight bearing, it is necessary to begin carefully. It is best to avoid immobilization as much as possible.

Tendons, capsules, and ligaments are just as affected by inactivity as muscles and cartilage. It has been demonstrated that after 8 weeks, 40% of strength, and 30% of stiffness in the tendons is lost.

Principles for Rehabilitating Sports Injuries

The goal of rehabilitation is to bring the patient back to the desired activity level. Hence, it is necessary to eliminate pain and reestablish range of motion, technique, and coordination, while avoiding the loss of muscle strength and endurance, during the period the athlete cannot train maximally.

Rehabilitation can be divided into three stages:

• Acute stage–lasts a few days to weeks
• Rehabilitation stage–lasts from weeks to months
• Training stage–lasts a few weeks to months

The stages often overlap. What determines when an athlete passes from one stage into another is not the time that has elapsed but the progress the patient has made.

Acute Stage

The main goal of the acute stage is to avoid having the injury worsen, and consequently the athlete often has to reduce or completely stop participating in routine training or competition. The type of injury that the athlete sustains and the sport in which the athlete is involved will determine how long she will have to stay away from sport. For acute injuries, the principles of PRICE therapy (described earlier) apply, often with brief or total immobilization and initial unloading. If the patient has an overuse injury, partially unloading the injured structure may also be necessary to begin with. Complete unloading is rarely necessary when treating overuse injuries. Some patients may correct malalignment by using specially adjusted insoles in their running shoes—for example, to provide medial support to correct overpronation. Unloading may also be accomplished by choosing appropriate shoes, by using shock-absorbing soles or heel cups, or possibly by relieving pressure with felt pads or similar devices. Protection against blows or impact can be achieved with the help of specially fitted braces.

When the causes and triggering factors that predispose an athlete to injuries are documented, the athlete will be able to resume all activity that does not contribute to worsening the injury. Then it is necessary to plan a way to eliminate factors that could provoke symptoms. During this stage, if the athlete is limited by inflammation or pain, the use of nonsteroidal anti-inflammatory drugs (NSAIDs) or other anti-inflammatory therapy may be indicated.

Rehabilitation Stage

During this stage the main goals are to prepare the athlete to train normally and in full. That is, it is necessary to ensure:

• normal range of motion
• normal strength
• normal neuromuscular function
• normal aerobic capacity

Pain and swelling are the main considerations when determining how much and what types of training to use during rehabilitation. The usual rule is to train at a level that does not cause pain. However, this is debatable. Many factors indicate that it is necessary to tolerate some pain, at least as long as pain or swelling does not worsen from one training session to the next. Gradual progressive pain or swelling is a sign that the training load needs to be reduced or that the patient may need to consider other types of training.

The best way to reestablish normal range of motion is for the patient to use active stretching exercises. This may not succeed at first. If it does not, the patient will need to train with passive stretching or stretch with the assistance of equipment or a therapist. Normal range of motion is key, because it is a prerequisite for returning the athlete to normal technique. In addition, reduced range of motion may limit the patient's ability to do strength training. For example, a patient who does not have full extension in her knee may not be able to train her vastus medialis muscle, and, consequently, it will not be possible to optimize her knee function. Specific stretching of the injured tissue can be completed according to the same principles with frequent light stretching during the early rehabilitation stage and more forceful and longer stretching later in the rehabilitation period.

To maintain general strength and muscular endurance, alternative forms of training are used that do not load the injured area. Examples of this are bicycling, swimming, or running in water (figure 2.3). Well-performed alternative training will allow the athlete to return to the playing field sooner. In addition to alternative training, the athlete can engage in the parts of the regular training program that do not load the injured part of the body. For example, a wrestler can train for upper body, abdominal, and back strength, even if he has a knee injury that prevents him from running or training for wrestling. It is often possible for the athlete to train unaffected areas more during this stage than he would have done if he had not been injured.

In addition to alternative training, the athlete must also engage in specific training—that is, training that affects the injured structures. The amount (including intensity, frequency, and duration) of training stimuli will depend on the location of the injury, which tissue is injured, how long the patient has had the injury, and any surgical intervention. In this connection, the practitioner should remember that all training is specific. The athlete improves only in what he trains for. When an athlete retrains after an overuse injury, it is necessary to place the greatest emphasis on exercises that train for both the type of strength (concentric, eccentric, or isometric) and for the muscle groups that the athlete requires for his sport. The specific training will be highly repetitive—numerous repetitions of the same movement in several series, several times a day. For example, the athlete may increase the amount of training once a week or every other week, preferably in consultation with a physical therapist.

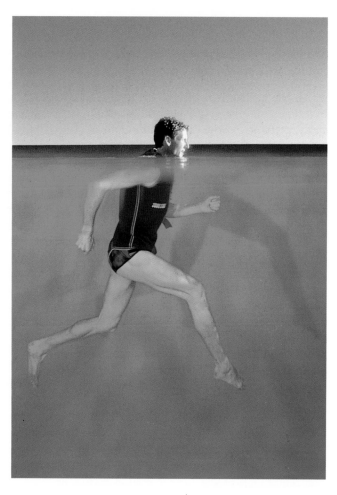

Figure 2.3 Alternative training: running in water while wearing a wet vest.

To the extent possible, technique and coordination are monitored and trained parallel to specific training for a particular sport. It is necessary to ensure that an athlete has regained at least 85% to 90% of his original strength before he is allowed to participate in competition again.

All athletes who must remain completely or partially at rest in connection with an injury will lose endurance. Aerobic capacity needs to be restored for the athlete to return to the level he was at before the injury. It is often necessary to select slightly different types of training, because the injury limits the possibility for customary training. For example, a runner with Achilles tendinosis will not be able to run on the ground, but he or she will often be able to bicycle or to run in water without pain.

Many assume that the rehabilitation is completed when pain is gone; when mobility, strength, and neuromuscular function have been regained; and when lost endurance has been restored. This can be true for nonathletes. The injured body part functions again, and the patient may return to his normal level of activity. This is not necessarily the case for a competitive athlete. The rehabilitation stage has enabled the athlete to train at a nearly normal level, but some work probably still remains before the athlete's ability to perform is back to normal.

Specific exercises to regain normal neuromuscular function are vital to the rehabilitation of patients, whether they have an overuse injury or an acute injury. Painful conditions may result in reflex inhibition. This causes changes in the recruitment pattern of muscles around an injured joint, thereby resulting in a change in technique, which may contribute to maintaining an unfavorable loading pattern. Acute ligament injuries may also result in reduced joint position sense and coordination, which may contribute to the involved joint being more vulnerable to new injuries. Specific neuromuscular exercises that challenge coordination and the ability to balance, to transfer weight, and to react quickly to changes of position are key elements of training that help an individual avoid new injuries.

Training Stage

The goal of the training stage is to ensure that the athlete regains her normal ability to perform in sport, to tolerate the loading that is unavoidable in competition, and to tolerate normal amounts of training before being allowed to compete again. The training stage is a critical phase for top athletes. A previous injury is the chief risk factor for sustaining a new injury, probably because many athletes return to competitive sport before they are completely rehabilitated after previous injuries.

During this stage, it is important for the athlete and the coach to ensure a gradual transition from controlled rehabilitation to exercises that are more and more like the sport itself. The role of the physician and the physical therapist is to ensure that the athlete undergoes practical testing to determine whether he can tolerate the anticipated loading required for competitive activity. This is often difficult, because pressure is maximal only during actual competition. However, the test situation should come as close as possible to emulating a competitive situation. Only after the athlete has completed this type of test, and is mentally prepared to resume competition, should he be allowed to participate again.

An athlete must be highly disciplined, and strong motivation is often required from the athlete as well as the physician and physical therapists to achieve the desired result. It is crucial for the athlete to be continuously instructed and, if necessary, to keep a training and pain diary to record and monitor his response to training. With injuries that require a prolonged rehabilitation period, health care personnel can be considered more like coaches than caregivers. Some claim that the rehabilitation of overuse injuries is more a matter of instructing than it is of providing treatment.

Methods of Supportive Therapy

Anti-inflammatory and pain-relieving therapy may be important as supportive therapy for athletes with acute or overuse injuries, but it is rarely sufficient as the only therapy. Exercises alone can have an effect on inflammation and pain, but a number of adjunct therapies are available that have a more or less well-documented effect, including medication, heat treatment, cold treatment, and various forms of electrotherapy. Anti-inflammatory and pain-relieving therapy can be important to enable the patient to begin rehabilitation exercises, thus avoiding atrophy, reduced coordination, and reduced muscular endurance and strength. Acute injuries usually cause tissue damage that results in bleeding and inflammation. Some patients with overuse injuries experience an acute onset of symptoms with obvious signs of inflammation; others experience this stage in connection with an acute worsening of the chronic condition. Anti-inflammatory and pain-relieving therapy may be used to minimize inflammation in newly formed, relatively vascular scar tissue after acute injuries, to minimize acute symptoms of inflammation in patients with acute bursitis or paratenonitis, or strictly for the purpose of relieving symptoms of chronic overuse injuries.

Drug Therapy

Pain is almost always a prominent symptom in sports injuries—in both acute and overuse injuries. Pain may be due to chemical irritation of the nerve endings as a result of inflammation of the surrounding tissue or strictly caused by mechanical irritation. Pain is also the prominent symptom of tendinosis.

Pain can be treated with a number of drugs that have a peripheral effect, including acetominophen, acetylsalicylic acid, or other NSAIDs (see below), or with centrally-acting analgesics such as codeine, propoxyphene, and tramadol. In low doses acetylsalicylic acid has a pain-relieving effect for peripheral pain, in addition to an antipyretic effect, and in high doses it also has an anti-inflammatory effect. However, because acetylsalicylic acid inhibits platelet aggregation and, therefore, may result in an increased bleeding tendency, the drug has limited use for sports injuries. Acetominophen has a pain-relieving effect and is antipyretic, but it does not have an anti-inflammatory effect, and it has no effect on blood platelets. Therefore, acetominophen can be used to relieve pain for acute injuries.

Non-steroidal anti-inflammatory drugs (NSAIDs) are widely used for treating sports injuries. They are available as tablets, in gel form (for local application), and for injection. The preparations have anti-inflammatory, analgesic, and antipyretic properties, and they work by inhibiting the enzyme cyclooxygenase, thus inhibiting the release of prostaglandin, an important mediator in the local inflammatory injuries (figure 1.6). There is no documentation to indicate that any specific NSAID preparation is more effective or has less side-effects than others. The choice of a drug seems to be largely dependent on pharmacokinetics. Fast-acting preparations may be preferable for acute injuries.

Cyclooxygenase exists in two isoforms, COX1 (which is expressed in the mucosal membranes of the stomach and kidneys) and COX2 (which is expressed during inflammation). The prostaglandins in the mucosal membranes have a protective effect, and inhibition of these prostaglandins via inhibition of COX1 increases the risk of ulcers. Therefore, NSAIDs that inhibit COX1 as well as COX2 (traditional NSAIDs) increase the risk of gastric ulcers, particularly after long-term use. However, it also occurs with short-term use, such as that for acute sports injuries. To avoid this side effect, so-called COX2 specific inhibitors have recently been developed. These drugs do not inhibit prostaglandin synthesis in the mucosal membranes and therefore have a lower frequency of gastrointestinal side effects.

NSAID/COX2-inhibitor treatment also seems to contribute to more-rapid mobilization of the patient after acute injuries, such as ankle sprains, even though better research-based documentation is desirable. It is also unclear as to whether this is due to their analgesic effect, which allows early mobilization, or if the anti-inflammatory effect is also important. In acute cases, oral treatment should be started as soon as possible using maximal doses, and it should be continued for 4 to 5 days. For overuse injuries, there is little evidence to indicate that anti-inflammatory treatment provides anything more than temporary relief from symptoms. This is true of oral treatment, local application in gel form, and injections.

Since the 1950s, the injection of corticosteroids has been a popular method of treating rheumatoid arthritis. This type of treatment also has a long tradition in sports medicine, even though there is no convincing documentation of a causal effect of the therapy, neither for oral treatment nor for injections. This is primarily because of the lack of placebo-controlled studies. Corticosteroids are usually given in combination with local anesthesia, and the actual cause of the therapeutic effect is unknown. Despite the lack of satisfactory documentation, injections are often used for overuse injuries, particularly bursitis, synovitis, and peritendinitis.

Cortisone and other corticosteroids block the earliest step in the inflammation cascade (the release of arachidonic acid) and, consequently, have significant effects (figure 1.6). In addition to inhibiting undesired inflammatory effects, corticosteroids can also inhibit and delay the formation and maturation of granulation tissue. In addition, unanticipated effects, such as osteoporosis, weight gain, reduced glucose tolerance, euphoria, and an increased risk of infection, can occur. The risk of side effects is related primarily to long-term oral treatment, and this type of treatment is not indicated for sports injuries. The risk of side effects is considerably lower for single injections or short term (4 to 5 days) oral treatment. However, tendon ruptures are a feared side effect from injections into or close to the tendons. Therefore, these types of injections should be avoided.

If an injection of corticosteroids is necessary, it should not be performed into or around tendons. Corticosteroid injections are not recommended for the treatment of acute injuries, nor are they recommended in children. After an injection, at least 2 weeks of relative rest or unloading is recommended. Multiple injections are given only if the first injection has a noticeable effect, and, in all cases, treatment should be limited to three injections at intervals of a few weeks.

Cold Therapy

Cold treatment is an important part of PRICE therapy for acute injuries, as described earlier. During the acute stage, cold treatment primarily has a pain-relieving effect. Later in the course of treatment for acute injuries and for overuse injuries, cold treatment will also result in vasoconstriction and will thereby reduce the blood flow into the superficial tissue (2 to 4 cm down). Cold also reduces metabolism via reduced enzyme function. In addition, cold treatment reduces or eliminates the transfer of impulses from peripheral pain fibers, and cold also has a favorable effect on muscle spasms. In the periphery, particularly in the fingers and toes, reflex cold-induced vasodilation occurs after cold treatment. This is the explanation for the painful erythema a patient may experience after strong exposure to cold.

Cold treatment, therefore, can be used before training to reduce pain and spasms during the early stages or after training to counteract pain or swelling as a result of training. Cold treatment can be administered in many different ways, such as disposable cold packs, multi-use gel packs, ice or snow packed into a wet cloth, running water, or an ice bath. The optimal cold effect is achieved after 20 to 30 minutes of treatment; beyond that, the application of cold does not appear to have any additional effect and increases the risk of cold injuries. It is necessary to be especially aware of the danger of cold injuries to the skin or superficial nerves near the joints, such as the ulnar nerve or the peroneal nerve.

Heat Therapy

Heat treatment should be avoided during the acute stage of acute injuries, but it can otherwise be an effective method of improving collagen tissue elasticity, increasing joint mobility, reducing muscle spasm, and minimizing pain. Heat treatment causes peripheral vasodilation and, consequently, increases local blood flow. In addition, vein and lymph drainage increases in response to heat treatment, as does the supply of oxygen, tissue metabolism, and the numbers of leukocytes and phagocytes. An undesired effect of heat treatment may be increased vascular permeability, which causes leakage of intravascular fluid, thereby increasing the tendency for edema.

The analgesic effect of heat is assumed to be caused by an increased pain threshold in the peripheral fibers and in the free nerve endings, a positive effect on the muscle spindles, and removal of mediator substances that cause pain. Through a combination of these types of effects, heat treatment suppresses the undesired development of a pain-spasm-pain cycle. Heat treatment may be administered in several forms, from hot baths and heat packs to various types of electrotherapy, laser, light, and ultrasound therapy. Because they can be used during training, neoprene and similar heat bandages are particularly useful aids in the rehabilitation and prevention of new injuries.

Preventing Sports Injuries

Roald Bahr

Introduction

A physically active lifestyle and active participation in sport are undoubtedly important for persons of all ages. However, individual motives for choosing an active lifestyle may vary. Common motives include the pleasure and sense of well-being that come from being physically active, innate competitiveness, a desire for social interaction, and a goal of maintaining or improving physical condition and health. However, participation in sport involves the risk of both overuse and acute injuries, and although uncommon, sport-related injuries may rarely result in permanent disability or even death. Of course, not all injuries in all sports are equally serious, but some sports—such as basketball, soccer, and team handball, have been documented to have a disturbingly high incidence of more serious injuries, particularly anterior cruciate ligament injuries. These injuries result in a long-term absence from work and sport and, despite the development of increasingly advanced treatment methods, increase the risk of early osteoarthritis in the affected joint. Consequently, sports injuries constitute a significant problem for sports, society, and for the affected individuals. However, sports injuries clearly represent a less serious burden to society than do traffic injuries and industrial accidents, the two personal injury categories that result in the greatest costs to society.

Nevertheless, many reports indicate that the health benefits from regular physical activity exceed the risk of injury associated with sport, even for elite athletes. Studies from Finland show that former national team athletes in endurance and team sports live to an older age than do nonathletes, largely because they have a lower incidence of cancer, lung disease, and heart and vascular disease. Former elite athletes also have a lower rate of hospitalization, although they are at greater risk for musculoskeletal and skeletal problems (primarily osteoarthritis in the knees and hips) than are nonathletes or recreational athletes.

Although the net health gains from regular physical activity include an increased life expectancy and a lower risk of cardiovascular disease and diabetes, we should not overlook the need to further reduce the risk of sports injury through prevention programs. This chapter begins with a description of the epidemiology of sports injuries, with an emphasis on the occurrence and severity of sports injuries. Next, causes and risk factors are described. Finally, prevention of sports injuries is discussed.

One of the greatest risk factors for any type of injury is a previous similar injury. Measures for avoiding reinjury (secondary prevention) are included in the sections on rehabilitation in chapters 4-15. Because injury prevention measures differ among sports, it is not possible to provide a complete description of all measures for all sports here. Therefore, the principles of prevention are described first, using examples of measures for three of the most common types of injuries—ankle injuries, knee injuries, and hamstring strains.

Incidence and Severity of Sports Injuries

Soccer, various skiing activities, and team handball cause the greatest portion of injuries in Norway. Overall, 33% of all injuries occur in soccer, 20% in skiing, and 12% in team handball (table 3.1). However, this does not mean that athletes in these sports are at the greatest risk of injury, since so many people ski and play soccer and team handball in Norway. The injuries are also unevenly distributed between the sexes: men sustain 84% of the injuries in soccer; women 62% of all injuries in team handball. This reflects the gender difference in participation rates for these sports. About one-fourth of all injuries sustained by children are sport related.

	13 to 17-year-olds	18 to 24-year-olds	25 to 64-year-olds	Persons older than 64 years
Soccer	30	36	33	3
Team handball	13	12	11	2
Volleyball	2	3	3	—
Basketball	8	5	1	2
Ball sports (unspecified)	7	6	6	4
Slalom/downhill skiing	5	6	5	1
Cross-country skiing	2	3	20	40
Ski jumping	2	2	4	—
Telemark skiing	3	2	2	1
Other ski sports including snow-boarding	2	1	—	—
Skating	1	1	1	—
Ice hockey	2	2	1	—
Gymnastics/martial arts	8	9	4	9
Track and field/jogging	3	4	6	11
Boating and water sports	2	1	2	3
Horseback riding	3	1	1	1
Other	3	3	6	16
Unspecified	2	2	3	7
Total (%)	100	100	100	100

Table 3.1 Injury distribution at outpatient clinics by sport and sex (n = 244,000). The distribution is based on figures from the Norwegian Public Health Registration at five Norwegian hospitals (1989-1997, Lereim 2000). Totals do not add up to 100 because of rounding off.

To compare the risk of injuries between various sports, the injury rate should be expressed as "incidence" or "prevalence." Incidence is best suited for describing the rate of acute injuries. It can be defined as the number of new injuries within a given time in a given population. It is usually expressed as the number of injuries per 1000 participation hours. For example, a soccer team with 16 players who train 8 hours a week during a 40-week season will have a combined exposure time of 5120 participation hours. If the team sustains a combined total of 46 injuries during the same period, the incidence is 9 injuries per 1000 participation hours (46/5120 × 1000). Injury rates are frequently broken down into the rate of injuries occurring during practice and the rate during competition. Incidence can also be expressed in other ways, such as the number of injuries per 1000 skier days, which is usually used to describe the incidence of injuries in downhill skiing.

Prevalence is the best way of describing the occurrence of overuse injuries. Prevalence can be defined as the percentage of athletes in a given population with an injury at a given time. For example, the prevalence is 30% if 3 out of 10 javelin throwers state that they have elbow pain.

Comparing the incidence between different sports or types of injuries presumes that the same definition of injury is used. Usually, only those injuries that result in a defined absence from training or competition (usually ≥ 1 day) are counted. If other less severe injuries that nevertheless required treatment were included, the incidence would be significantly higher. Limited information is available about some sports, but comparable figures exist for many team sports. As table 3.2 shows, the incidence of injuries occurring during competition is higher than that observed during training. This is to be expected, because the intensity is higher during competition and because much training time is used for warm-up exercises and technical training, during which the risk of injuries is low. The difference in incidence during games versus during practice can be considerable, particularly in sports with a high frequency of competition, such as ice hockey, where much of the training time is used strictly for recovery exercises.

The incidence of certain injury types of special interest can be calculated in a similar manner. For example, the frequency of anterior cruciate ligament injuries occurring during competition is about 0.1 injuries per 1000 hours among female soccer players and about 0.9 injuries per 1000 hours among female team handball players. This means that a typical Norwegian elite handball team can expect to lose one player every season as a result of a cruciate ligament injury. Another sport that causes concern because of a high proportion of serious knee injuries is downhill skiing, but incidence data that could be used to compare it with the risk of injuries in soccer and team handball are unavailable.

Sport	Incidence (number of injuries per 1000 participation hours)	
	In competition	In training
Basketball	2-3	5-6
Soccer	11-35	2-8
Team handball	14	1-2
Ice hockey	29-79	1-3
Volleyball	3-6	1-4

Table 3.2 Incidence of acute injuries during competition and training in selected team sports based on studies of Scandinavian elite sports.

To fully understand the risk related to participation in sport, one must consider not only the incidence of injuries but also their severity. The severity of an injury can be described in terms of the type and location of the injury, the type and duration of treatment required, expected absence from sport or work, resultant permanent disability, or direct or indirect costs. For example, the incidence of ankle injuries in volleyball is about the same as for anterior cruciate ligament injuries in team handball among women. However, because an anterior cruciate ligament injury carries with it a higher risk for future functional limitation than does an ankle sprain injury, injuries and their prevention tend to be a greater concern in team handball than in volleyball. The severity of an anterior cruciate ligament injury is reflected in the need for more comprehensive medical treatment when compared to an ankle sprain, longer absence from sport and work, a greater degree of medical disability, and higher direct and indirect treatment costs. Preventive measures should therefore assume particular importance and emphasis in sports that have a high incidence of serious injuries. Knee injuries have served as the focus of the above discussion, but head and neck injuries may warrant even more serious consideration.

Causes and Risk Factors

Prevention of sports injuries demands a thorough understanding of the cause(s) of the injuries. Even in cases in which the cause of an injury appears to be very obvious, such as a direct kick on the shin causing a transverse tibial fracture, in reality the cause may be quite complex. In this example, contributing factors could include shin guards that were too short, a pre-existing subclinical stress fracture in the area, an osteoporotic skeleton (e.g., due to an eating disorder), or simply that the athlete was fatigued at the end of a tough match and may have consequently been inattentive or too slow to avoid the contact.

Because the causes of sports injuries are often complex, more complete models have been developed to describe the multicausal relationships that also take into consideration the chain of events that result in an injury (figure 3.1). The Meeuwisse multifactorial causal model classifies intrinsic or athlete-related factors as predisposing factors that may be necessary, but are rarely sufficient, to trigger an injury. Examples of intrinsic risk factors include age, reduced range of motion, previous injuries that reduce neuromuscular function or cause mechanical instability, and osteoporosis. The existence of one or more intrinsic factors may predispose an athlete to injury. Extrinsic risk factors affect the athlete from the outside environment. Examples include playing team handball on flooring where the friction is too high or too low, playing soccer on an uneven grassy surface,

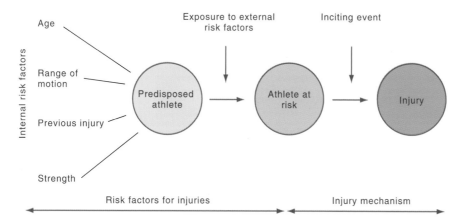

Figure 3.1 Causes of sport injuries. Meeuwisse's dynamic, multifactorial model of athletic injury etiology divides the causes into intrinsic and extrinsic risk factors and describes the injury mechanism in the inciting event.

sprint training in cold weather, and running on hard asphalt or running with bad shoes. Both intrinsic and extrinsic factors are usually separated in time from the moment the injury occurs and in isolation are rarely sufficient to cause injuries. However, the combination of, and the interaction between, risk factors renders the athlete vulnerable to injury.

To be able to both prevent injuries and provide effective treatment advice, the practitioner must understand the causes. This is particularly true of overuse injuries, which often recur if the athlete is unable to modify his loading pattern.

The inciting event is the last in a series of events that result in injury, and as a result the patient can usually describe the mechanism of injury (e.g., trauma to the lateral side of the knee that results in a medial ligament injury). Because an injury can often be described in simple kinematic terms, there is a danger that the description of the injury mechanism may draw attention away from important internal or external risk factors. Even though it is often difficult, the athlete's relevant risk factors must also be accurately identified to facilitate successful treatment and prevention of sports injuries. Although the Meeuwisse model provides a basis for an expanded understanding of the causes of injuries, it is not complete. One limitation is that the description of the injury mechanism alone may not provide sufficient information to permit planning and implementation of comprehensive preventive measures. The circumstances that lead up to the moment of injury may be just as important as the final mechanism, because certain characteristic playing situations may exist that carry with them a high risk of injuries. Another limitation is that the model does not take the team's training routine and competitive schedule into consideration as key injury risk factors.

Risk Analysis

It is possible to perform a risk analysis to document the parts of the season during which athletes are at the greatest risk for sustaining injuries as a result of the training or competitive programs (figure 3.2). Well-accepted examples of situations in which the risk of injury increases include switching from one training surface to another (e.g., from grass to gravel) or to new types of training (e.g., at the start

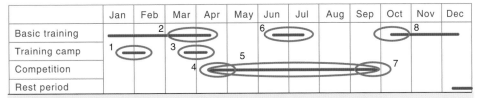

1. Change of surface, climate, and running tempo during training camp in Portugal.

2. Transition to greater training loads and high-intensity training, combined with several practice games indoors and on artificial turf.

3. Final training camp to polish up on form before beginning the competitive season, including practice games on hard grassy playing fields on Cyprus. Competition for a spot on the team increases the intensity during competition and training.

4. Start of the competitive season. A high tempo and packed competitive schedule to which the athlete is unaccustomed. Change of surface to soft grass.

5. High risk of acute injuries during the competitive season, featuring a packed competitive schedule at full intensity.

6. Period of hard basic training, including resistance training to which the athlete is unaccustomed, and more running than normal.

7. The end of the competitive season. Worn out and tired players?

8. Transition to basic training period, with running on gravel.

Figure 3.2 Risk profile. Examples of periods of the season when there is an increased risk of injury among members of a senior-level soccer team. Comments regarding the circled risk periods are listed under the chart.

of a strength-training period). This type of analysis is an important basis for planning preventive measures, particularly those designed to limit overuse injuries. The analysis is based on the idea that the risk of injuries is greater during transitional periods and that each stage has certain characteristics that may increase risk. The risk profile usually varies from sport to sport. Health care personnel responsible for teams or training groups should undertake this type of analysis in collaboration with the coaches and athletes and create a plan for relevant preventive measures, based on the risk analysis.

Principles for Preventing Sports Injuries

Ideally, injury prevention measures are developed on the basis of research information about the risk factors and the injury mechanisms in various sports. Because risk factors and injury mechanisms may be extremely different in different sports, it is not possible to describe specific measures for individual sports here. Instead, Haddon's matrix, a general model that may form the basis for developing preventive measures for various sports, is described first. Next, training methods that were developed to prevent some common injury types are described.

Originally developed primarily for motor vehicle accidents, Haddon's matrix is an injury prevention model that can be adapted to sports injuries (table 3.3). The model is two-dimensional. The first dimension divides injury prevention measures into three stages: precrash, crash, and postcrash. When the model is applied to sport, the second dimension can be divided into at least three groups; factors related to the athlete, the equipment, and the environment. Table 3.3 gives examples of how the model can be applied to develop injury prevention measures within various sports. The measures in the model assume sound understanding of the causes of injury, but whereas there is detailed information about the risk factors and injury mechanisms for some sports and the associated types of injury, the information for other sports and injuries is insufficient.

Measures related to the precrash stage have been developed to counteract potential injury-causing situations, by preventing accidents altogether. Precrash measures may focus on the athlete: for example, a downhill skier can improve his skiing technique to prevent falls or a team handball player can develop enhanced neuromuscular control of the knee to prevent landing with the knee in a vulnerable position. Precrash measures related to the surroundings might include optimizing playing surface conditions (e.g., if floor friction is too high it could increase the risk of injury to the knees and ankles, while if it is too low the athlete may slip and fall), or modifying the rules to

	Precrash	Crash	Postcrash
Athlete	Technique Neuromuscular function	Training status Falling techniques	Rehabilitation
Surroundings	Floor friction Playing rules	Safety nets	Emergency medical coverage
Equipment	Shoe friction	Tape or brace Ski bindings Leg padding	First aid equipment Ambulance

Table 3.3 Haddon's matrix applied to sport injury prevention: measures effective in preventing sport injuries.

prevent risky play (e.g., penalties for dangerous checking from behind in ice hockey or tackling from behind in soccer). Equipment-related examples of precrash measures could include changing footwear in accordance with the playing surface: for example, shoes should be worn with cleats that are the appropriate length for the weather conditions and type of playing surface (e.g., artificial turf vs grass).

Measures related to the second stage, the crash stage, have been developed to protect the athlete if a potentially injurious situation arises. Well-known examples of crash measures from traffic medicine are the use of seat belts and airbags in cars and laws requiring that protective helmets be worn by cyclists. Crash measures for sports injuries place special emphasis on athlete conditioning to train muscles, ligaments, and skeletal structures so that they can tolerate the forces resulting from accidents or collisions. Most injury prevention measures that have been developed to date have focused on sporting equipment, including release bindings on downhill skis, shin guards for soccer players, helmets for a number of different sports, taping or bracing to protect knee and ankle joints, and protective eyewear for racket sports and ice hockey.

Postcrash measures focus on reducing the consequences of an injury. These measures deal primarily with the medical treatment sequence, from first-aid interventions to hospital transport to injury rehabilitation protocols and techniques. This is an area in which medical personnel who assume responsibility for acute medical coverage during a sporting event have a special obligation.

General Injury Prevention Measures

Although different sports tend to have unique injury patterns, with different causes of and risk factors for the more commonly occurring injuries, a few general principles of injury prevention apply to sport in general.

Warm-up and stretching. Proper warm-up before all training and competition is a prerequisite for peak performance and for injury avoidance. Warm-up should begin with a general exercise at moderate intensity (such as jogging), in order to increase body temperature, and should be followed by stretching to prepare muscles and joints for maximal exertion. Stretching programs should include static stretching exercises, each lasting 10 to 15 seconds in duration, repeated at least three times for each muscle group. This type of stretching (which is for the purpose of preparing the muscle and joint for maximal efforts) should be distinguished from flexibility training (which is for the purpose of increasing the maximum joint range of motion). All relevant muscle groups essential for sport performance should be included. Additional specialized exercises adapted to a particular sport should be included to gradually approach the desired intensity. Whether stretching is effective in preventing injuries in endurance sports is controversial.

Proper progression of training. One of the most important risk factors for overuse injuries is increasing the training load too rapidly. However, if an athlete is going to improve his performance, he must increase his training load beyond that to which he is accustomed. To achieve this goal, the intensity, duration, or frequency of training may be increased or new types of training may be selected. Experience has shown that the risk of injuries is greatest in connection with changes in the training program–for example, at training camp, where the total amount of training may reach twice the normal level. Changes in training load should be well-planned, and special attention should be paid to the risk of overuse injuries. This is particularly true of team sports where some athletes may require more time to adjust to changes in training load than others. Similarly, the practitioner should be aware that a change in surface (e.g., from a soft surface like grass or gravel to a hard field surface) may result in changes in the loading pattern that can lead to injuries.

Protective gear. Protective gear is one of the most well-documented injury prevention measures in sports. When worn by athletes (e.g., glasses, helmets, mouth guards, braces and leg or arm padding), it is crucial that it fits properly. Protective gear on the playing field (e.g., the placement of safety nets on a downhill ski trail and padded referee stands in volleyball) must also be closely examined. Playing surfaces need to be evaluated. For example, globs of hand resin on a team handball court may create areas of extremely high friction. A poorly maintained soccer field may have divots or uneven areas that are potentially dangerous. A key job of the team doctor is to ensure that potentially dangerous elements are removed from the competitive field or court and that it is padded in a responsible manner. Worn or damaged protective gear should be replaced.

Fair play. The playing rules and equipment for various sports have been modified to accommodate developing or disabled athletes. Some playing rules have been instituted specifically for the purpose of preventing dangerous situations from arising, such as stricter penalties for illegally tackling from behind in soccer, checking from behind in ice hockey, and high-sticking and hooking in hockey. In many cases, the rules of play have evolved to include requirements for wearing safety gear, such as leg padding, visors, or helmets. Enforcement of the rules of play is the responsibility of the referees, and recognition and awareness of safety factors should be a central part of referee training. Nevertheless, it is even more vital for coaches and trainers to be aware of their responsibility and to clearly communicate attitudes toward fair play and respect for the rules of the sport. This includes being aware of signs of doping among athletes.

Physical exams. Routine preparticipation physical exams for healthy athletes cannot be generally recommended, as the costs are too high in comparison to the health benefits accrued. However, individuals with a known disease or injury should be examined, to assess the potential risk and make the necessary adjustment in their training program. This is particularly true of patients with known cardiovascular disease or patients with cardiopulmonary symptoms (e.g., angina pectoris or dyspnea) or findings such as hypercholesterolemia or hypertension that indicate an increased risk of cardiac events. Nevertheless, physical exams can play a key role for health personnel who are responsible for a specific team or a training group. An examination before the beginning of the season may uncover potential problems that may increase the athlete's risk of injury, such as sequelae from a previous injury, joint instability, generalized deconditioning, or biomechanical considerations (e.g., malalignment). This type of screening may be accomplished by means of a single clinical examination, or it may include advanced physiological tests for high-level athletes, where access to laboratory testing and resources allow it.

Preventing Ankle Injuries

Injury mechanisms and risk factors. Ankle injuries are typically caused by internal rotation and supination of the ankle when landing in plantar flexion, such as when running or landing on an uneven surface. In team sports such as basketball and volleyball, ankle injuries often result from one athlete landing on the foot of another, whereas ankle injuries in soccer may be caused by a combination of landing and tackling. The main intrinsic risk factor for ankle injuries is a history of previous ankle injury, particularly a relatively recent injury. Ankle sprains may result in mechanical instability if the lateral ligaments do not heal, or they may impair neuromuscular function—that is, the ability to register and correct the position of the foot. Some athletes with previous injuries have both mechanical instability and reduced neuromuscular function. Athletes may be at a higher risk for ankle injuries because of poor technique (beginners) or poor ability to register where teammates and oppo-

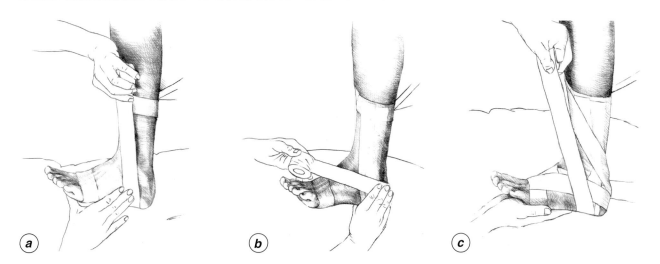

(a) (b) (c)

nents are located on the field. Extrinsic risk factors include the sporting surface, which may range from an uneven surface–which causes numerous ankle injuries in orienteering–to a hard surface to which the athlete is unaccustomed. This might occur, for example, when a soccer player makes the transition from training on grass to training on gravel or when a track and field athlete switches from training on grass and gravel in running shoes to running on a track with spiked shoes.

Preventive measures. Teaching appropriate technique is an important preventive measure. It is crucial to take the athlete's skill level into consideration when introducing risky exercises. There are several sports in which it is worthwhile to take time to perform exercises that emphasize basic movement skills, such as lateral movements, takeoffs, and landings, as a supplement to more sport-specific training. It is not known how helpful balance exercises are for improving ankle control and for preventing injuries in people who have not previously injured their ankle. However, for athletes who have had prior ankle injuries and have developed secondary instability, neuromuscular training has been shown to have a significant effect on ankle function while reducing the incidence of new injuries. For athletes with a history of prior ankle sprain, the use of ankle tape or a brace has also been proven to be an effective preventive measure. The reason may be that ankle braces work not by providing mechanical support but by stimulating neuromuscular function. Therefore, there is reason to recommend that athletes with a previous ankle injury and generally reduced neuromuscular function use tape (figure 3.3, a-c) or a brace (figure 3.4, a-b) to reduce the risk of recurrent injury. In that case, ankle support should be used until an appropriate neuromuscular training program has been completed.

Figure 3.3 One of many ankle taping techniques that can be used. Three alternate turns are made as "stirrups" under the heel *(a)* and around the forefoot *(b)*. Finally, the tape is locked using half *(c)* or whole figure eights around the heel.

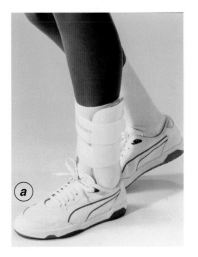
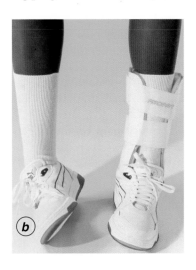

(a) (b)

Figure 3.4 Use the ankle brace. The brace is designed to allow free mobility for plantar/dorsal flexion *(a)*, while simultaneously providing support for supination *(b)*.

Ankle Program

Athletes with previous ankle injuries should complete a balance training program on a wobble board according to the "10-5-10" rule (i.e., 10 minutes, 5 times a week, for 10 weeks). This type of training may also be useful for preventing injuries in people with "healthy" ankles. In the basic position, the athlete stands on one leg while the other leg is lifted in the air with the knee bent at 90° (figure 3.5). The arms are crossed in front of the chest, and the goal is primarily to use an "ankle strategy" to maintain balance—that is, to attempt to make all balance corrections using the dynamic ankle joint stabilizers only, while repositioning the arms, hips, and knees as little as possible. At first, balancing on the floor may represent an adequate challenge, particularly if the athlete has her eyes closed. The difficulty of the training program can be progressively increased by having the patient stand on an unstable balance mat or on a balance board. As the athlete progresses, ball or partner exercises may be added to make training more challenging and fun.

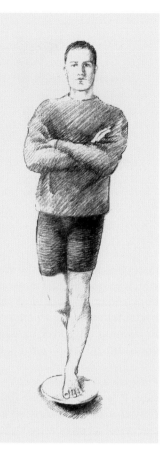

Figure 3.5 Balance exercises—ankle training. The basic position is with the arms crossed over the chest and the knee extended. The goal is to correct balance using the ankle alone.

Preventing Knee Injuries

Injury mechanisms and risk factors. The mechanisms that cause knee injuries are described in detail in chapter 12, and for the sake of simplicity they are classified here as contact injuries and noncontact injuries. Contact injuries result from collisions with other athletes or objects; noncontact injuries result from landings or cutting maneuvers that place the knee in a vulnerable position, where the stabilizing ligaments, particularly the anterior cruciate ligament, can be torn. The most common noncontact mechanism for knee injury seems to be sudden, powerful foot plant on a nearly extended knee that then collapses into a valgus position. Analysis of the risk factors for anterior cruciate ligament injury suggests that it occurs three to five times more frequently among women than among men in comparable sports. Several theories have been advanced to explain this gender difference in injury incidence—including narrower cruciate ligaments in females, narrower intercondylar notches in addition to other anatomical differences, hormonal effects on ligaments, poorer neuromuscular control among women, reduced strength, or inappropriate stopping and landing techniques. Ultimately, however, the cause is still unknown. The principle extrinsic risk factor for ACL injury may be the effect of friction between the athlete's shoe and the surface. Excessively high friction is thought to increase the risk of injuries by causing the foot to abruptly stop while planting or landing, causing the knee to twist suddenly.

Preventive measures. Because most ACL injuries (particularly in team handball) occur when attempting a fake or in a landing situation, it is natural to focus preventive measures on changing the faking and landing technique. This may be accomplished

Knee Program

BALANCE EXERCISES

The main exercise is a balance exercise that emphasizes knee control, keeping the "knee over the toes" (figure 3.6). The goal is primarily to use a "knee strategy" to maintain balance—that is, to attempt to correct balance in the knee joint as much as possible and to minimize the use of arms, hips, and ankles. The exercises are normally done standing on a balance board or on an unstable balance pad, with the knee slightly flexed. Ball or partner exercises may also be included to make the training more challenging and fun. The exercises can be adjusted to the relevant sport, incorporating faking and landing exercises that imitate the requirements of the sport, while continually emphasizing knee control. The exercises are well suited for use as part of a warm-up program. During an initial training period of at least 5 weeks, the exercise should be done at least 3 times per week, training 10 to 15 minutes at each session. Maintenance training is done once or twice a week throughout the competitive season.

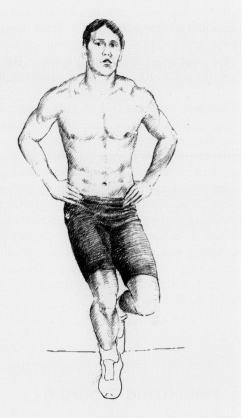

Figure 3.6 Balance exercises—knee control. The basic position is with the hands on the hips and the knee slightly bent. The goal is to make all balance corrections using the knee.

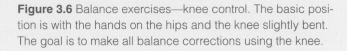

by teaching the players to land on two legs instead of one. Two-legged landings will reduce the forces affecting the knee, thus reducing the load on the anterior cruciate ligament. It has also been suggested that athletes should practice faking and landing with the knees bent even more, thereby distributing the forces that act on the knee over a larger range of motion and reducing the maximum force that transmitted to the anterior cruciate ligament. An individualized program emphasizing neuromuscular training of the knee has been demonstrated to reduce the risk of anterior cruciate ligament injuries. This program used balance exercises to enhance control over and awareness of knee positioning during fakes and landings. The goal is to train athletes to avoid situations in which the knees are subject to valgus loading. Use of a knee orthosis is known to prevent knee injuries, particularly medial and lateral collateral ligament injuries in contact sports like football. Such orthoses have not been proven to be effective in noncontact sports in general or for anterior cruciate ligament injuries in particular.

Preventing Hamstring Strain

Injury mechanisms and risk factors. Hamstring strains (incomplete tears or ruptures of the semimembranosus, semitendinosus, and the biceps femoris muscles), typically occur at the myotendinous junction. The hamstring muscles are two joint muscles that extend the hip joint and flex the knee joint. The injuries usually occur during maximum sprinting, when resisting knee extension, or at foot strike, when the muscle is close to its maximum length and eccentric power generation is at its maximum. Hamstring strains are the most common injury among soccer players and sprinters. An important risk factor is poor warm-up (e.g., a soccer player who begins training with maximal sprints or by shooting at the goal instead of first warming up). Two less well-documented risk factors for hamstring strains are reduced range of motion and poor strength. In some individuals, a previous strain that caused scar tissue to form in the hamstring musculature may result in reduced range of motion. If the quadriceps musculature is strong but the hamstring muscles are weak in relation, the risk of hamstring strains is also increased.

Preventive measures. The most important step in preventing hamstring strains is to warm up thoroughly–in particular, to stretch out the posterior side of the thigh before maximal sprinting–so that the muscles are prepared for maximum loads. This is especially true if the weather is cold. In cold weather, athletes should dress warmly, and it may be advisable to avoid maximal sprint training altogether, depending on the conditions. Note that the type of stretching performed is not for the purpose of increasing range of motion, but rather to prepare for maximal effort. This type of pre-exercise stretching is not sufficient if the athlete wishes to improve flexibility and range of motion. To achieve this latter goal, the athlete must also engage in separate systematic stretching sessions, preferably at the end of the regular training session. In addition, athletes should strengthen the posterior musculature, particularly emphasizing eccentric muscle action. Figures 3.7 through 3.9 show an exercise program for preventing hamstring injuries.

Hamstring Program

Warm-up Exercises

During warm-up before every single training session and game, stretch your hamstring musculature *before* beginning sprinting or shooting exercises (figure 3.7). Use support, preferably from another player. Allow your ankle to relax. Press your heel against the ground for 5 to 10 seconds, to activate the hamstring muscles, then relax and use your hand to straighten out your knee. Hold the stretch for about 20 seconds. If necessary, bend forward slightly at your hip until you feel the stretch in the hamstrings, but be sure to keep your back straight. Stretch each leg three times.

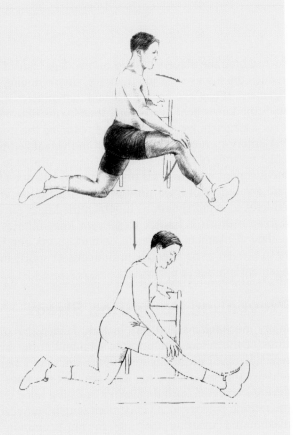

Figure 3.7 Warm-up exercises—hamstring stretching. The goal is to prepare for maximal effort.

PREVENTING SPORTS INJURIES

FLEXIBILITY TRAINING

If your range of motion is limited, stretch your hamstring muscles regularly for 5 to 10 minutes at a time, at least three times a week during the preseason period and twice a week during the competitive season (figure 3.8). Your partner lifts your leg with the knee slightly bent, until you feel stretching on the posterior side of your thigh. Hold this position for a while before actively pressing your leg against your partner's shoulder, so that your knee straightens out. Hold for 10 seconds. Then relax completely while your partner carefully stretches, by leaning forward. Hold that position for at least 45 seconds. It is important to relax your ankle, so you stretch the posterior side of the thigh, and not the lower leg. Stretch each leg three times.

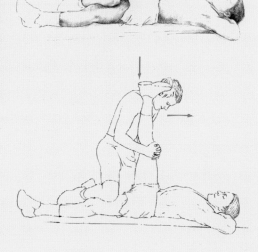

Figure 3.8 Flexibility training—hamstring stretching. The goal is to increase range of motion in the hip joint.

STRENGTH TRAINING

Perform eccentric strength training for the hamstring group regularly, at least three times a week during the preseason period and twice a week during the competitive season (figure 3.9). Some American football and European soccer teams have successfully used this type of eccentric strength training. The resistance exercises are partner exercises, in which your partner stabilizes your legs. Lean forward in a smooth movement, keep your back and hips extended, and work at resisting the forward fall with your hamstring muscles as long as possible until you land on your hands. Go all the way down so that your chest touches the ground and push off immediately with your arms until the hamstring muscles can take over and you can straighten up into a kneeling position again.

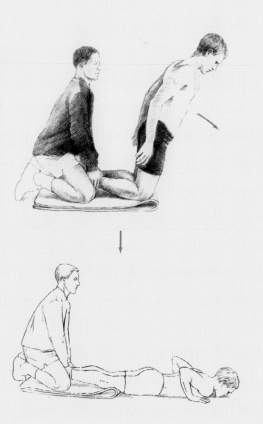

Figure 3.9 Eccentric strength training for the hamstrings. The goal is to hold the descent as long as possible, to achieve maximal eccentric loading of the hamstrings.

Head Injuries

Paul McCrory and Ingunn R. Rise

Clinicians must be able to recognize and manage brain injuries ranging from mild concussion to fatal penetrating brain trauma. The most common form of brain injury is concussion. Sports medicine physicians, trainers, and others involved in athletic care need to have a thorough understanding of the early management of the concussed athlete and the potential sequelae of such injuries that may affect the athlete's ability to return to sport. This chapter deals only with sport-related head injury (see table 4.1).

Definition

Head trauma is the broad description applied to injuries to the brain or its coverings, skull bones, soft tissues, and vascular structures of the head and neck. In this chapter, when considering such injuries, the term traumatic brain injury will be applied to the injuries of the brain or central nervous system, and head injury to incorporate injuries to other structures of the head.

Occurrence

Traumatic brain injury is one of the leading causes of morbidity and mortality worldwide. The crude incidence for all traumatic brain injuries is estimated at 300 per 100,000 inhabitants per year. Males are more than twice as likely to suffer a traumatic brain injury than females, with a peak incidence among the 15- to 24-year-old population. Mild traumatic brain injury accounts for 80% of all brain injuries, with moderate and severe injury each accounting for 10%. Concussion, which is a subset of mild brain injury, requires appropriate management to avoid potential long-term problems. In the United States, approximately 300,000 sport-related concussions occur annually.

Most common	Less common	Must not be overlooked ❗
Concussion (p. 63)	Migraine	Skull fracture (p. 65)
		Diffuse cerebral swelling (p. 65)
		Postconcussion syndrome (p. 66)
		Acute subdural hematoma (p. 67)
		Extradural hematoma (p. 68)
		Traumatic intracranial hematoma/contusion (p. 69)
		Traumatic subarachnoid hemorrhage (p. 70)

Table 4.1 Overview of the differential diagnosis of acute head injuries.

In hospital-based surveys of brain trauma, sports injuries contribute to approximately 10% to 15% of all cases. The sports most commonly associated with severe brain injuries were golf, horse riding, and mountain climbing. Sport-related deaths due to brain injury are rare, although these injuries have not been rigorously studied outside American and Australian football.

Differential Diagnosis

In moderate to severe brain injury, the differential diagnosis is limited, and the fact that an athlete has sustained a significant brain injury is usually obvious. The diagnostic problem in this situation is that of sorting out the different types of injury (e.g., subdural hematoma, extradural hematoma) and then determining the appropriate management priorities.

In mild brain injury and, in particular, the subset of concussion, the diagnosis is often missed because the symptoms are subtle, the athlete does not seek medical attention, or the athlete recovers rapidly before a full assessment can be made. Most sport-related head injuries occur without loss of consciousness. In this situation, the most common differential diagnosis is that of posttraumatic migraine, which may manifest similar early symptoms. The key clinical symptom of concussion used in establishing the presence of this injury is memory disturbance. The key differential diagnosis not to be missed is that of an expanding intracranial hematoma, which may mimic the symptoms of concussion in its early stages.

Diagnostic Thinking

The key objectives when assessing any athlete who has sustained a traumatic brain injury are

- to institute an appropriate first aid sideline assessment of the injured athlete;
- to make an accurate diagnosis and rule out an expanding intracranial hematoma; and
- to manage the injury appropriately, minimizing the risk of any secondary injury such as might be seen with coexistent hypoxia or hypotension.

Although many general classification schemes for traumatic brain injury have been proposed, the most widely used system is the Glasgow Coma Scale (GCS) (table 4.2). This scale has two distinct uses: to measure brain injury status and to separate traumatic brain injury into a prognostically useful injury severity grading. In the former role, an immediate GCS is performed at the time of the initial assessment of an injured patient and then continuously to monitor progress. In the second role, the separation of mild, moderate, and traumatic brain injury is based on a scoring system using eye opening, verbal response, and motor response to standard stimuli and is measured at 6 hours postinjury after resuscitation has been completed. It is important to note that the term *concussion* (or *commotio cerebri*) refers to a different injury construct and is not synonymous with the term mild traumatic brain injury.

The treating clinician must also face the decision of who should be referred to a hospital emergency facility or neurosurgical center. Table 4.3 lists some urgent indications. Even though some of these indications are based on anecdotal rather than evidence-based information, they are widely accepted. Referral to a neurosurgical center also depends on the experience, ability, and competence of the physician at hand. The clinical referral pathways will be different for the team physician who happens to be a neurologist or neurosurgeon experienced in brain injury management and for a family practitioner called to assist at a football match after an injury has occurred. The overall approach should be "when in doubt, refer." If no physician is present, and the

Category	Response	Score
Eye opening response (E)	Spontaneous	4
	To speech	3
	To pain	2
	No response	1
Verbal response (V)	Oriented	5
	Confused, disoriented	4
	Inappropriate words	3
	Incomprehensible sounds	2
	No response	1
Motor response (M)	Obeys commands	6
	Localizes	5
	Withdraws (flexion)	4
	Abnormal flexion (posturing)	3
	Extension (posturing)	2
	No response	1

Table 4.2 Glasgow Coma Scale. Score = E + M + V (maximum 15).

Any player who has or develops the following:

- Fractured skull
- Penetrating skull trauma
- Deterioration in conscious state after injury
- Focal neurological signs
- Confusion or impairment of consciousness >30 minutes
- Loss of consciousness >5 minutes
- Persistent vomiting or increasing headache postinjury
- Any convulsive movements
- More than one episode of concussive injury in a session
- Where there is assessment difficulty (e.g., an intoxicated patient)
- Children with head injuries
- High risk patients (e.g., hemophilia, anticoagulant use)
- Inadequate postinjury supervision
- High risk injury mechanism (e.g., high velocity impact)

Table 4.3 Indications for urgent hospital referral.

management is in the hands of an athletic trainer, physical therapist, or paramedically trained individual, then medical referral should be considered mandatory in all cases of head injury.

Clinical History

The fact that an athlete has suffered a head injury is usually obvious to the team medical staff. Head injuries in collision sports are usually the result of direct trauma

Time and place of injury
Mechanism of injury (eyewitness or video)
Presence or duration of loss of consciousness
Postinjury behavior
Presence of convulsions postinjury
Past medical history
Medication use

Table 4.4 Early assessment of concussion—history.

to the athlete's head but may also be caused by falls or whiplash-type head movement during all types of sport activities. Witness information or videotape of the episode, where available, is vital in understanding the nature of the injury, especially if the athlete is unconscious. Information about the event and about the immediate clinical findings must be directly conveyed to the hospital staff. Table 4.4 lists the kind of relevant data they will need.

The clinical symptoms of head injury can vary enormously. In more severe cases, loss of consciousness is the rule, although in mild brain injury and concussion this is rarely the case. More severe types of brain injury are also typically associated with focal signs or symptoms such as paralysis, speech disturbance, double vision, or sensory disturbance. When focal symptoms are present, careful neurological examination is required to separate spinal cord injury from brain injury. In milder cases, the symptoms may be nonspecific, such as headache or blurred vision, but associated cognitive disturbance such as memory loss or confusion is invariably present. These cognitive symptoms may be transient in nature but should be sought in all cases.

Sideline or First Aid Management

Sideline management occurs when the clinician is at a sporting event and is called on to manage an acute brain injury. The major priorities at this early stage are the basic principles of first aid. The letters DR ABC are a simple and useful mnemonic device (table 4.5).

Once the basic aspects of first aid care have been achieved and the athlete is stabilized, consideration of removal of the athlete from the field to an appropriate facility is then necessary. Only trained individuals should remove the athlete's helmet.

D	Danger	Ensure that there are no immediate environmental dangers that may potentially injure the patient or treatment team. This may involve stopping play in a football match or marshalling cars on a motor racetrack.
R	Response	Is the patient conscious? Can he talk?
A	Airway	Ensure a clear and unobstructed airway. Remove any mouthguard or dental device that may be present.
B	Breathing	Ensure the patient is breathing adequately.
C	Circulation	Ensure an adequate circulation.

Table 4.5 Basic principles of first aid.

Careful assessment for the presence of a cervical spine injury or other injury is necessary. Neck bracing and transport on a suitable spinal frame are required if an alert athlete complains of neck pain, has evidence of neck tenderness or deformity, or has neurological signs suggestive of a spinal injury (see chapter 5). If the athlete is unconscious, a cervical injury should be assumed until proven otherwise. Airway protection takes precedence over any potential spine injury.

The clinical management may involve the treatment of a disoriented, confused, unconscious, uncooperative, or convulsing patient. The immediate treatment priorities remain the basic first aid principles of ABC (airway, breathing, and circulation). Once these have been established and the patient has been stabilized, a full medical and neurological assessment exam should be performed. On-site physicians are in an ideal position to initiate the critical early steps of medical care to ensure optimal recovery from a head injury.

Clinical Examination

The clinician should perform a full neurological examination on an athlete with a head injury. Because the major management priorities at this stage are to establish an accurate diagnosis and exclude a catastrophic intracranial injury, this part of the examination should be particularly thorough.

The neurological exam should include a baseline measurement of the Glasgow Coma Score. The initial neurological exam serves as a reference to which other repeated neurological examinations may be compared. It is necessary to record findings so that an overall trend in improving or deteriorating mental function can be clearly and objectively documented. In addition, skull palpation should be a quick and simple component of every physical exam in head trauma. The exam also should include a check for CSF leak from the nose or ears. Fluid that runs from the nose or ears can be clear or mixed with blood. A positive glucose stick test indicates that the fluid is cerebrospinal fluid. The assessment of cognitive function in this situation is covered in the section on concussion management (see page 63).

Vital signs must be recorded after an injury. Although head injury produces several types of respiratory patterns, an acute rise in intracranial pressure with central herniation usually manifests rising blood pressure and falling pulse rate (the Cushing response). Hypotension is rarely due to brain injury, except as a terminal event, and alternate sources for the drop in blood pressure should be aggressively sought and treated. Restlessness is a frequent accompaniment of brain injury or cerebral hypoxia. If the patient is unconscious but restless, attention should be given to the possibility of increased cerebral hypoxia, a distended bladder, or painful injuries elsewhere. Only when these causes have been ruled out should drug sedation be considered. This point cannot be underestimated because cerebral hypotension and hypoxia are the main determinants of outcome following brain injury and are treatable factors.

When time permits, a more thorough physical exam should be performed to exclude coexistent injuries and to detect the late-developing signs of skull injury (e.g., Battle sign). In recent times the application of simple neuropsychological tests has created considerable interest as a means to objectively assess the cognitive function of athletes with concussions. The standard approach of asking the orientation items (e.g., day, date, year, time, and date of birth) has been shown to be unreliable following concussive injury. This aspect of memory remains relatively intact in the face of concussive injury, so the orientation test should not be used. More useful in making a diagnosis of concussion, as demonstrated in prospective studies, are questions of recent memory. A typical question battery (Maddock's questions) is shown in table 4.6. An alternative

Which field are we at?
Which team are we playing today?
Who is your opponent at present?
Which quarter is it?
How far into the quarter is it?
Which side scored the last goal?
Which team did we play last week?
Did we win last week?

Table 4.6 Postconcussion memory assessment (Maddock's questions).

valid assessment strategy would be the SAC (standardized assessment of concussion). This is a 5- to 10-minute written test that has been shown to be valid in the trainer's diagnosis of concussion. The SAC is a far less practical tool than the Maddock's questions, which are designed for rapid on-field assessment.

If the presence of a concussive injury has been determined, the athlete needs to be continuously monitored until full recovery ensues. If the athlete is sent home after recovery, he should be in the care of a responsible adult. The patient and his attendant should be given a head injury advice card at the time of discharge.

Supplemental Examinations

Indications for emergent cranial CT imaging in the initial evaluation of the athlete with a head injury are listed in table 4.7.

Computed tomography (CT). CT evaluation should proceed as soon as the patient is hemodynamically stable and all immediately life-threatening injuries have been addressed. Because the incidence of delayed extradural hematoma formation following head trauma is substantial, any deterioration in the neurological examination warrants prompt evaluation by CT, even if a previous study was normal. Delayed onset of extradural hematoma has been reported in patients whose initial CT scans were normal. Performing a CT scan on children may present practical difficulties, so young children may need to be sedated or anesthetized for an optimum scan.

Depressed level of consciousness
Focal neurological deficit
Deteriorating neurological status
Skull fracture
Progressive or severe headache
Persistent nausea or vomiting
Posttraumatic seizure
Mechanism of injury suggesting high risk of intracranial hemorrhage
Examination obscured by alcohol, drugs, metabolic derangement, or postictal state
Patient inaccessibility for serial neurological examinations
Coagulopathy and other high-risk medical conditions

Table 4.7 Indications for emergent neuroimaging—for any player who has or develops the conditions listed above.

Magnetic resonance imaging (MRI). The role of MR imaging in the evaluation of acute head trauma is limited. Compared to CT, MRI is time consuming, expensive, and less sensitive to acute hemorrhage. Moreover, access to critically ill or unconscious patients is restricted during lengthy periods of image acquisition, and the strong magnetic fields generated by the scanner necessitate the use of nonferromagnetic resuscitative equipment. Currently, MR imaging is best suited for electively defining associated parenchymal injuries after the acute event.

Plain X ray examination. Other, more traditional diagnostic tools have largely been supplanted by cranial CT in the initial assessment of the head-injured patient. Plain skull radiographs are inexpensive and easily obtained and often reveal fractures in patients with extradural hemorrhage. However, the predictive value of such films is poor, because one finding is not requisite for the other. Lateral shift of the pineal gland, indicative of hemispheric mass effect, is a nonspecific and highly variable finding.

Neuropsychological testing. Neuropsychological testing to determine recovery and guide return to play is accepted worldwide. In Australian football, such strategies have been used since 1985. More recently, American professional football and ice hockey (NHL) have followed similar strategies. Computerized test platforms such as CogSport (www.cogsport.com) have largely replaced the traditional "pen and paper" assessments for screening large numbers of athletes. Postinjury tests are usually compared to a player's baseline or preseason performance. The most important conceptual point is the understanding that these tests are not designed as a diagnostic test for concussion in the acute situation but rather are a means of objectively measuring return to baseline level of function and hence guide the timing of return to play.

Specific Diagnoses—Common Injuries

Brain Concussion—Commotio Cerebri

The most widely used definition of concussion was proposed by the Congress of Neurological Surgeons (now the American Association of Neurological Surgeons). It states that concussion is ". . . a clinical syndrome characterized by the immediate and transient posttraumatic impairment of neural function such as alteration of consciousness, disturbance of vision or equilibrium due to mechanical forces." Because of the obvious limitations in this definition, the Vienna Consensus Group in 2002 proposed a new definition of concussion that has now become the standard. The key points of this definition include the following:

- Concussion may be caused either by a direct blow to the head or elsewhere on the body with an "impulsive" force transmitted to the head.
- Concussion results in an immediate and short-lived impairment of neurological function.
- Concussion may result in neuropathological changes; however, the acute clinical symptoms largely reflect a functional disturbance rather than structural injury.
- Concussion may result in a graded set of clinical syndromes that may or may not involve loss of consciousness. Resolution of the clinical and cognitive symptoms typically follows a sequential stereotyped course.
- Concussion typically has normal conventional (CT and MR scanning) neuroimaging studies.

The classification of concussion injury severity is a complex and controversial area of injury management. More than 40 published concussion grading schemes exist, none of which have been scientifically validated. The Vienna Consensus Group recently recommended that all grading schemes be abandoned and management be directed at measuring individual recovery using a combination of clinical symptoms and cognitive assessment.

- Symptoms and signs–early management: This refers to the situation in which an injured athlete has been brought for assessment to the medical room or alternatively to an emergency department or medical facility. Assessment of injury severity is best performed in a quiet medical room rather than in the middle of a football field in front of 100,000 screaming fans. During assessment of the acutely concussed player, various aspects of the history and examination are important. The symptoms of acute concussion include loss of consciousness, headache, dizziness, blurred vision, balance disturbance, and nausea. It is worth noting that the presence of headache is not confined to concussion; up to 20% of athletes report exercise-related headache. Given that much emphasis is placed on headache as an important symptom of concussion, medical assessment must be accurate in ascertaining the nature and cause of the player's symptoms. Loss of consciousness, an important aspect of concussion, has been repeatedly emphasized in published studies. Although an important symptom of concussion in its own right, loss of consciousness has no prognostic significance in this setting. As such its presence or absence should not be the basis on which diagnosis, further investigation, or management is determined. In a brain concussion, unlike severe traumatic brain injury, the duration of the loss of consciousness has no predictive value in determining injury outcome.
- Symptoms and signs–late management: This refers to the situation in which a player has sustained a concussive injury previously and is now presenting for advice or clearance before resuming sport. The main management priorities at this stage are the assessment of recovery and the application of the appropriate return to sport guidelines.
- Management of posttraumatic seizures: Impact seizures or concussive convulsions are a rare but well-recognized sequelae of head impact. These are not epileptic and require no specific management beyond the treatment of the underlying concussive injury. By contrast, posttraumatic epilepsy may also occur and is more common with increasing severity of brain injury. A convulsing patient is at increased risk of hypoxia with resultant exacerbation of the underlying brain injury. Maintenance of cerebral oxygenation and perfusion pressure (blood pressure) is critical in the management of such patients. Management of posttraumatic seizures is determined by the timing of their occurrence in relation to the head injury. Because of the potential for convulsions to cause a dramatic increase in intracranial pressure, intense efforts should be made to prevent seizures during the recovery phase of the acute head injury. Phenytoin (or fosphenytoin) is usually the drug of choice in this situation because a loading dose can be administered intravenously to rapidly achieve therapeutic concentrations and because phenytoin does not impair consciousness. Benzodiazepines (e.g., lorazepam, clonazepam, diazepam) can be used for the acute treatment of posttraumatic seizures, but they will produce at least transient impairment of consciousness. Neither phenytoin, any of the benzodiazepines, nor any other antiepileptic drug has been shown to be effective for preventing the development of posttraumatic epilepsy. After recovery from the acute head injury, posttraumatic epilepsy should be managed in the same manner as symptomatic focal epilepsy from any etiology.
- Prognosis: Criteria for return to sport after a concussion remains the most contentious area of debate. Although the traditional approach is to advocate a mandatory arbitrary exclusion period from sport, the use of neuropsychological testing in conjunction with clinical assessment opens the door to the possibility of objective and scientifically valid testing of patient recovery. Where any doubt exists, clinical judgment should prevail. The guiding policy should be that until

completely symptom free, concussed athletes should not resume any training or competition. All athletes sustaining a concussion require a medical clearance, which may include neuropsychological testing, before resumption of their sport. Once the acute concussive symptoms resolve, a graduated plan of return to low-level aerobic training followed by noncontact drills and finally contact play will allow close monitoring of the development of any adverse symptoms. Persisting or newly developing symptoms necessitate further follow-up and detailed medical evaluation.

Other Specific Diagnoses

Cranial Fracture—Skull Fracture *!*

All types of sport activity in which trauma to the head occurs have the potential to cause a cranial fracture. Cranial fractures are divided into two categories: linear fractures and depressed fractures. Most linear fractures are uncomplicated, although a coexistent extradural hematoma may be seen particularly in children. A depressed fracture caused by a blow to the head from a relatively small object causes the bone fragments to impact or tear the dura mater of the brain.

- Symptoms and signs: Athletes with a cranial fracture usually have a headache and may or may not have symptoms of an underlying brain injury. Local soft tissue swelling may also indicate an underlying fracture, and palpation of the skull should be a mandatory part of the clinical assessment of all head injuries. Percussion of the skull may result in a characteristic "cracked pot" sound. Rhinorrhea and otorrhea are classic signs of skull fracture with torn dural membranes. If a glucose stick test of nasal or ear fluid leak is positive, the fluid is cerebrospinal fluid.
- Diagnosis: The diagnosis is usually made with a CT scan of the head or plain skull X ray.
- Management: In all cases of skull fracture, especially if a CSF leak is present, an urgent neurosurgical consultation is required. When a skull fracture is suspected, the patient should always be hospitalized for observation and neurosurgical evaluation. The physician should cover the injured area of an open cranial fracture with a sterile dressing.
- Prognosis: Linear fractures heal in a few months to a year; if no additional injury occurs, the athlete can often return to her sport. The grade of brain injury will usually determine the outcome. The prognosis is often good when the brain and membranes are uninjured.

Diffuse Cerebral Swelling—Second Impact Syndrome *!*

Diffuse cerebral swelling (figure 4.1) is a rare but well-recognized complication of mild traumatic brain injury that occurs predominantly in children and teenagers. The impact, however trivial, sets in train the rapid development of cerebral swelling due to increased cerebral blood volume, which usually results in brainstem herniation and death. Its cause is unknown but is thought to involve disordered cerebral vascular autoregulation control mechanisms.

The injured brain has long been known to swell within the cranial cavity. This increase in brain volume, whatever its cause or nature, will eventually be associated with an increase in intracranial pressure (ICP). In the first few hours and days following severe head injury, ICP is often raised because of alterations in the volume of the cerebrovascular bed, whereas brain swelling subsequent to this time is due to an increase in brain tissue water content. CT scanning and anecdotal evidence show massive traumatic cerebral edema, which occurs within 20 minutes of cerebral injury.

The second impact syndrome is a label attributed to the finding of cerebral swelling after head injury where repeated concussive injuries have been proposed as the cause of this syndrome. This has been scientifically examined, and the published evidence for the existence of this phenomenon is not compelling. It is more likely that a single impact of any severity may result in the rare complication of diffuse cerebral swelling as outlined previously. However, participation in sport often draws attention to concussive injuries in this setting.

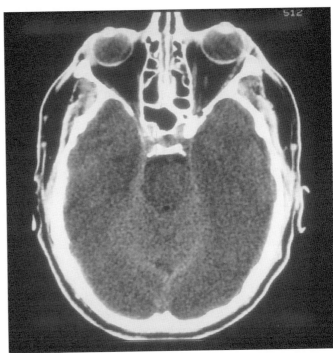

Figure 4.1 Axial CT images of the brain demonstrating diffuse cerebral swelling with sulcal effacement and loss of ventricular and cisternal spaces.

- Symptoms and signs: Downward displacement of the cerebrum caused by increased intracranial pressure results in compression of the diencephalon and midbrain through the tentorial notch. During this process, the ipsilateral third cranial nerve and the posterior cerebral artery are compressed by the uncus and edge of the tentorium. Herniation can also compress the posterior cerebral artery to cause occipital lobe ischemia.
- Treatment: If cerebral swelling is suspected or noted on imaging studies an urgent neurosurgical consultation is required. Treatment for elevated intracranial pressure due to edema relies on several modalities. The goal is to normalize elevated intracranial pressure by restricting cerebral blood flow or fluid to the brain tissue. Treatments that are currently used include hyperventilation, diuresis, fluid restriction, blood pressure control, steroids or surgery when indicated, and drug therapy.
- Prognosis: In cases of cerebral herniation complicated by ischemia, patients may suffer permanent neurological sequelae. It has also been found that individuals with absent pupillary light reflexes never regained independent daily function, but the early onset after the initial insult of incomprehensible speech, orienting spontaneous eye movements, or the ability to follow commands was indicative of a good outcome. Measurement of intracranial pressure also has been linked with prognosis. Most patients with a maximum intracranial pressure increase of less than 30 mm Hg experience good recovery. Others have noted that aggressive treatment based on intracranial pressure monitoring can significantly reduce mortality when applied to patients with cerebral swelling secondary to head injury.

The Postconcussion Syndrome !

The issue of a constellation of physical and cognitive symptoms labeled the postconcussive syndrome (PCS) remains as controversial today as when it was first proposed in the 19th century.

- Symptoms and signs: Symptoms may include headache, vertigo, dizziness, nausea, memory complaints, blurred vision, noise and light sensitivity, difficulty concentrating, fatigue, depression, sleep disturbance, loss of appetite, anxiety, loss of coordination, and hallucinations. It is worth noting that these symptoms are not the same as the acute symptoms of concussion that typically resolve over several days but are instead a difficult-to-characterize symptom complex that blurs into the acute recovery period, which then remains persistent. Two distinct schools of thought have arisen regarding the pathophysiology of this condition. The first proposes that the symptoms associated with PCS are a direct consequence of brain injury, whereas the second proposes that the symptoms are functional and represent psychological or emotional sequelae of the brain injury. The issue of malingering and compensible litigation is also often proposed as a mechanism for symptom prolongation. At this time the relative contribution of these two mechanisms remains unclear.

- Treatment: No specific treatment is available for this condition.
- Prognosis: This condition is usually noted several months after injury and may be the basis for ongoing difficulties. As such its investigation and management is elective in nature. In broad terms, PCS is uncommon in most collision and contact sport situations, although relatively few studies have followed sporting populations for significant lengths of time. Whether this relates to different impact forces as compared to motor vehicle crash studies remains speculative. In general terms, the incidence decreases with time with approximately 75% resolution by 12 months postinjury.

Acute Subdural Hematoma !

Subdural hematomas (figure 4.2) can be the result of either nonpenetrating or penetrating trauma to the head. In both scenarios, extravasation of blood into the subdural space is the mechanism for hematoma formation caused by arterial bleeding from the surface of the brain. These injuries are typically seen after falls on hard surfaces or assaults with nondeformable objects rather than from low-velocity injuries.

- Symptoms and signs: Clinical signs and symptoms depend on the size and location of the subdural hematoma as well as the rapidity of its development. As a rule, the more severe the head injury, the more likely the presence of a subdural hematoma. In most cases, at least a brief period of confusion or loss of consciousness is reported. Only one-third of the patients remain lucid throughout their course. Impaired alertness and cognitive function are found frequently during initial examination. Soft tissue injuries are seen at the site of impact. Other signs of significant head trauma, which can result in subdural hematomas, include periorbital and postauricular ecchymoses, hemotympanum, CSF otorrhea/rhinorrhea, and facial fractures. The focal neurological deficits depend on the location and size of the lesion. Enlargement of the hematoma or an increase in edema surrounding the hematoma produces additional mass effect, with further depression of the patient's level of consciousness, increases in motor or

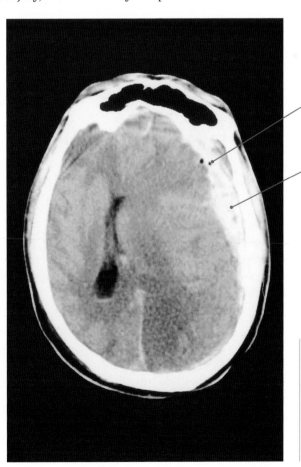

Air bubbles

Subdural hematoma

Figure 4.2 Subdural hematoma with cerebral edema. Left-side subdural hematoma with air bubbles as a sign of skull fracture and torn dura, cerebral edema, and midline shift.

speech deficit, and eventually ipsilateral compression of the third nerve and midbrain.

• Treatment: Medical management of subdural hematoma is the same as for intracerebral hematomas. An urgent neurosurgical consultation is required. Although some hematomas may be managed conservatively with mannitol, corticosteroids, or both, some authors advocate evacuating all hematomas to eliminate the mass effect and vasoactive substances released by the hematoma that may promote further ischemia. Operative treatment is directed toward evacuation of the entire subdural hematoma; control of the source of hemorrhage; resection of contused, nonviable brain; and removal of confluent intraparenchymal hemorrhage.

• Prognosis: Frequently, the impact that produces acute subdural hematoma also causes severe injury to the cerebral parenchyma. This coexisting severe brain injury explains, in large part, the superior outcome in these other entities (e.g., extradural hematomas) when compared with acute subdural hematoma. Indeed, in most cases of acute subdural hematoma, it is likely that the extra-axial collection is less important in determining outcome than the parenchymal injury sustained at the time of impact.

Extradural Hematoma ❗

Irrespective of the nature of inciting trauma, a direct blow to the head is essential for extradural hematoma formation. As the skull is deformed by the impact and the adherent dura forcefully detached, hemorrhage may occur into the preformed extradural space (figure 4.3). The source of bleeding is arterial, the arteries most often being ruptured by a fracture. In the supratentorial compartment, hemorrhage from the middle meningeal artery contributes to most extradural hematomas.

• Symptoms and signs: The clinical variability associated with extradural hemorrhage is remarkable. Rarely, extradural hematomas may be asymptomatic; most, however, present with nonspecific signs and symptoms referable to an intracranial mass lesion. The mode of presentation may be correlated with the size and site of the hematoma, the rate of expansion, and the presence of associated intradural pathology. Extradural hematomas involving the temporal lobe may cause a more precipitous decline than those at other sites because of their proximity to the brainstem. Alteration in consciousness is a hallmark manifestation of extradural hematoma but can be quite variable in extent and duration. The "lucid interval" occurs in less than one third of patients, and thus is not a sensitive diagnostic discriminator.

• Treatment: Rapid diagnosis and prompt surgical evacuation afford the best chance for optimizing outcome.

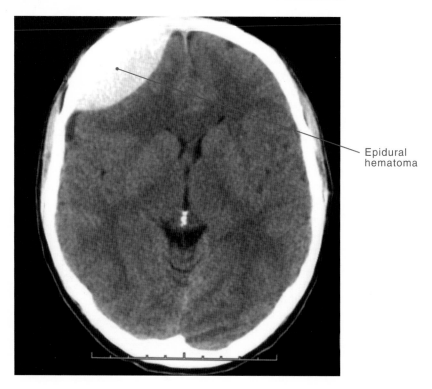

Figure 4.3 Epidural hematoma.

Epidural hematoma

• Prognosis: If this condition is suspected or diagnosed on imaging studies, an urgent neurosurgical consultation is required. If treatment is instituted before obtundation, pupillary dysfunction, or vegetative motor posturing, the probability of full functional recovery is high. The natural history of large traumatic extradural hematomas is dismal if the lesion is unrecognized or untreated. In the vast majority of cases, progressive neurological dysfunction is precipitated by the expanding mass lesion, ultimately resulting in transtentorial or uncal herniation, brainstem compression and ischemia, and death. The expanding extradural lesion only partially accounts for the neurological morbidity observed with extradural hematomas. Coincident intradural pathology is encountered in up to 50% of cases and is associated with lower admission Glasgow Coma Score, more substantial and prolonged intracranial pressure elevation, and higher mortality. In general, it is the sequelae of these lesions that dictate the degree of residual functional impairment in patients who survive extradural hematoma.

Traumatic Intracerebral Hematoma/Contusion !

Traumatic intracerebral hematomas are divided into acute or delayed types. Acute traumatic intracerebral hematomas occur at the time of the initial head injury and are present on early CT images (figure 4.4). Delayed traumatic intracerebral hemorrhages, which are more common, have been reported to occur from as early as 6 hours after injury to as long as several weeks.

• Symptoms and signs: Clinical signs and symptoms depend on the size and location of the intracerebral hematoma as well as the rapidity of its development. As a rule, the more severe the head injury, the more likely the presence of an intracerebral hematoma. In most cases, at least a brief period of confusion or loss of consciousness is reported. Only one third of the patients remain lucid throughout their course. Impaired alertness and cognitive function are found frequently on initial examination. Direct rupture of intrinsic cerebral vessels at the moment of injury is the most identifiable cause of the acute intracerebral hematomas. Many intracerebral hematomas are formed later from the coalescence of blood in the area of brain contusion.

• Treatment: If this condition is suspected or diagnosed on imaging studies, an urgent neurosurgical consultation is required. Medical management of intracerebral hematomas is directed primarily at reducing posttraumatic edema and ischemia. Treatment involves establishing

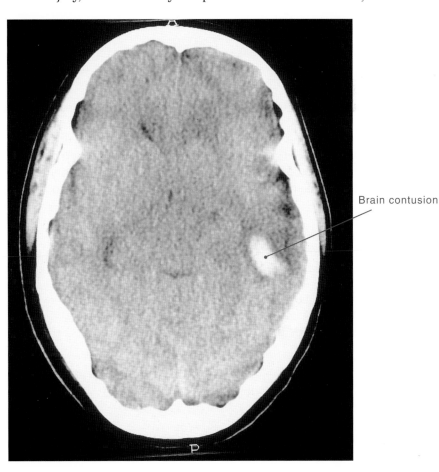

Figure 4.4 Brain contusion. Left-side brain contusion in the temporal lobe, resulting from a fall from a bicycle.

Brain contusion

adequate circulation and ventilation, aggressive monitoring of blood pressure and intercranial pressure to ensure adequate cerebral perfusion pressures, close intensive care monitoring, correction of any coagulopathies or electrolyte abnormalities, seizure prophylaxis, and corticosteroids if a significant amount of edema is associated with the hematoma. Head-injured patients should be monitored for coagulopathy for at least 24 to 48 hours after injury. Coagulopathics are treated aggressively with transfusions of fresh frozen plasma, cryoprecipitate, or platelets as needed. Interventions to control elevated intracranial pressure include sedation, osmotic diuresis, and emergency ventriculostomies. The alert patient with a focal neurological deficit and a small intracerebral hematoma can be observed closely. Some advocate evacuating all hematomas to eliminate the mass effect and vasoactive substances released by the hematoma that may promote further ischemia. A deteriorating neurological status, intracranial pressure elevations unresponsive to medical treatment, and midline shift on CT scan of more than 1 cm are indications for operative evacuation. Postoperative care usually involves repeated CT and continued aggressive management of persistent intracranial hypertension. Implementation of osmotic diuresis, seizure prophylaxis, and sedation is often critical to optimize outcome. Any postoperative deterioration warrants immediate repeat neuroimaging to elucidate the etiology.

- Prognosis: The overall cognitive impairment and the speed and quality of recovery are strongly related to the associated diffuse axonal injury. When occurring in isolation and when the volume is less than 30 cc, an intracerebral hematoma is compatible with a favorable recovery. Brainstem compression and loss of consciousness significantly worsen prognosis regardless of treatment. Overall, mortality rates are in the range of 25% to 30%.

Traumatic Subarachnoid Hemorrhage ❗

Traumatic subarachnoid hemorrhage is usually a consequence of bleeding from contused brain tissue or vertebral artery injury, either a tear or dissection, although it may also be due to tearing of meningeal vessels.

- Symptoms and signs: Subarachnoid bleeding typically presents with florid meningeal symptoms such as headache, neck stiffness, and photophobia. The most common initial symptoms in vertebral artery injury are neck pain and occipital headache that may precede the onset of neurological symptoms from seconds to weeks. It has been noted that headache symptoms in the majority of cases are ipsilateral to the vascular injury and that the pain usually radiates to the temporal region, frontal area, eye or ear. None of the reported cases had cervical tenderness or objective restriction of neck movement although a subjective exacerbation of pain did occur with neck movement.
- Treatment: If this condition is suspected or diagnosed on imaging studies, an urgent neurosurgical consultation is required. Early angiography is usually performed to assess the site of the bleeding and to rule out an aneurysmal bleed. Consultation with a neurosurgeon is recommended and surgery may or may not be indicated depending on the site of bleeding.
- Prognosis: The prognosis is extremely variable with many cases being diagnosed only post mortem.

Facial Injuries

Stein Tveten, Ingunn R. Rise, and Per Skjelbred

Occurrence

Sport activities, traffic accidents, and violence are the three most prevalent causes of facial injuries. Injuries to the head account for approximately 10% to 30% of all sporting injuries with the face being the major site of these. Facial injuries are caused by direct contact between athletes or sport equipment, such as hockey sticks, shoe spikes, goal posts, or railings. The shoulder and upper limb and the head of an opponent are the body parts that most frequently cause injuries to the face.

In amateur boxing, ice hockey, bandy, horseback riding, motorcycle sports, martial arts, and American football, mandatory protective equipment has indirectly reduced the number of facial injuries. Athletes in several sports wear mouthguards to prevent dental and orofacial injuries.

Differential Diagnosis

Soft-tissue injuries are the most common type of facial injuries in sport (see table 4.8). Next come facial fractures and tooth injuries. It is easy to confuse facial fractures with soft-tissue injuries at the time the accident occurs.

Diagnostic Thinking

Sport-related facial injuries are seldom life threatening. However, the increased use of new sport equipment, such as in-line skates, snowboards, and all-terrain bicycles, has increased the complexity of the injury pattern. The result is that primary caregivers are more frequently confronted with serious injuries. If these injuries are not

Most common	Less common	Must not be overlooked
Grazes (p. 75)	Soft-tissue loss (p. 79)	Maxilla fractures (p. 82)
Soft tissue contusions (p. 75)	Intraoral soft-tissue injuries (p. 80)	Nasoethmoidal fractures (p. 82)
Cuts (p. 76)	Frontal fractures (p. 80)	Panfacial fractures (p. 83)
Nasal fractures (p. 76)	Orbital fractures (p. 81)	Corneal erosion (p. 84)
Mandibular fractures (p. 77)	Alveolar ridge fractures (p. 83)	Contusion of the eyeball (p. 85)
Zygomatic fractures (p. 78)	Tooth fractures (p. 79)	Perforation of the eyeball (p. 85)
Tooth luxation (p. 78)		Septum hematoma (p. 76)
		Foreign object in the eye (p. 84)

Table 4.8 Overview of the differential diagnosis of facial injuries.

treated properly, they may have cosmetic or functional sequelae. A clinical examination is necessary to determine whether a patient with a facial injury needs to be sent for diagnostic imaging to exclude fractures.

The goal of the clinical examination during the acute phase is to evaluate whether there is a soft-tissue injury or a more complex injury that requires treatment by a specialist. In general, patients with suspected fractures must be sent to the emergency room for imaging. A dentist must treat all patients with dento-alveolar injuries immediately. If the most important differential diagnoses can be excluded by means of a clinical evaluation, additional examinations for this purpose are unnecessary.

If the patient has a severe facial injury, the airway may be obstructed by a foreign body, a blood clot, loose tissue, bone parts, a tooth, or a dislodged mouthguard. On-site treatment includes securing a clear airway and hemostasis. If attempts to secure a clear airway after foreign objects are removed are unsuccessful, the patient must be intubated. A tracheotomy is used only in rare cases when intubation is not possible because of soft-tissue swelling or a soft-tissue injury. A cricothyrotomy may be used as an emergency procedure.

Pressure bandages are used to stop bleeding. Bleeding from arteries (e.g., facial or temporal arteries) can be stopped by surgical ligation if uncontrolled. It may be difficult to control bleeding from the throat, nose, and mouth. Various methods, including nasal tamponade, epistaxis catheter, and compresses, may be used for internal tamponade.

The injury mechanism is used as a basis for making the proper diagnosis and for determining the extent of the injury (see figure 4.5). In most cases of facial injuries, the injured athlete is able to account for the injury mechanism. Most case histories are one of two types: Either the patient hit himself in the face or he got hit. The observations of fellow players may be important in making a proper diagnosis. Injuries to the oral cavity are often caused by direct trauma to the lips or teeth, caused by a blow or kick from an opposing player or by sport equipment, such as hockey stick, ice hockey puck, bandy ball or a ski pole.

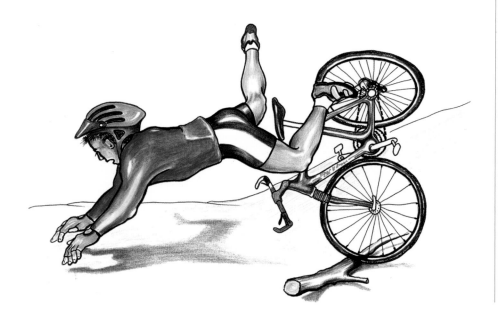

Figure 4.5 Injury mechanisms for facial injuries. Falls from bicycles often result in soft-tissue injuries, tooth injuries, and facial fractures.

Clinical Examination

Inspection. The examination should take place as soon as possible after the injury. However, often the patient is not examined until several hours after the event. Swelling and pain may make the examination difficult. All wounds should be washed and cleaned. Then the patient's face is systematically examined. Depression fractures may be visible in the forehead. The bridge of the nose and the nasal septum are checked for deviation. Fractures in the nasoethmoidal area increase the distance between medial corners of the eyes (telecanthus), cause the tip of the nose to turn upwards, and change the palpebral aperture (round doll's eye) on the affected side. A depressed zygomatic complex causes the contour of the cheekbone to become flattened. Injuries in the orbital area may cause changes in the position of the eyeball, such as proptosis (protrusion of the eyeball), hypophthalmos (inferiorly positioned eyeball) and enophthalmos (recessed eyeball), double vision, and reduced ocular movement. A depressed, elongated, widened midface indicates a fracture with dislocation (see figure 4.6). Open occlusion often occurs. Malocclusion may be caused by fractures to both the upper and the lower jaw. Injuries to the lacrimal canal cause annoying tearing.

Palpation. If the patient has hematoma and a swollen face, thorough palpation of the underlying structures and the surrounding areas is necessary to exclude fractures in the area (see figure 4.7). The facial skeleton is palpated for "depressions" or discontinuity. A depression in the middle lower section of the forehead, a loose nasal pyramid, and steps in the orbital margin are typical signs of fractures. Levels I-III Le Fort fractures cause the upper jaw or midface to be mobile. The temporomandibular joint spaces can be palpated, and an injury will usually cause pain here. In addition, the patient's mouth-opening range will be conspicuously reduced. Pathological movement when the lower jaw is bimanually palpated is an indication of fractures in the area. Irregularities in occlusion and in the dental arch are findings that require follow-up.

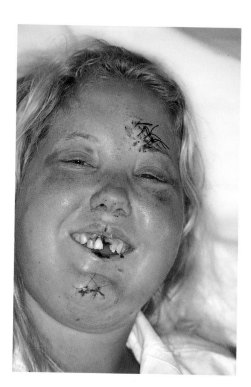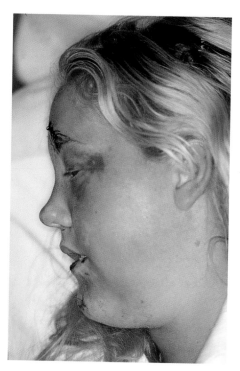

Figure 4.6 Midface fracture. Note that the midface is depressed and widened.

Jaw movement. The normal mouth-opening range of an adult is between 45 and 60 mm, measured between the incisive teeth in the upper and lower jaws.

The distance that the lower jaw can be moved forward varies from 2 to 6 mm in adults (measured in the area of the incisive teeth). Lateral movements range between 3 and 7 mm (measured in the canine-tooth region). If the patient has an acute injury, the mouth-opening range and the distance it can be moved forward and laterally may be conspicuously reduced. Temporomandibular joint dislocations cause malocclusion, so the patient is unable to close the mouth. These dislocations also cause the lower jaw to deviate toward the contralateral side of the dislocation.

Neuromuscular function. Facial fractures can cause deficit in the sensory nerve branches (all three trigeminal branches). Injuries to the supraorbital nerve reduce sensation in the forehead. Injuries to the infraorbital nerve reduce sensation in the midface, whereas injuries to the inferior alveolar nerve and the mental nerve reduce feeling in the lower jaw and lower lip. Traumatic facial paresis rarely occurs in isolation, although it may be a complication of an underlying skull fracture.

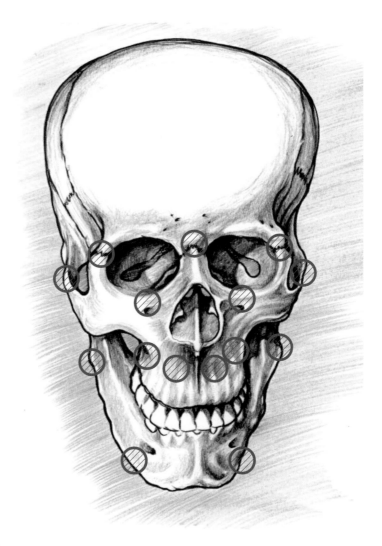

Figure 4.7 Common facial fractive areas. Key palpation points are marked.

Supplemental Examinations

Radiographic examinations. A plain radiograph is recommended as the first examination for facial skeleton fractures. An orthopantogram (OPG), combined with frontal and lateral images of the lower jaw and midface, is recommended for most lower jaw fractures. If tooth fractures, tooth luxation, or fractures of the alveolar process are suspected, the OPG should be supplemented with dental X rays. Nasal fractures are diagnosed using lateral X rays, but decisions regarding the need for surgery on a nasal fracture depend on the clinical evaluation. If fractures are found, additional CT scans are often indicated.

CT scans. As a rule, a specialist should order diagnostic imaging examinations. Images in both the coronal and axial planes are important. Coronal plane images are necessary to demonstrate the extent of isolated orbital floor fractures. For Le Fort-type extensive midface fractures, all possible types of CT scan projections (i.e., axial, coronal, and sagittal, as well as three-dimensional reconstruction) should be used in the preoperative work to obtain the best possible overview of the extent of the fracture. Newer CT machines may completely replace conventional radiographic examinations, because both OPG and dental X rays are possible.

MRI. An MRI is not used for standard facial injury examinations. It may, however, provide useful information about injuries to the eye and to the surrounding soft tissue.

Specific Diagnoses—Common Injuries

Grazes

Grazes occur frequently.

- Symptoms and signs: Superficial wounds limited to the epidermis and dermis are caused by falls on a rough surface (see figure 4.8).
- Diagnosis: The diagnosis is made clinically by inspection and palpation of the injured area after dirt has been removed.
- Treatment by physician: Abrasions are partial damage to the skin. Abrasions heal by re-epithelialization. Wounds that are penetrated by dirt particles often heal with permanent tattooing if the particles are not removed. If the graze has much dirt, cleaning is a painful procedure, and sometimes it must be done under general anesthesia.
- Prognosis: Healing is usually uncomplicated if the wound is protected by a thin layer of antibiotic ointment and cleaned daily to remove exudative residue. Occlusive dressings have been shown to improve healing of skin lesions rather than the traditional approach of open or dry wound dressing.

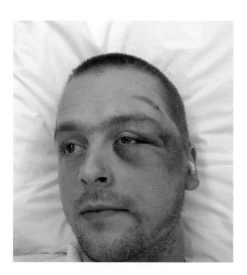 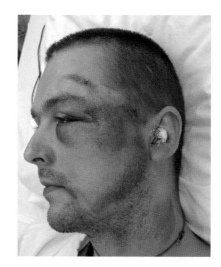

Figure 4.8 Abrasion. Facial grazes after falling while rollerblading.

Soft Tissue Contusions

Blows and pinching injuries are among the most frequent soft-tissue injuries in sport.

- Symptoms and signs: Ruptures of small veins, with bleeding in the skin, cause redness and variable degrees of hematoma formation in the affected area.
- Diagnosis: The diagnosis is made clinically by inspection and palpation of the injured area, after dirt has been removed.
- Treatment by physician: After underlying fractures have been excluded, the most important task is to reduce inflammatory reactions. Elevation of the head and ice packs during the first 2 to 4 hours will counteract swelling and discomfort. After 48 hours, the acute inflammatory phase begins to subside. Paracetamol preparations and glucocorticoids have been documented to reduce swelling and pain in the facial area.
- Prognosis: Most contusion injuries require no further treatment after 48 hours and heal spontaneously in 1 to 2 weeks.

Lacerations/Cuts

Cuts include tears and puncture wounds that are often caused by sport equipment penetrating the skin. For example, cuts are often caused by knobs on soccer shoes, spiked shoes, and sharp edges on ski equipment.

- Symptoms and signs: Less complicated cuts and punctures are usually superficial.
- Diagnosis: If the wound is deep, a neurological examination must be performed, so that nerve damage can be ruled out.
- Treatment by physician: Superficial tears and puncture wounds are treated with skin sutures and taping. The use of 5.0 and 6.0 sutures is recommended.
- Prognosis: The patient must be informed that it takes several months before facial scars are finally mature. Martial arts practitioners, in particular, must be informed that resuming the sport too soon after the injury may lead to complications during the healing period. For the first 6 months, scars must be protected from the sun by applying sun block or bandages, because exposure to the sun may cause hyperpigmentation.

Nasal Fractures

Fractures of the nasal skeleton are among the most frequent types of sports injuries to the face.

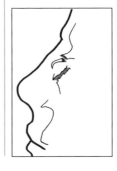

- Symptoms and signs: Symptoms and signs of nasal fractures are malalignment of the nasal skeleton, hematoma, and soft-tissue swelling.
- Diagnosis: For a proper diagnosis, the practitioner must evaluate the following: blows to the nasal area, mobility and crepitation of the nasal skeleton, bleeding, swelling, hematoma, and reduced air flow in the nose. Nasal fractures are diagnosed radiographically, using lateral images, but the need to surgically treat a nasal injury depends on the clinical evaluation (see figure 4.9, a-c).
- Treatment by physician: The patient should be referred to an ear, nose, and throat specialist. Septum hematoma must be evacuated. Closed nasal bone reposition

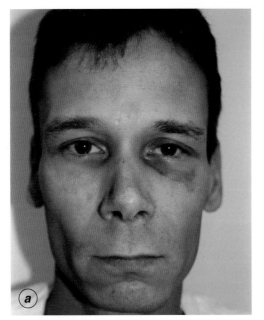
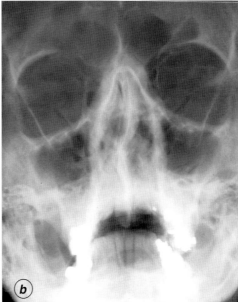
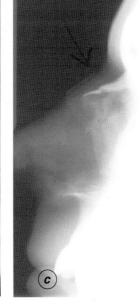

Figure 4.9 Nasal fracture with deviation of the bridge of the nose (a). The frontal view demonstrates traumatic septum deviation (b). The sagittal view shows a nasal bone fracture (c).

is the most common treatment. This should be done either immediately after the injury or 3 to 7 days later, when the swelling is reduced.

• Prognosis: The prognosis is good. The patient should wear a protective splint or face mask for 4 weeks when participating in training or competition.

Mandibular Fractures

Mandibular fractures are the second most common group (13% to 45%) of sport-related facial injuries. They are usually caused by a blow to the lower jaw, such as may occur in fighting and team sports. Falls in which the lower jaw or the chin hits a hard surface are another common injury mechanism.

• Symptoms and signs: Symptoms and signs of lower jaw fractures are swelling and hematoma, problems with occlusion, mucous membrane tears, differences in the level of the tooth row, mobility in the area of the fracture, and hypoesthesia with nerve damage in the mental nerve area.

• Diagnosis: Definite signs of a fracture are changes in occlusion resulting from differences in the level of the tooth row and mobility in the area of the fracture. The standard radiographic examination is an OPG (see figure 4.10, a and b).

• Treatment by physician: Most lower jaw fractures should be treated by a specialist. To achieve proper occlusion, the fractured fragments must be anatomically reduced and then fixed using mini titanium plates. Intermaxillary fixation is always used intraoperatively but is seldom needed after surgery. Soft food is recommended for 4 to 6 weeks. Temporomandibular joint fractures with fracture lines in the joint area are difficult to operate on and are therefore treated conservatively by intermaxillary fixation for 3 to 6 weeks.

• Prognosis: The prognosis depends on the extent and the location of the fracture. If proper occlusion is achieved after the operation, the prognosis is good. For temporomandibular joint fractures for which surgery is not indicated because the fracture is close to the joint, problems with occlusion and the reduced ability to open the mouth wide may be the outcome.

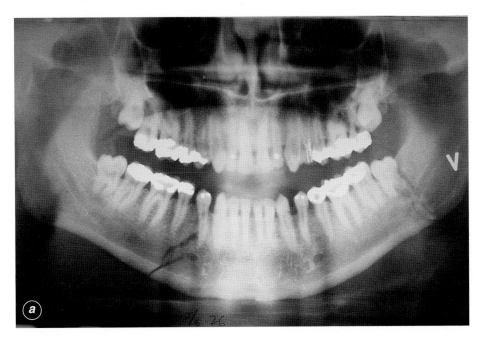

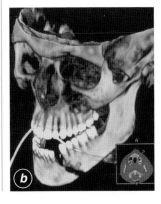

Figure 4.10 Mandibular fracture. The orthopantogram demonstrates a right-side subcondylar fracture, a left-side angulus fracture, and a right-side body fracture *(a)*. The three-dimensional reconstructed CT image illustrates a paramedial mandibular fracture *(b)*.

Zygomatic Fracture

Typical cheekbone fractures involve fractures to the weakest structures of the zygomaticomaxillary complex: the infraorbital rim, the orbital floor, and the lateral orbital rim (see figure 4.11, a and b). Cheekbone fractures are the third most common sports injury to the face. In case of an impending injury, the athlete will often turn her head to the side, making her cheekbone more vulnerable to injury.

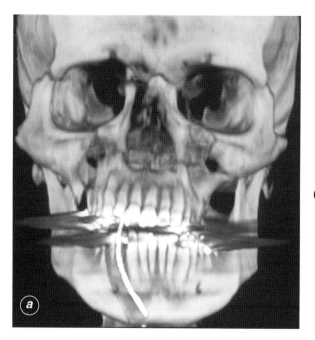

(a)

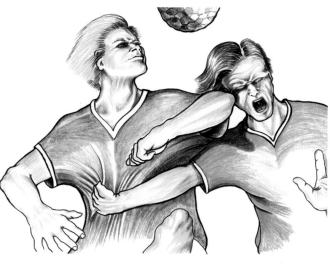

(b)

Figure 4.11 Zygomatic fracture. Dislocated right-side zygomatic fracture (a). A common injury mechanism is trauma to the cheekbone (b).

- Symptoms and signs: The clinical presentation of a cheekbone fracture is a flattening of the prominence of the cheekbone. If the cheekbone is pressed inward, it may be difficult for the patient to open the mouth wide. Double vision and nerve injury corresponding to the infraorbital nerve are symptoms of a fracture in the orbital floor.
- Diagnosis: Dislocations and broken edges that can be palpated on the infraorbital rim, the intraoral zygomaticomaxillary buttresses, and the lateral orbital rim are definite signs of a fracture. A CT scan with axial and coronal views provides the best imaging.
- Treatment by physician: Treatment consists of open reposition and plate osteosynthesis. In addition, the herniated orbital content is reduced and the orbital floor is reconstructed. A facial injury specialist should treat these injuries.
- Prognosis: The extent of the fracture and the possibility for surgery immediately after the injury determine the result. Secondary corrections are difficult.

Tooth Luxation

Tooth luxations (dislocations) are divided into subtotal and total luxations. Subluxation often occurs when the alveolus is fractured, causing the tooth to be luxated out of normal position. Total luxation is complete avulsion of the tooth.

- Symptoms and signs: The tooth is subluxated or completely knocked out of the alveolus.
- Diagnosis: Diagnosis is made through a clinical examination.
- Treatment by dentist: The treatment of subtotal luxations consists of reposition in the proper anatomic position and fixation with the help of an arch bar. The fixation period is 4 weeks. For total luxation, vital tissue on the root surface must be treated

carefully. The outcome of the treatment depends on how long the tooth is outside the alveolus and in which medium it is stored. Ideally, the tooth should be put back in the alveolus immediately and held in place with the patient's mouthguard or a foil splint until an urgent dental consultation is achieved. The ultimate prognosis of tooth survival depends on its time out of the mouth. If the tooth is contaminated, it should be carefully cleaned in sterile saline. It must not be scrubbed or cleaned with cotton or lint as the cells critical for healing may be irrevocable damaged thus impairing tooth viability. The best temporary storage media are sterile saline, saliva, and milk. The tooth is reimplanted as quickly as possible and fixed using an arch bar for 1 to 2 weeks. In case of total luxations and alveolar fractures, fixation time is 4 weeks. Prophylactic antibiotic treatment is recommended.

- Prognosis: Teeth that have not completed root growth may be revitalized. If root growth is complete, root canal treatment should be undertaken 7 to 10 days after luxation.

Tooth Fracture

Tooth fractures are divided into crown fractures and root fractures (see figure 4.12, a and b).

- Symptoms and signs: Crown fractures without pulp opening are a sign of tooth fracture. If the crown of the tooth is bleeding, the pulp is open. Malalignment of the crown of the tooth is another sign.
- Diagnosis: Diagnosis is made by clinical examination and radiography (dental X rays).
- Treatment by dentist: Normally, crown fractures are reconstructed using synthetic fillings. If the pulp is open, root canal filling is usually necessary. In children, however, because the growth of the root of the tooth is not complete, only the upper portion of the pulp is removed. Split or longitudinal fractures result in extraction of the tooth. Root fractures are treated by exact repositioning of the crown of the tooth using a stable arch bar. The brace should be worn for 2 to 3 months.
- Prognosis: The aesthetic result is often very good for crown fractures without opening of the pulp. Pulp opening and subsequent root filling may cause varying degrees of discoloration of the tooth. The prognosis for root fractures is good if the fracture ends are slightly displaced. If dislocation of the crown fragments is substantial, fracture healing is not very likely. Root filling of these teeth must be done early.

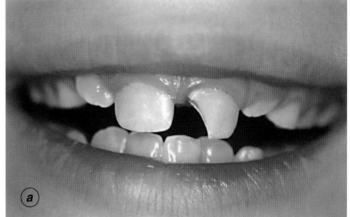

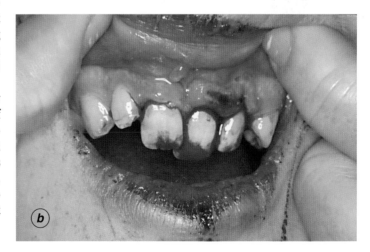

Other Specific Diagnoses

Soft-Tissue Loss

Extensive facial injuries with tissue loss are rare in sport. They occasionally occur as a result of horseback riding, skiing, and bicycling accidents (see figure 4.13).

Figure 4.12 Crown and root fractures. Crown fracture with exposed pulp (a). Root fracture with a dislocated crown fragment (b).

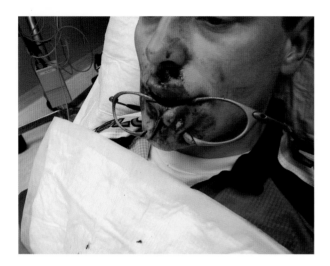 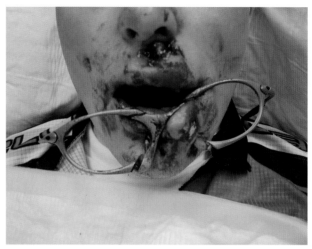

Figure 4.13 Soft-tissue injury. A bicyclist who got his own glasses stuck in his lower lip.

- Symptoms and signs: Extensive soft-tissue injuries are often combinations of lacerations, abrasions, and contusions.
- Diagnosis: Initially, this type of injury is examined carefully after a thorough cleaning. If palpation indicates an injury to the underlying bone structure, the athlete must be sent for radiographic clarification. If the underlying tissue is damaged, the trigeminal nerve and facial nerve must be tested for skin sensation and motor innervation.
- Treatment by physician: Debridement must be conservative for star-shaped wounds, so that enough tissue is kept to allow closing, thus preventing displacement of neighboring structures. Major defects require plastic reconstructive techniques.
- Prognosis: This treatment often has a surprisingly good outcome, with few disfiguring scars.

Soft-Tissue Injuries in the Oral Cavity

The most frequent injuries occur to the lips and the anterior part of the mucous membrane of the mouth. Injuries to the buccal mucosa and to the roof of the mouth are rare.

- Symptoms and signs: Symptoms and signs are bleeding from the oral cavity and lips and, frequently, hematoma and swelling shortly after the injury occurs.
- Diagnosis: The physician must thoroughly inspect and palpate the injured area. This requires good light and suction.
- Treatment by physician: The principles that apply for extraoral soft-tissue injuries also apply for intraoral injuries. The use of ointments and bandages is unnecessary. Suturing with 3.0 resorbable sutures is recommended. In the lip area, single 5.0 sutures are recommended. Precise suturing of the red-white lip line is key. The sutures are removed after 7 days. Good oral hygiene is maintained by rinsing with chlorhexidine gluconate, because it may be difficult for the patient to brush the teeth.
- Prognosis: Normally, wounds in the oral cavity heal without complications or lasting harm.

Frontal Bone Fracture

Fractures of the forehead are often caused by a blow to the lower portion of the forehead and are typically the result of being kicked by a horse or of head duels in soccer. These fractures are rare: They represent only 2% of sport-related injuries to the face.

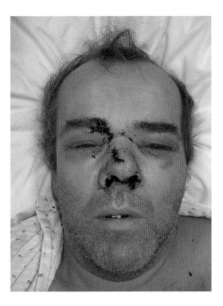 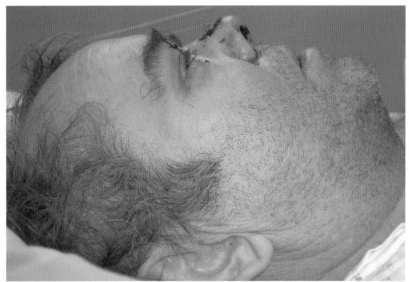

- Symptoms and signs: Visible or palpable depressions in the area above the frontal sinus indicate frontal bone fracture (see figure 4.14).
- Diagnoiss: A definite sign of a fracture is a palpable depression with crepitation in the anterior wall of the frontal sinus. Sensory deficit in the area of innervation of the supraorbital nerve is also considered a sign of a fracture in this area. To exclude a frontobasal injury, the doctor must always order a CT scan.
- Treatment by physician: If there is a fracture of the posterior wall of the frontal sinus, with air intracranially and liquorrhea as signs of dura damage, further treatment must be given, in collaboration with a neurosurgeon.
- Prognosis: The prognosis is good. For larger injuries, the prognosis depends on additional intracranial injuries.

Figure 4.14 Impression fracture of the forehead. Direct trauma to the root of the nose can cause a frontonasoethmoidal fracture.

Orbital Fracture—Eye Socket Fracture

Fractures in the orbita are divided into fractures of the orbital margin and fractures of the orbital floor, walls, and roof. Blunt trauma to the bulb of the eye refers force to the orbital walls and the orbital floor, which is the weakest bone structure in the orbital complex. Blowout fractures are among the least common sports injuries. The classic causes are tennis or squash balls hitting the eye. The most common orbital floor fractures seen are those caused by running into elbows or fists during team sports. Fractures of the infraorbital rim are a relatively common result of this type of injury.

- Symptoms and signs: Findings that indicate fractures are periorbital swelling, monocle hematomas, subconjunctival bleeding, recessed eyeball (enophthalmos), inferiorly positioned eyeball (hypophthalmos), sensory deficit in the area of the infraorbital nerve, limited ocular movements, and double vision. Swelling, hematoma, and increased volume in the orbit cause diplopia and limit movement.
- Diagnosis: A CT scan of the orbit with coronal sections provides a good overview of fractures in the orbital floor (see figure 4.15, a and b).
- Treatment by physician: Indications for surgical intervention are a recessed eyeball (enophthalmos), an inferiorly positioned eyeball (hypophthalmos), a disorder of ocular movement, and double vision.
- Prognosis: The extent of the fracture and the possibility of surgery immediately after the injury determine the outcome. Secondary corrections are difficult to make, and the results are not as good as they are for immediate surgery.

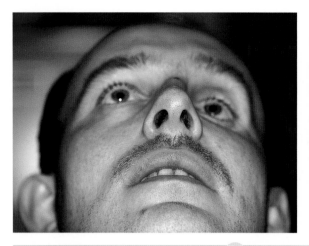
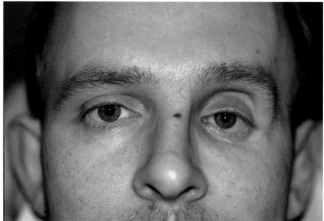

Maxillary Fracture—Midface Fracture !

Maxillary fractures result from trauma to the midface. The result is a loosening of (1) the upper jaw (Le Fort I); (2) the upper jaw with the nasal bone (Le Fort II); or (3) the entire midface with the upper jaw, cheekbone, and nasal bones (Le Fort III) (see figure 4.16). Sport-related Le Fort fractures are rare and make up only 1% to 3% of all sports injuries to the face. The most common injury mechanisms are falls from great heights, high-speed trauma, winter sport trauma, and bicycling and climbing accidents.

- Symptoms and signs: Malocclusion combined with problems involving movement of the upper jaw or the central or entire midface are characteristic of all Le Fort fractures. Typical symptoms are periorbital hematoma (raccoon eyes), rhinorrhea, and backward and downward dislocation of the midface (dish face).
- Diagnosis: Definite signs of fracture are changes in occlusion combined with mobility in the upper jaw or midface. A CT scan between the axial and coronal section provides the best overview.
- Treatment by physician: Maxillary injuries should be treated by a facial injury specialist. Dislocated fragments are reduced and fixed using titanium plates.
- Prognosis: The extent of the fracture and the possibility for surgical intervention immediately after the injury determine the result. Secondary corrections are difficult to make, and the results are not as good as the results of immediate correction.

Figure 4.15 Orbital fracture with enophthalmos and hypophthalmos. Injury to the orbital margin may lower the position of the bulb, whereas a fracture in the floor and walls increases the volume of the orbit and causes a recessed eyeball.

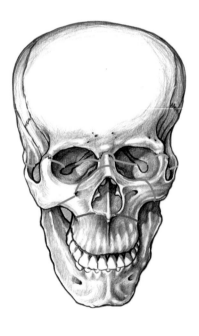

Figure 4.16 Le Fort I-III fractures. These are the most common fracture lines in the midface.

Nasoethmoidal Fracture—Combined Nose and Lacrimal Bone Fractures !

Nasoethmoidal fractures are localized to the area between the eyes, consisting of the nasal bone and the lacrimal bone (see figure 4.17). The lacrimal bone is thin and fractures easily. Therefore, parts of the nasal complex can be pushed posteriorly. This may cause damage to the lacrimal canal and eyelids. The medial attachment of the eyelids may become loose and may be drawn out laterally.

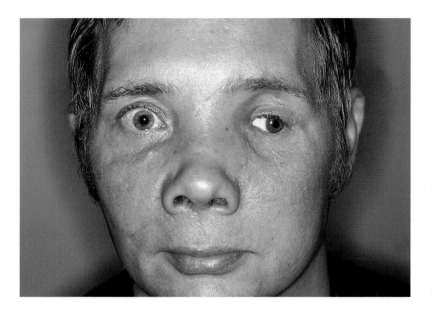

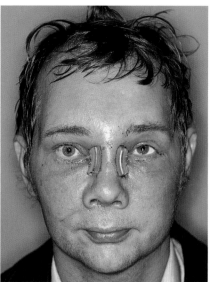

- Symptoms and signs: Symptoms and signs include the depressed bridge of the nose, an increased distance between the medial canthi (telecanthus), a changed palpebral aperture (doll's eye), and a turned-up apex of the nose.
- Diagnosis: Diagnosis is made using a CT scan and is indicated by an increased distance between the canthi combined with a fracture of the nasal skeleton.
- Treatment by a physician: A specialist in facial injuries should treat this type of injury.
- Prognosis: The prognosis depends on the complexity of the fracture. A good outcome depends on surgery immediately after the injury occurs, with exact repositioning of the bone fragments and canthal ligaments (canthopexy). Secondary corrections are difficult, and the results are not as good as the results of immediate correction.

Figure 4.17 Nasoethmoidal fracture. The typically depressed root of the nose, turned up apex of the nose, telecanthus, and doll's eye.

Panfacial Fractures—Multiple Fractures in the Facial Skeleton !

Panfacial fractures are caused by major trauma to the face. They include multiple fractures in the facial skeleton (i.e., the forehead, cheekbone, nose, upper jaw, and lower jaw).

- Symptoms and signs: Symptoms and signs are total crushing of the face, with pathological movement of the fragments; and flattened, widened, and lengthened midface, combined with occlusion problems.
- Diagnosis: Clinical examination includes axial, sagittal, and coronal CT sections of the facial skeleton.
- Treatment by a physician: A facial injury specialist must treat this type of fracture. Treatment is by plate osteosynthesis surgery.
- Prognosis: Prognosis is good when the fragments are properly reduced.

Alveolar Ridge Fracture

Alveolar ridge fractures are segment fractures in the tooth-bearing portion of the upper and lower jaw, where a segment contains a group of two or more teeth (see figure 4.18).

- Symptoms and signs: Symptoms and signs are abnormal mobility of the tooth segment, changes in occlusion, differences in the level of the tooth row, bleeding, and injuries to the mucous membrane.

- Diagnosis: The diagnosis is made radiologically, with OPG and tooth X rays; and clinically, by mobility of the tooth segment.
- Treatment by physician: The physician performs repositioning and fixation of the fractured fragment with the help of arch bars. The bars are used for 4 weeks. If insufficient stability is achieved using labial arches, the patient must

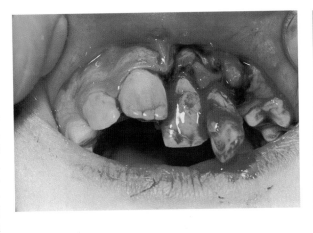

Figure 4.18 Alveolar ridge fracture. Fracture of the tooth alveolus with subluxation of the teeth.

have intermaxillary fixation for a few weeks. Open reposition using plates may cause healing problems in the form of poor circulation to the reduced fragments and is seldom used.
- Prognosis: The result depends on reduction of the injured fragments. If this is done correctly, permanent changes in bite are avoided. A dentist must evaluate the tooth with respect to the need for root canal treatment.

Foreign Object in the Eye !

Specks of dust often get stuck in the tarsal sulcus on the inside of the upper eyelid.

Blinking is painful and may cause epithelium damage on the cornea.

- Symptoms and signs: Symptoms and signs are pain, red eye, and tearing.
- Diagnosis: The foreign object is visible when the eyelid is examined by turning it inside out.
- Treatment by physician: Foreign objects are removed, possibly after anesthetization with oxybuprocaine eye drops. Antibiotic ointment for 3 or 4 days is recommended as an infection prophylactic.

Corneal Erosion !

Contact with branches, fingernails, or other objects often cause wounds on the cornea (see figure 4.19).

- Symptoms and signs: Strong pain, tearing, eyelid cramps (blepharospasm), sensitivity to light, and blurred vision are symptoms and signs of corneal erosion.
- Diagnosis: Diagnosis is made by fluorescein solution, which colors erosion.
- Treatment by physician: Local antibiotics, such as chloramphenicol ointment over night, and per oral analgesics are used. Diclofenac eye drops may be tried.
- Prognosis: In most cases healing occurs within 24 hours.

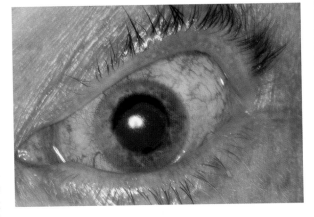

Figure 4.19 Corneal erosion. Fluorescein-colored corneal erosion.

Contusion of the Eyeball !

Contusion of the eyeball (see figure 4.20) may be caused by direct blows to the eye (boxing), a ball in the eye (squash), crashing into a hard object, and falling accidents.

- Symptoms and signs: Tearing, light sensitivity, and blepharospasm (cramps of the eyelid) are signs and symptoms of contusion of the eyeball.
- Diagnosis: Diagnosis is made if any of the following have occurred: swelling and bleeding in the eyelid, subconjunctival bleeding, corneal edema, corneal damage, bleeding in the

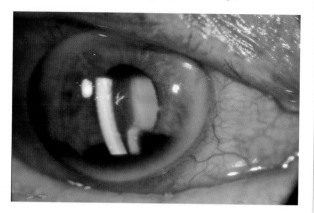

Figure 4.20 Contusion of the eyeball. Bleeding in the anterior chamber and the iris.

anterior chamber (hyphema), separation of the iris (iridodialysis), traumatic paresis of the pupil (mydriasis, oval pupil), accommodation paresis, lens damage or dislocation, bleeding in the vitreous, retinal damage (bleeding or edema), or damage to the optic nerve.
- Treatment by physician: The physician should examine the eye while it is under surface anesthesia, and refer the patient to an ophthalmologist. Blunt trauma to the eyeball may have serious consequences. The diagnosis may be difficult to make because several areas of the eye may be injured. For this reason, the threshold for referral to an ophthalmologist should be low.
- Prognosis: Prognosis depends on the extent of the injury and the possibility of treatment by an ophthalmologist.

Perforation of the Eyeball !

Ski poles in the eye, bow and arrow shooting accidents, and accidents with other sharp objects frequently cause eye perforation (see figure 4.21). Ruptures of the eye may also be caused by powerful blunt contusion trauma. In that case, the eye ruptures at the weak points (along the limbus and the optic nerve).

- Symptoms and signs: The case history is crucial. Perforation may be difficult to see. If perforation is suspected, the patient should be sent to the nearest ophthalmology department. The parenteral use of an antibiotic prophylactic (e.g., benzylpenicillin) may be necessary if transport will take a long time. It is critical that the patient avoids straining or cough-

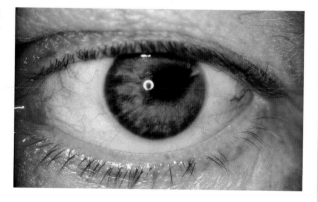

Figure 4.21 Perforation of the eyeball. Perforated eye that is not circular. Contusion changes of the pupil.

ing, otherwise extrusion of the intra-ocular contents may result. Consideration of the use of a parenteral antiemetic during transport is recommended.
- Diagnosis: A specialist confirms the diagnosis.
- Treatment by physician: Treatment of a perforated eyeball must be done by a specialist.
- Prognosis: Prognosis depends on the extent of the injury.

Rehabilitation of Head Injuries

Paul McCrory and Ingunn R. Rise

Goals and Principles

Table 4.9 follows the principles for and lays out the goals of head injury rehabilitation.

The functional outcome in patients who have sustained an acute head injury varies greatly. Fortunately in sport most injuries are mild and recover rapidly without any lasting sequelae. In contrast, moderate and severe traumatic brain injuries have a variable and unpredictable outcome. Lasting problems include both mental (such as personality changes and memory deficit) and physical (such as hemiparesis and speech disturbance).

The goal of rehabilitation of patients with severe head injuries is to get the patient back to a level of function in which he is as independent of others as possible. In the best case, the patient will return to the level he was at before the injury. In principle, rehabilitation of patients with serious head injuries begins at the hospital immediately after the injury or operation. Most rehabilitation occurs during the first 6 months after the injury, but it is not until a year later that there is any degree of certainty about which level the patient will attain. However, the rehabilitation potential of many patients extends beyond one year. Physical therapy and occupational therapy are not only vital in reducing contractures and improving strength in the extremities, but also for stimulating the patient's own motivation.

Return to Sport

Concussion. Once the athlete's symptoms and cognitive deficits have fully resolved, then return to play is appropriate. A player should never return to play while symptomatic. "When in doubt, sit them out!" In professional sport, with experienced and trained sports medicine clinicians on the sideline, return on the day of injury is possible once recovery has ensued.

	Goals	Measures
Phase 1	Prevent secondary brain damage	Acute treatment at the proper level of care
Phase 2	Mobilization and regaining primary functions	Practical help from physical and occupational therapists
Phase 3	Complete recovery of lost functions	Specialized rehabilitation program

Table 4.9 Goals and measures for rehabilitation of head injuries.

In most other situations, however, return to play is usually the next match for the injured athletes. Ideally this follows a medically supervised process in accordance with the Vienna consensus guidelines:

1. No activity, complete rest; once the athlete is asymptomatic, proceed to the next level
2. Light aerobic exercise such as walking or stationary cycling
3. Sport-specific training (e.g., skating in hockey, running in soccer)
4. Noncontact training drills
5. Full contact training after medical clearance
6. Game play

With this progression, the athlete should continue to proceed to the next level if asymptomatic at the current level. If any postconcussion symptoms occur, the patient should drop back to the previous asymptomatic level and try to progress again after 24 hours.

It is widely believed that having sustained a concussive injury, one is then more prone to future concussive injury. The evidence for this contention is limited at best. It would seem obvious that in any collision or contact sport the risk of concussion is directly proportional to the amount of time playing the sport. In other words, the more games played the more chance of an injury occurring. Therefore the likelihood of repeat injury may simply reflect the level of exposure to injury risk. The association of an increased risk of subsequent concussions reported in players with a past history of concussion is thought to reflect a player's style of play where his risk of injury may be increased by utilizing dangerous game strategies and illegal tackling techniques. Apart from boxing-related head injuries, the most widely cited studies of the cumulative effects of concussion have studied patients with injuries sustained in motor vehicle accidents that were severe enough to warrant presentation to a hospital. It is widely acknowledged that boxing carries a high risk of neurological injury. Boxing, however, should not be considered as a model for cumulative head injury seen in other sports since it presents unique risks to the athlete in terms of the frequency of repetitive head trauma. There are significant methodological problems with the published studies suggesting a cumulative effect of repeated concussion. More recent prospective studies have not found convincing evidence of a cumulative effect of recurrent brain trauma. Similarly well-performed animal studies have failed to demonstrate cumulative damage from repeated trauma. At the present time, no consensus exists suggesting the long-term risk from concussive injuries outside of sports such as boxing.

Recent research in boxers has suggested that chronic traumatic encephalopathy or "punch drunk syndrome" in boxers may be associated with a particular genetic predisposition. The apolipoprotein E epsilon-4 gene (ApoE), a susceptibility gene for late onset familial and sporadic Alzheimer's disease, may be associated with an increased risk of chronic traumatic encephalopathy in boxers. In a nonboxing population, ApoE polymorphism was significantly associated with death and adverse outcomes following all levels of acute traumatic brain injury. Although only in the early stages of the understanding of these issues, the interaction between genetic and environmental factors may be critical in the development of the postconcussive phenomena or concussive sequelae.

Life threatening or severe head injury. Return to sport following a severe or potentially life threatening brain injury is controversial, and few guidelines exist for the clinician to follow. There are some situations where the athlete could place himself at an unacceptably high risk of sustaining further injury and hence should

Persistent postconcussional or postinjury symptoms
Permanent neurological sequelae (hemiplegia, visual deficit, dementia or cognitive impairment)
Hydrocephalus with or without shunting
Spontaneous subarachnoid hemorrhage from any cause
Symptomatic neurological or pain-producing abnormalities about the foramen magnum
Craniotomy for evacuation of intracerebral or subdural hematoma

Table 4.10 Conditions contraindicating return to contact sport.

be counselled against participation in collision sport (table 4.10). In such situations, common sense should prevail.

Although sports physicians should keep an open mind when assessing neurological recovery from severe brain injuries, nevertheless it is recommended that at least 12 months pass before such a decision is contemplated.

Thoughtful deliberation and analysis of all the available medical evidence should occur when making such a decision. The counsel of a neurologist or neurosurgeon experienced in sporting head injury management should be sought. This is an important point because a number of individuals who suffer a moderate to severe traumatic brain injury may be left with a lack of insight and impaired judgment over and above their other neurological injuries. This in turn may make such an individual unreliable in gauging recovery. The use of neuropsychological assessment as well as information from family and friends may assist the clinician in his deliberation. The assessment of cognitive performance or clinical symptoms when fatigued is often useful.

Return to collision sport is relatively contraindicated in almost any situation where surgical craniotomy is performed. In such situations, the subarachnoid space is traumatized, thus setting up scarring of the pia-arachnoid of the brain to the dura with both loss of the normal cushioning effect of the cerebro spinal fluid and vascular adhesions that may subsequently bleed if torn during head impact. Even if neurological recovery is complete, a craniotomy for anything other than an extradural hematoma effectively precludes return to collision sport.

With an extradural hematoma without brain injury or other condition where surgery is not required, return to sport may be contemplated in selected cases as per the previous discussion after a minimum of 12 months assuming neurological recovery is complete.

Soft-tissue injuries. In most cases, athletes with grazes and contusions may begin training and participate in competition shortly after the injury occurs. For cuts and extensive soft-tissue injuries with tissue loss, the practitioner must tape sutured wounds for support, so that healing is not interfered with and scars do not form. In some cases this means that the athlete must continue to take it easy until after the sutures have been removed, normally 7 days postoperatively.

Dentoalveolar injuries. All tooth injuries that result in loosening of one or more teeth or tooth-bearing fragments require fixation with an arch bar. The bar is used for 1 week for luxated teeth without alveolar fractures, for 4 weeks for subluxated teeth with alveolar fractures, and for 8 weeks for root fractures. During that period, the athlete may train and compete in sports, except for martial arts and other sports where blows to the mouth and face occur. Consideration of the use of a mouthguard with improved dental protection is worthwhile. An example of this would be a custom-moulded laminated guard with or without a hard inset anteriorly, depending on the sport involved.

Fractures of the facial skeleton. All facial fractures take 4 to 6 weeks to heal. The question of whether the athlete may train or compete depends entirely on the extent of the injury and must be evaluated in every single case. In most cases, light training is possible as early as 1 week after the injury. In some cases, the athlete may participate in the sport only if he wears a special face mask. In most cases, the athlete is not able to compete until 3 to 4 weeks later.

Preventing Reinjury

When assessing an injured player, details regarding protective equipment employed at the time of injury should be sought. The benefit of this approach allows for modification and optimization of protective behavior and an opportunity for head injury education.

Relatively few methods exist by which brain injury may be minimized in sport. The brain is not an organ that can be conditioned to withstand injury. Thus, extrinsic mechanisms of injury prevention must be sought. Helmets have been proposed as a means of protecting the head and theoretically reducing the risk of brain injury. In sports where the potential exists for high speed collisions, missile injuries (e.g., baseball), or for falls onto hard surfaces (e.g., gridiron football and ice hockey), published evidence has shown the effectiveness of sport-specific helmets in reducing head injuries. For other sports such as soccer and rugby no sport-specific helmets have been shown to be of proven benefit in reducing rates of head injury. Some believe that the use of protective equipment may alter playing behavior deleteriously so that the athlete actually increases his or her risk of brain injury. This is particularly true of child and teen athletes.

Although the use of correctly fitting mouth guards can reduce the rate of dental oro-facial and mandibular injuries, the evidence that they reduce cerebral injuries is largely theoretical with no evidence for reducing concussion.

Consideration of rule changes (e.g., no head checking in ice hockey) to reduce the head injury rate may be appropriate where a clear-cut mechanism is implicated in a particular sport. Similarly, rule enforcement is a critical aspect of such approaches, and referees play an important role.

Neck muscle conditioning may be of value in reducing impact forces transmitted to the brain. Biomechanical concepts dictate that the energy from an impacting object is dispersed over the greater mass of an athlete if the head is held rigidly. Although attractive from a theoretical standpoint, there is little scientific evidence to demonstrate the effectiveness of such measures.

As the ability to treat or reduce the effects of concussive injury after the event is minimal, education of athletes, colleagues and those working with them as well as the general public is a mainstay of progress in this field. Athletes and their health care providers must be educated regarding the detection of concussion, its clinical features, assessment techniques and principles of safe return to play. Methods to improve education including various web-based resources (for example www.concussionsafety.com), educational videos, outreach programs, concussion working groups, and the support and endorsement of enlightened sport groups must be pursued vigorously.

Acute Neck and Back Injuries

Jens Ivar Brox and Roger Sørensen

Definition

The occurrence, diagnosis, and treatment of acute neck and back injuries are discussed in this chapter (see table 5.1). Disk herniations are not usually caused by an acute injury, and so this topic is discussed in the sections on neck and back pain.

Occurrence

In North America, the annual occurrence of spinal cord injuries resulting from sport-related accidents is about 30 per one million inhabitants. Sport activity is the fourth most common cause of spinal column fractures and, after traffic accidents, is the most common cause of spinal cord injury. About half of all sport-related spinal cord injuries result in complete quadriplegia. Therefore, the consequences for those who are affected, and for society as a whole, are significant. More than 30% of all vertebral column fractures and more than 50% of all fractures/dislocations of the cervical spine are caused by diving accidents during unorganized sport activity. Serious back injuries also occur in sports, including horseback riding, motorized sports (especially snowmobiling), parachuting, hang gliding, paragliding, climbing, ice hockey, bicycling, snowboarding, downhill skiing, and ski jumping. A recent Canadian study stated that the incidence of spinal column fracture was 0.01 and 0.04 per 1,000 ski days for downhill skiers and snowboarders, respectively. Most snowboarding injuries occurred in connection with jumps. Most skiing injuries occurred as a result of falls. Compression or crush injuries accounted for more than 70% of the fractures, with the majority of fractures involving the T11 and L1 vertebral bodies. Nine percent of the injured snowboarders and 24% of the injured downhill skiers had neurological deficits, about half of which were secondary to spinal cord injuries.

The annual incidence of neck and back injuries among American high school athletes has been reported to be 0.7 per 100,000 football players and 2.6 per 100,000 hockey players. The most common serious neck injuries are crush fractures and dislocations,

Most common	Less common	Must not be overlooked !
Muscle contusions and strains (p. 100)	Fractures of transverse or spinous processes (p. 105)	Spinal cord injuries (p. 101)
	Stable thoracolumbar vertebral body fractures (p. 103)	Unstable fractures (p. 102)
		Inner organ injuries (see chapter 7)

Table 5.1 Overview of the differential diagnosis of acute neck and back injuries.

with about half the accidents resulting in spinal cord injury. In Canadian ice hockey, 11- to 20-year-olds sustain more than 60% of all spinal cord injuries. Most of the injuries are caused by head-first collisions with the sideboard, after being checked from behind. Helmets protect the head, but do not prevent the neck from bending forward slightly, and it is that position in which the individual is most vulnerable to neck injuries. There is no empirical basis for maintaining that the mandatory use of helmets reduces the occurrence of serious neck injuries. Stricter enforcement of the regulations regarding checking from behind would probably be a more effective preventive measure.

In a Finnish study, 9% of all soccer injuries were found to involve the neck and head. Most of these injuries involved conditions that did not require specific treatment. However, the prevalence of neck pain in retired soccer players is higher than in the rest of the population.

Differential Diagnosis

Table 5.1 contains an overview of the differential diagnosis for acute neck pain. Direct trauma to the back may cause intense pain, which is fortunately related to relatively insignificant muscle contusions in most cases. Falling with or without twisting may cause muscle strains, ligament damage, and/or fractures, and, less frequently, disk injuries.

The practitioner must evaluate the forces contributing to a specific injury and the possible consequences of that injury. Spinal trauma may cause spinal cord injury. To avoid catastrophic worsening of a back injury, the injured athlete must be moved from the scene of the injury in the proper manner.

If the patient has an injury that was caused by a collision, the physician must examine the abdominal organs– particularly the kidneys and spleen (see chapter 6)–to exclude damage to these vital structures. Such injuries may be acutely life threatening due to heavy internal bleeding and secondary hypotension.

Diagnostic Thinking

About 80% of all spinal cord injuries occur in connection with polytrauma. Therefore, polytrauma patients must have both an initial neurological examination and repeated and extended evaluations to exclude spinal cord injuries. Many patients who sustain spinal cord injuries due to accidents have no neurological deficit when examined at the scene of the accident. It is tragic when a patient is paraplegic on arrival at the hospital when the initial examination findings indicated that the patient was able to move both his arms and legs before being transported. Good knowledge of, and practical training in, emergency care is the only way to avoid this type of *unnecessary* catastrophe.

An athlete with a possible neck injury must not be moved from the sport facility before a competent examiner has completed a neurological examination to assess whether there is evidence of possible spinal cord injury or an unstable fracture which may precipitate a spinal cord injury if left unattended. If serious injuries of this type cannot be excluded, the patient's neck must be stabilized before he is moved (figure 5.1, a-f).

Dysesthesias and numbness in the legs, in connection with a neck injury, should be treated as a sign of possible spinal cord injury until proven otherwise. Awkward positioning or reflex tension in the neck may be the only protection a conscious patient

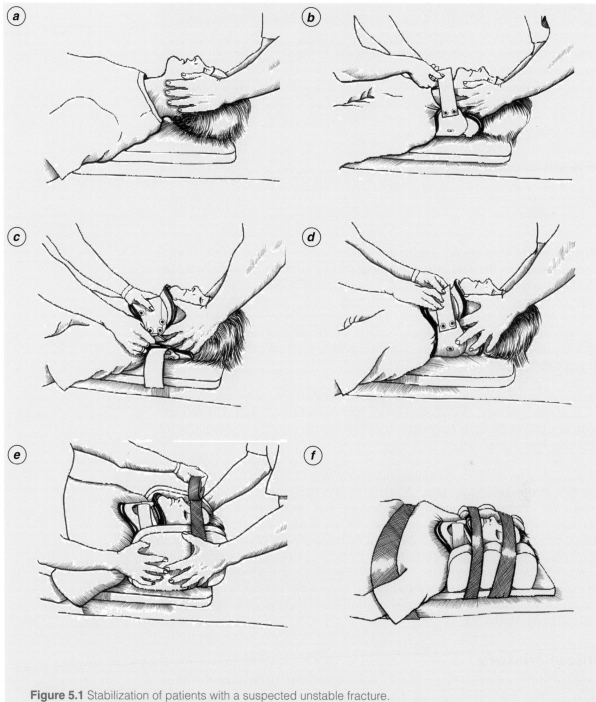

Figure 5.1 Stabilization of patients with a suspected unstable fracture.

- Stabilize the head and neck (a).
- Put on the back part of the collar (b).
- Put on the front part of the collar (c).
- Secure the collar (d).
- Roll the patient onto a stiff board or stretcher.
- Center the patient on the board.
- Place two blanket rolls or foam blocks on the board.
- Anchor the blocks around the patient's head (e).
- Anchor the blocks to the board (f).

Establish an open airway and control any bleeding.
Stabilize the head; do not correct the position of a patient who is conscious.
Perform an initial neurological examination.
Call an ambulance.
Put the patient in a stable side position: The neck of an unconscious patient must be stabilized.
Repeat the initial examination.
Make sure that the patient is adequately stabilized.
Direct the ambulance driver to drive carefully.

Table 5.2 Emergency care of patients with possible spinal cord injury.

has against spinal cord injury, and no attempt should be made to "correct" such abnormal postures in the field. An unconscious patient must not be moved until she is appropriately positioned and stabilized. Unanticipated dislocation of an unstable cervical spine may cause permanent spinal cord injury in a patient who has no symptoms or signs of this type of injury during the preliminary examination. Table 5.2 outlines the guidelines for emergency care of a patient with a suspected vertebral column fracture. The most experienced person on site must take charge of the situation when this type of injury occurs.

Patients with vertebral column fractures must be referred for appropriate orthopedic or neurosurgical care, evaluated in detail, and treated accordingly. The patient's primary health care provider can treat less serious injuries after the evaluation at the hospital has been completed.

Most patients who come to the emergency room with neck pain have been rear-ended in a motor vehicle accident. Skeletal X rays are usually negative but are necessary for insurance purposes. If the history and clinical examination point to nerve root irritation or radiculopathy, a cervical MRI is indicated. Most individuals who present to the emergency room with complaints of neck pain due to a sport-related accident, such as a fall while bicycling or skiing, probably did not have much neck protection at the time of the accident. Therefore, the cervical spine may have been subjected to significant force. Immediate referral for appropriate care is indicated if the patient has neurological damage and/or numbness and paresthesias in the legs.

Clinical History

Knowledge of the individual sport should make it easier to understand the injury mechanism. The practitioner should determine whether there was sudden strong rotation in connection with an injury sustained during a collision with the ground or with an opponent. Acute back pain triggered by a throwing motion may result from an avulsion fracture of the transverse processes and/or a muscle strain (possibly with associated hemorrhage) in the quadratus lumborum muscle and/or the iliopsoas muscle. The pain will usually radiate out toward the iliac crest, the groin, and/or the thigh in a referred pattern of pain.

The actual mechanism of injury may be compression of the head or neck, such as that caused by hitting a sideboard in ice hockey (figure 5.2). Other possible

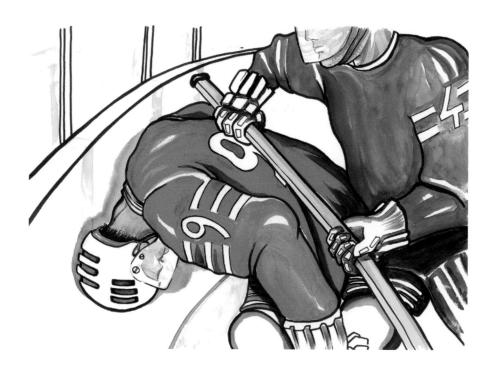

Figure 5.2 Injury mechanism. Serious neck injuries may result from crashing into the sideboard after being checked from behind. The helmet protects the head but does not prevent the neck from bending forward. Stricter enforcement of the rules can prevent fatal injuries.

mechanisms include being fallen on by another player during collision sports, falling from a great height when snowboarding, a forceful blow to the neck in contact sports, or strong involuntary movement of the neck as the result of a motor vehicle accident. Risk factors for injuries are equipment failure, violation of regulations (such as checking from behind in ice hockey), or a lack of skill (e.g., when jumping on a snowboard or trampoline). Cervical extension may be caused by a hard blow to the forehead and may result in rupture of the anterior longitudinal ligament, forward avulsion of a bone fragment on a vertebral body, or spondylolysis.

Classification systems for both cervical and thoracolumbar fractures are based on the clinical history and the injury mechanism and may improve the understanding of the consequences of various types of injuries (figure 5.3). When viewed in the sagittal plane, the vertebral column may be divided into three columns. The anterior column consists of the anterior longitudinal ligament, the anterior half of the intervertebral disk, and the vertebral body. The middle column consists of the posterior longitudinal ligament, the posterior half of the intervertebral disk, and the vertebral body. The posterior column consists of the posterior arch with the laminae, the transverse processes, the facet joints, the ligamentum flavum, the supraspinal ligament (from the C7 nuchal ligament), and the interspinal ligament. If at least two columns are involved radiographically, the fracture is assumed to be unstable.

Compression fractures usually involve only one column and are stable. Combined discoligamentous injuries caused by flexion and extension forces are usually unstable two-column injuries. Rotational trauma (figure 5.4) causes the highest proportion of neurological injuries. Table 5.3 shows injuries divided according to the degree of severity based on the clinical history and radiographs.

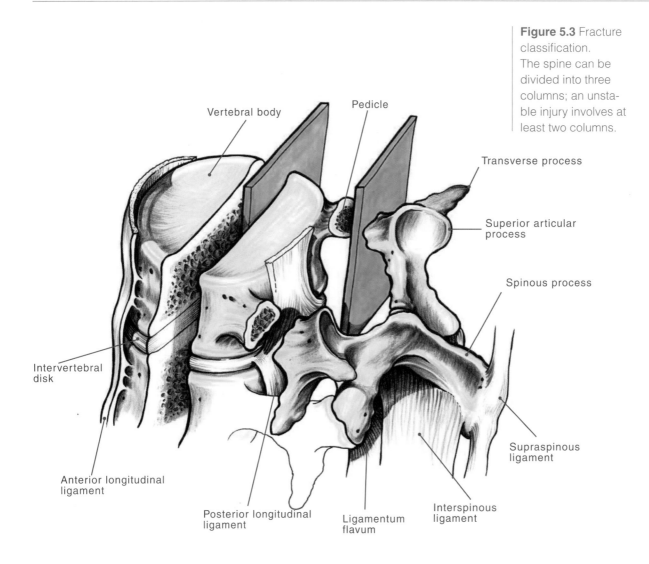

Figure 5.3 Fracture classification. The spine can be divided into three columns; an unstable injury involves at least two columns.

Vertebral body

Pedicle

Transverse process

Superior articular process

Spinous process

Intervertebral disk

Anterior longitudinal ligament

Posterior longitudinal ligament

Ligamentum flavum

Interspinous ligament

Supraspinous ligament

Clinical Examination

When a serious injury/fracture to the vertebral column is suspected, the physician must first evaluate the patient's circulation, respiration, and level of consciousness. Next, the patient's neurological status must be evaluated. Can the patient move his hands and feet? Fractures, dislocations, and discoligamentous injuries, with significant deformity and/or instability, may be present without initial neurological deficit. A careful search by palpation of the spinous processes may indicate a rupture of the interspinal ligament. Numbness and dysesthesias, and/or loss of proprioceptive awareness in the legs may be the only findings that point toward spinal cord involvement. Hyperreflexia is often masked by spinal shock. The segmental diagnostics are described in figure 5.5.

Supplemental Examinations

Radiographic examination. Frontal and lateral X rays should be taken of the indicated area. If the patient is unconscious, the neck must be examined, to exclude neck injuries. Because of overprojection of the shoulder section, it is difficult to obtain sufficient information about the cervicothoracic transition (C7/T1) using this

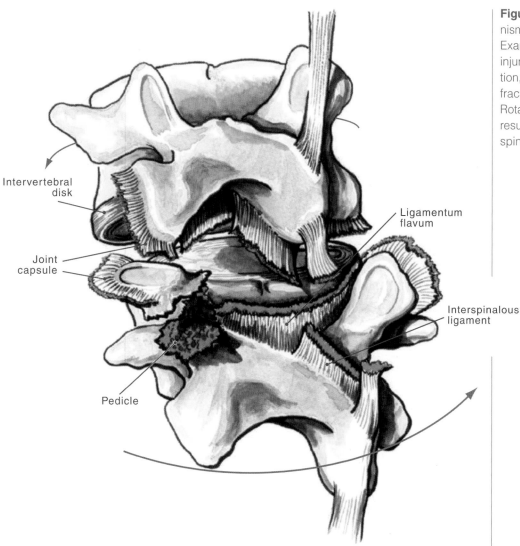

Intervertebral disk

Joint capsule

Pedicle

Ligamentum flavum

Interspinalous ligament

Figure 5.4 Injury mechanism involving rotation. Example of rotational injury causing dislocation, ligament rupture, fracture, and disk injury. Rotational injuries often result in nerve root or spinal cord injury.

Type	Injury mechanism	Neurologic damage, %
A	Compressive forces alone (compression fractures without ligament damage, such as falls on the buttocks or landing on the feet after parachute jumping or paragliding)	14
B	Stretching forces in flexion or extension (purely discoligamentous injuries, or like A, or posterior ligament rupture)	32
C	Rotational injuries alone or in combination with A or B	55

Table 5.3 Classification of fractures according to the AO-group. Each type can be divided into a hierarchy of groups and subgroups according to the increasing degree of seriousness (i.e., the degree of neurological damage).

examination. *A negative radiographic examination does not exclude an unstable neck injury.* Therefore, flexion and extension views of the cervical spine may be necessary, but a skilled professional must perform this examination.

Magnetic Resonance Imaging (MRI). MRI is the most sensitive means of examining the soft-tissue structures and the medulla. It is also the only test that can demonstrate, in detail, combined injuries of the intervertebral disk and ligament (discoligamentous

Level	Function	Reflex	Sensation
C3-5	Respiration (diaphragm)		
C5	Shoulder abduction (deltoid muscle)	Biceps	Lateral upper arm
C6	Elbow flexion	Brachioradialis	Lateral forearm
C7	Elbow extension	Triceps	Middle finger
C8	Finger flexion		Small and ring fingers
T1	Finger spreading		Medial forearm
L1-2	Hip flexion		
L3-4	Knee extension	Patellar	Medial thigh
L5	Big toe extension	Medial hamstring	Base, big toe
S1	Plantar flexion and toe flexion	Achilles	Lateral foot
S2-4	Sphincter function on rectal examination	Bulbocavernosus	

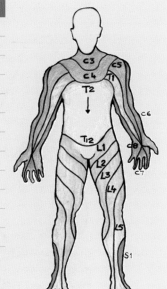

Figure 5.5 Segmental diagnostics, including dermatome chart.

injuries). Instability is evaluated by flexion and extension views on a plain X ray. If the MRI reveals ruptures of the interspinal ligament, the neck is potentially unstable and must be stabilized by surgery.

Computerized Tomography (CT). CT is an excellent method for evaluating the diameter of the spinal canal and the degree of bony collapse when the patient has a compression fracture. An isolated compression fracture with minor to moderate collapse is considered stable.

Common Injuries

Muscle Contusions and Strains

Muscle contusions occur frequently in various contact sports. Muscle strains occur most frequently in explosive sports. The injury is often localized to the erector muscles of the spine.

- Symptoms and signs: Palpation causes distinct pain that is usually unilateral. If the patient has a muscle strain, he often complains of cramping when bending forward and when rising. If isometric contraction does not provoke pain, the patient may have an isolated ligament injury.
- Diagnosis: The diagnosis is based on clinical history plus exclusion of other causes of pain after a clinical examination and possibly diagnostic imaging for a suspected fracture.
- Treatment by physician: Drug treatment is the same as for acute lumbago. If the patient has a muscle contusion, inform her that the prognosis is good and that she will probably be able to resume full activity in a few days. However, a strain injury may prevent her from participating in sport activity for a relatively long time. Mobilization may be indicated if the examination seems to reveal an isolated ligament injury and the injury has become chronic with limited segmental movement.

• Treatment by physical therapist or self-treatment: Ice and information are the first treatments offered. If the patient has a muscle strain, he should undergo alternative training after a few days. Gradual progression to a more competitive type of activity during a 3- to 8-week period is recommended.

Other Injuries

Spinal Cord Injuries !

Spinal cord injuries may be characterized as either complete or incomplete. A complete injury is defined as a loss of neuromuscular function below the level of the injury, including the most distal sacral segments, that lasts longer than 48 hours. Incomplete injuries are divided according to the long pathways that are affected. Depending on its location, the injury may be classified as anterior, lateral, dorsal longitudinal fasciculus, central, or conus (T12-L1), or as cauda equina syndrome (below L1). An unstable neck fracture (see figure 5.6) may place direct pressure on

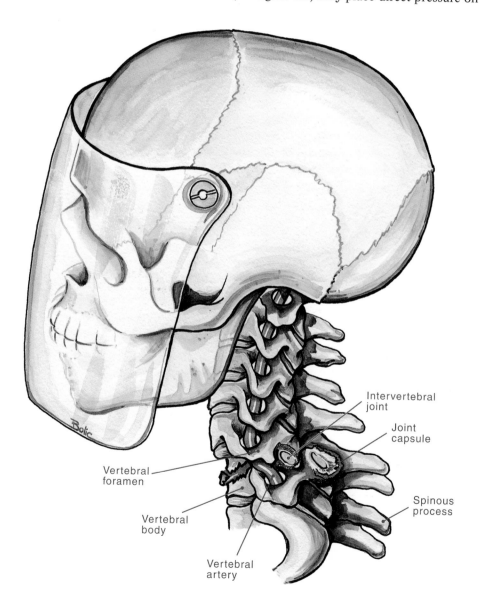

Intervertebral joint

Joint capsule

Vertebral foramen

Vertebral body

Vertebral artery

Spinous process

Figure 5.6 Unstable cervical fracture, which may cause a partial anterior spinal cord injury. The symptoms may be caused by direct pressure on the spinal column or compression of the vertebral artery.

the spinal cord or compress the vertebral artery. A mechanism of injury such as this can affect the pyramidal tracts and may result in an anterior cord syndrome–characterized by flaccid paralysis, as well as reduced sensitivity to pain and temperature distal to the site of the injury. Proprioceptive sensation is transmitted in the dorsal longitudinal fasciculus and is generally well preserved.

- Symptoms and signs: Symptoms and signs of spinal cord injuries include neck pain, numbness, dysesthesias, and motor dysfunction involving the hands and feet. An examination of sensation must include sensitivity to touch and pain (anterior spinothalamic tract), joint sensation (dorsal longitudinal fasiculus), and sensitivity to light touch (lateral corticospinal tract). Neuromuscular function should be graded from 0 (no contraction) to 5 (normal muscle strength). If the patient has neurological deficits, the level of injury is defined as the last normal level (i.e., preserved sensation and motor function > 3) (figure 5.5). Shallow respiration, hypotension with bradycardia, areflexia, lack of anal sphincter tone, priapism, and loss of sensitivity to pain distal to the injury are signs of spinal cord damage in an unconscious patient.
- Diagnosis: The diagnosis of spinal cord injury is primarily clinical. The patient must not be moved before being properly stabilized. The patient must be referred to a spine surgeon for further evaluation and treatment. A patient without symptoms and signs that indicate spinal cord injury may have an unstable fracture.
- Treatment: The patient must be transported to the hospital (figure 5.1). Drug therapy with methylprednisolone 30 mg/kg body weight must be given within 8 hours, with a maintenance dose of 5.4 mg/kg in 24 to 48 hours, to reduce the degree of permanent paralysis. Surgery consists of decompression and possibly fusion of two or more levels of the joint.
- Prognosis: Early drug treatment with methylprednisolone, as described, improves the prognosis. Signs of spinal activity during the first 72 hours after the injury predict walking function 1 year after a partial injury. Functional gait can be expected in about 50% of patients who have partially intact sensory function and in about 85% of those who show signs of motor activity. Lack of motor and sensory activity in the first 72 hours indicates that the patient likely will not regain the ability to walk. If the CT shows compression of the medulla when the patient has a partial spinal cord injury, the medulla must be decompressed, even if the paresis is not progressive, because decompression may reduce the degree of paresis. Performing surgery on patients with complete spinal cord injuries after the hyperacute phase does not improve the prognosis.

Unstable Fractures !

A fracture is stable if controlled movements do not cause neurological deficit. If the fracture is unstable, controlled movements may result in or may worsen a nerve root or spinal cord injury. The fracture may be classified according to the number of columns involved. If two or more columns are involved, the injury is considered unstable (figures 5.3 and 5.7, a and b).

- Symptoms and signs: A combination of high-energy trauma, abnormal positioning of the head caused by neck muscle contractions or reflex muscle spasm of the neck, or the inability of the patient to stand on her feet are signs of an unstable fracture.
- Diagnosis: The patient must be referred for appropriate neurosurgical or orthopedic care and should be treated as if he has an unstable fracture until the contrary has been proven. This applies regardless of whether the athlete is examined at the sport facility or in the emergency room. A complete neurological examination and a diagnostic imaging examination including a skeletal X ray (and MRI) are necessary to exclude the diagnosis.

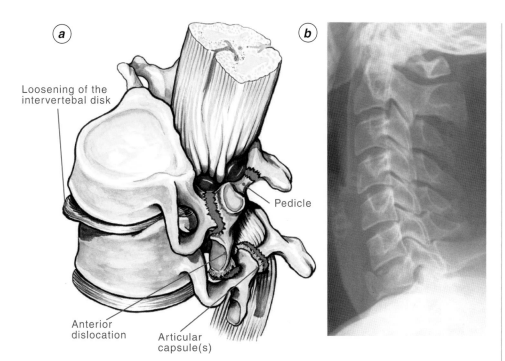

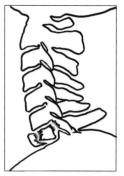

Figure 5.7 Unstable cervical fracture. The drawing *(a)* shows that all three columns are injured with rupture of the ligamentum flavum, anterior dislocation, fracture of the vertebral arch, loosening of the intervertebral disk, and spinal cord injury. The sagittal X ray view *(b)* demonstrates an injury of the anterior column and middle column, with a fracture of the vertebral body and arch.

- Treatment: Abnormal positioning of the head caused by neck muscle contractions or reflex muscle spasm of the neck may be secondary to vertebral fractures and/or spinal cord injuries and may be the only protection a conscious patient has against brainstem damage. Therefore, no attempt should be made to correct the position of the patient. The patient should be transported to the hospital using appropriate precautions (figure 5.1). If neurological deficit is present, treatment includes skull traction or surgery for unstable cervical fractures. The patient should wear a rigid cervical collar if a slight degree of malalignment and no neurological deficit are present. Surgery is indicated to treat unstable thoracolumbar fractures.
- Prognosis: The prognosis is good if an injury is suspected before complications (spinal cord damage) occur and the patient receives adequate transport and treatment.

Stable Thoracolumbar Vertebral Body Fractures— Crush Injuries of the Thoracic or Lumbar Vertebrae

Stable thoracolumbar vertebral body fractures (figure 5.8, a-c) include epiphyseal plate fractures and compression or crush injuries of the vertebral body. These are stable if the posterior column is not affected. Fractures that affect the epiphyseal plate are common among young people and the elderly and occur primarily in the thoracic and lumbar sections.

- Symptoms and signs: Symptoms depend on the injury mechanism and the location of the injury. Pain at the fracture site, possibly radiating to the dermatome that corresponds to the fracture, is the most common symptom. The patient has distinct sensitivity to pressure on the spinous process of the injured vertebra, and local muscle spasm is common.
- Treatment: Surgery is commonly performed if the anterior portion of the vertebral body is reduced by more than 40% when compared to the vertebrae above and below it. The basis for this strategy is that surgical fixation provides primary stabilization. This is the most secure method of preventing further collapse of the vertebra, and the fracture is stable for training within a few days.

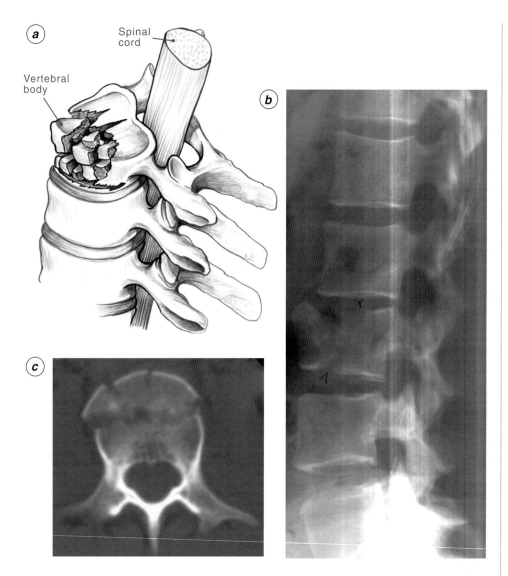

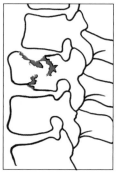

Figure 5.8 Stable compression fracture. Fractures of the end plates, collapse, and compression fractures of vertebral bodies are considered stable if the posterior column is not affected. Stable compression fractures may occur in the cervical, thoracic, and lumbar regions. The illustration *(a)* shows a stable cervical compression fracture, whereas the X ray view *(b)* shows a stable lumbar fracture, and the CT image *(c)* shows a stable thoracic compression fracture.

However, recent reports maintain that there is no indication for surgery on isolated thoracolumbar compression fractures, because the prognosis is similar without surgery. The relationship between the degree of kyphotic angulation caused by the fracture and symptoms is not definite. There is a need for randomized studies to evaluate the effect of thoracolumbar compression fracture treatment.

• Treatment by physical therapist: The most important step is to mobilize the patient gradually, beginning on the 1st day. Early mobilization reduces the risk of deep venous thrombosis and apparently does not increase kyphosis. Specific back and abdominal muscle exercises have not been shown to be more effective than early mobilization, so no restrictions are placed on the patient's level of activity. Nevertheless, the athlete should wait until healing of the fracture is radiographically verified before returning to full competitive sport activity. Treatment with a brace limits large movements of the trunk but not intervertebral movement. Hyperextension orthoses do not appear to affect the progression of the collapse of a compression fracture. Thus, the use of a brace has not been shown to stabilize the fracture, and bracing should be prescribed only if pain prevents the patient from being mobilized without it.

• Prognosis: Most patients recover or experience only minor pain. Some patients develop chronic pain and do not return to full competitive activity.

Fractures of the Transverse or Spinous Processes

Fractures of the spinous processes and transverse processes are rare (figure 5.9). Isolated fractures of the spinous process may be one of several injuries to result from flexion trauma. Fractures of the spinous process do not require any special treatment, but the physician must exclude any serious injury occurring simultaneously. Fractures of the transverse processes are far more common. Usually the fracture occurs in the lumbar section and affects the iliopsoas muscle and the quadratus lumborum muscle.

- Symptoms and signs: The patient usually has severe pain in connection with the trauma. If the patient has a fracture of the transverse processes in the lumbar spine, hip flexion and torsion make the pain worse. The patient will be sensitive to palpation: both paravertebrally and in the abdomen. Bleeding from the fracture site and musculature may result in anemia. Pain is often provoked by hip flexion (iliopsoas muscle) and by lateral flexion (quadratus lumborum muscle).
- Diagnosis: A radiographic examination demonstrates the avulsed processes. A CT scan provides the best overview and is indicated if the X ray is negative and the patient's history and clinical examination suggest a fracture.
- Treatment by physician: The patient should be referred immediately for appropriate orthopedic or neurosurgical care if concurrent serious injuries are suspected. Treatment of isolated fractures is conservative. Therefore, a primary care provider can evaluate and treat the patient. If pain does not allow rapid mobilization, the use of a brace may be helpful.
- Treatment by physical therapist: Functional training is recommended.
- Self-treatment: The patient can self-treat by gradually increasing activity.
- Prognosis: The prognosis is good. Healing usually takes place in 6 to 8 weeks, but an additional 3 or 4 weeks of gradually increasing training is usually recommended before full activity in contact sports is allowed.

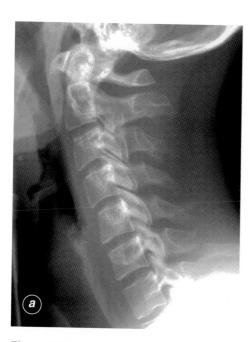
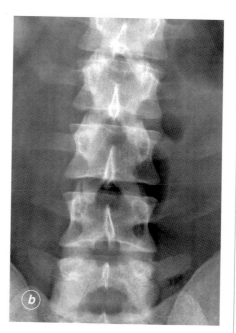
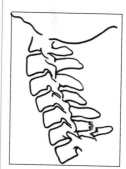
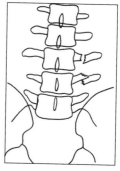

Figure 5.9 Fractures of the spinous process and the transverse process. Fracture of a cervical spinous process *(a)*. A simultaneous major injury must be excluded. Fracture of a lumbar transverse process *(b)*. The clinician should be alert to the possibility of simultaneous injury to the psoas muscle, which originates from the lumbar transverse processes.

Neck Pain

Jens Ivar Brox

Definition

Acute neck pain may develop without known trauma or in connection with a minor trauma. It may also result from trauma to the neck or head, or it may represent pain referred from another location, or due to another etiology.

Occurrence

Neck pain is a common symptom that occurs about as often as back pain, which affects almost 50% of the adult population each year. There are approximately 40 to 80 new cases of cervical nerve root pain per 100,000 per year.

Thirty percent of the retired Norwegian national soccer players suffer from chronic neck symptoms and limited neck movement. In a study of soccer players and a control group, disk degeneration was found to be significantly more common, and occurred 10 to 20 years earlier, in the soccer players than in the controls. Potential explanations for these differences include: (1) the combination of repeated compression and hyperextension loading when making contact with the soccer ball and (2) collisions with other players.

In Western countries, neck pain that results from being rear-ended in a motor vehicle accident occurs so frequently that it seems to be epidemic. The epidemic is difficult to explain from a biomechanical perspective. The patient seldom has definite pathophysiological changes or specific clinical signs. This type of complaint occurs to a small percentage of athletes who are frequently subjected to corresponding biomechanical forces. The way in which modern medicine and the legal system have focused on this type of complaint appears to have created a culture of disease and disability that contributes to unnecessary anxiety about physical activity being harmful to the neck.

Differential Diagnosis

Neck pain may be classified in various manners. It is common to distinguish between neck pain that radiates (cervicobrachialgia) and pain that does not radiate

Most common	Less common	Must not be overlooked
Cervicalgia (p. 110)	Cervicobrachialgia (p. 110)	Unstable fracture (p. 102)
	Cervical radiculopathy (p. 111)	Infection (p. 107)
	Acute torticollis (p. 110)	Tumor (p. 107)
	Thoracic outlet syndrome (p. 111)	

Table 5.4 Overview of the differential diagnosis of neck injuries.

to the upper extremities. The radiating pain may follow a nerve root pattern (cervical radiculopathy) or worsen by elevation of the arm and palpation of the brachial plexus (thoracic outlet syndrome). It may also be caused by entrapment of the peripheral nerves. A more common differential diagnostic approach to the problem is to distinguish between pain that radiates from the neck down into the shoulder and arm, and primary shoulder pain with secondary neck pain. Table 5.4 provides an overview of the most relevant differential diagnoses. Neck pain may also represent referred pain, such as when the patient has a throat infection or a cervical tumor. In the elderly, dizziness and neck pain may be caused by stenosis in the vertebral artery.

Diagnostic Thinking

The examiner must determine whether the pain is coming from the neck or originates elsewhere, whether there are neurological symptoms and signs, and whether the pain is due to a specific neck disorder or is nonspecific (figure 5.10). Acute neck pain can be very intense, accompanied by improper positioning (torticollis) and stiffness. This pain may make the patient anxious, further complicating the situation. Therefore, instilling confidence during the initial consultation has a good therapeutic effect. The natural history of neck pain is in most instances good, so comprehensive treatment is not generally recommended.

To understand, diagnose, and treat painful conditions in the neck, it is advisable to determine whether the patient has an illness that has no specific treatment or if the patient has a disease with obvious diagnostic characteristics and an anticipated course. An example of the latter type of condition is radiating neck pain and neurological deficit. Neck pain and stiffness without specific signs is defined as an illness. Degenerative changes revealed by radiographic or MRI examinations occur about as frequently in healthy asymptomatic people as in individuals with neck pain, and so the findings on imaging may be of little diagnostic value. If the pain continues, the physician should determine whether the pain has a significant organic characteristic or whether the symptoms indicate somatization. In individual cases, the history and clinical examination may suggest that the patient's symptoms and functional limitations are motivated by possible secondary gain in the form of

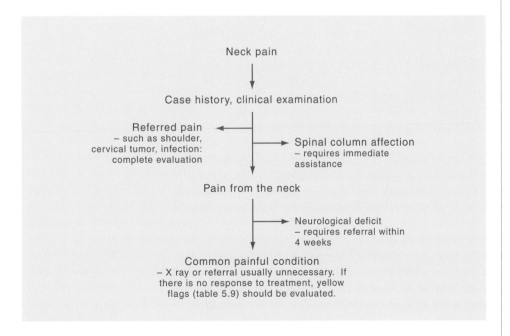

Figure 5.10 Algorithm for evaluating patients with acute neck pain.

insurance compensation. In this case, it may be useful to observe the patient outside the examining room. Diagnostic imaging is indicated if nerve root involvement is suspected or if there is atypical pain.

Clinical History

The patient's history must describe how the pain originated and what their main symptoms are. Did the pain originate in connection with an acute event or did it develop gradually?

The most essential part of taking the patient's history is to obtain an accurate description of the location of the pain and any accompanying symptoms, such as headache, a lapse in concentration, dizziness, nausea, and vision or hearing disturbances.

Is the pain diffuse or distinctly localized? Is the pain provoked by coughing or sneezing? Does it radiate only to the upper extremities, and if so, does the radiation have radicular characteristics? Muscle weakness may indicate nerve root involvement, but primary shoulder conditions and peripheral nerve entrapment must be excluded by means of a clinical examination. To refine the differential diagnosis, the practitioner must ask whether the patient has bladder dysfunction. Gait dysfunction or balance impairment may be a sign of myelopathy.

Clinical Examination

Inspection. Torticollis is the tilting of the head to one side, caused by contraction of the muscles on that side of the neck. The condition may be congenital, or may be due to a serious injury. Other potential etiologies include reflex muscle activity caused by disc herniation or facet joint dysfunction, muscular strain injury, or myofascial pain. The practitioner must evaluate the patient's muscle tension. Does the patient unconsciously shrug the shoulders? Cervical tumor should be ruled out.

Neurological examination. If the patient has pain that radiates beyond the shoulders, he should be given a neurological examination (figure 5.5).

Range of motion. Active and passive range of motion should be examined. The normal range of motion in the neck is 55° extension, 45° forward flexion, 45° lateral flexion, and 70° rotation. Normal variation is considerable, and a simple means of assessing range of motion is to ask the patient to put her chin on her chest and to see whether lateral flexion and rotation are symmetrical. If pain and neck stiffness are the primary problems, neck movement should be examined while the patient is sitting, standing, stooping, and lying. If muscle pain and stiffness are present, range of motion is significantly reduced when the patient is stooping but normal when the patient is supine.

Spurling test. A positive Spurling's maneuver (figure 5.11) indicates cervical nerve root involvement, but the test may be falsely negative. The test is based on dynamically narrowing the cervical neural foramina via neck extension, coupled with rotation and bending the head toward the affected side. If this reproduces the pain in the upper extremity, the test is positive.

Roos test. This test (figure 5.12) should be positive if the patient has thoracic outlet syndrome. For this test the patient repeatedly clenches the fist for 3 minutes while the arm is in an abducted, externally rotated position. If the symptoms are provoked on the affected side, or if the patient has problems clenching the fist, the test is positive.

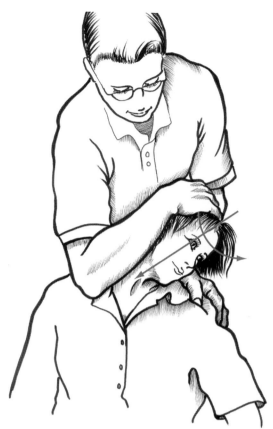

Figure 5.11 Spurling's maneuver. The space for the exiting nerve root is reduced when the examiner combines side flexion and rotation with axial cervical compression.

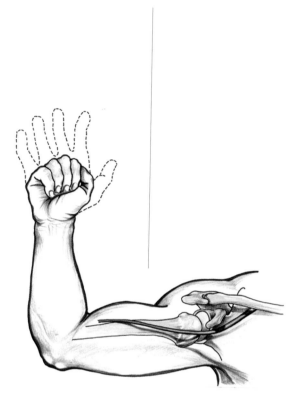

Figure 5.12 Roos test. Have the patient repeatedly clench and open his fist, as shown in the illustration. Impingement of nerves or vascular structures in the scalene port is assumed to be the cause of the symptoms.

Palpation. The practitioner should palpate the spinous process and the transverse processes, the suboccipital muscles, the trapezius muscle, the levator scapulae, the scalene, and the sternocleidomastoid muscles bilaterally and supraclavicularly. Palpatory findings are often difficult to interpret but may be important if the tenderness is unilateral or localized.

Supplemental Examinations

X rays of the cervical spine with oblique projections are indicated for atypical pain and to evaluate the intervertebral foramina when there is radicular pain.

MRI is the first choice for clinical symptoms and signs that suggest nerve root involvement. The examination is not indicated during the acute phase if drug therapy has an adequate effect on the patient.

EMG and nerve stimulation studies are seldom used but may be helpful (1) in cases in which the patient may have peripheral or central pathology, (2) when differentiating between radiculopathy and peripheral nerve entrapment or (3) when differentiating between disorders of nerve or muscle. Electrodiagnostic testing should normally be requested by a specialist.

Common Painful Conditions

Cervicalgia/Cervicobrachialgia

It is common to classify neck pain that does not radiate to the upper extremities as cervicalgia and neck pain with diffusely disseminating radiation as cervicobrachialgia. A distinction must be made between cervicobrachialgia and cervical radiculopathy (a condition in which the radiating pain follows a nerve root pattern). Unilateral monotonous loading and psychosocial conditions are contributing factors. Pain may be vertebrogenic, discogenic, or muscular. Often more than one structure is involved.

- Symptoms and signs: Symptoms and signs include neck pain that may or may not radiate to the shoulder and upper arm, difficulty moving the neck, and normal or slightly reduced passive range of motion. Accompanying symptoms, such as fatigue, lapses in concentration, dizziness, tinnitus, and nausea indicate stress-related neck pain.
- Diagnosis: The diagnosis is made clinically by excluding nerve root pain and pain referred from other organs. A simple clinical examination, without supplemental diagnostic imaging, is sufficient for the initial examination.
- Treatment by physician: Over-the-counter analgesics or nonsteroidal anti-inflammatory drugs (NSAIDs) for 3 to 7 days reduce the duration of the acute pain. More potent analgesics may be necessary for sleep disturbance. Treatment for chronic pain depends on whether the pain seems to be organic or is mostly stress related. The periodic use of a cervical collar may provide relief and alleviate symptoms of organic pain in elderly patients.
- Treatment by physical therapist: The effects of the various forms of available treatment are not well documented. Mobilization and manipulation appear to be better than no treatment. Manipulation of the neck is not recommended because the therapeutic effect is typically minor in comparison to the few serious complications that have been reported. Several studies indicate that electromagnetic therapy may have an analgesic effect. Active exercises and stretching are recommended for chronic pain. If treatment is not effective, the status of the indication should be reevaluated. The patient should continue with general training.
- Prognosis: The prognosis is usually good, but repeated injuries to patients who participate in contact sports may force the athlete to end his sport career.

Other Painful Conditions

Acute Torticollis

Torticollis is a condition of acute neck pain characterized by improper positioning of the neck, usually lateral flexion combined with rotation.

- Symptoms and signs: The patient often states that their pain began suddenly, often following a specific movement—for example, while sleeping—after which the neck gradually became stiffer and more painful. Generally, cervical range of motion is significantly reduced, and the neck is stiff and tilts to one side. When range of motion is tested, pain is often asymmetric.
- Diagnosis: The diagnosis is based on the clinical history. Physical examination should attempt to rule out other causes of acute torticollis, such as trauma, disc injury (with or without radiculopathy), throat infection, and tumors. The physician should perform diagnostic imaging if the pain has lasted more than 14 days.
- Treatment by physician: Recommended treatments are muscle relaxants, NSAIDs, or acetominophen. The prognosis is good and patients are normally able to resume full activity after a few days.
- Treatment by physical therapist or self-treatment: Ice, information, and mobilization of the neck.

Cervical Radiculopathy

Radiculopathy is most commonly caused by a herniated disk in patients 40 years or younger. However, in the elderly, pain is more often caused by degenerative changes that reduce the height of the intervertebral disk and cause facet joint arthropathy that contribute to the relative stenosis of the intervertebral foramina. The prevalence of disk herniation and degenerative changes demonstrated on diagnostic imaging is actually quite high among asymptomatic people. Therefore, a cervical disc herniation may not be associated with nerve root pain.

- Symptoms and signs: Common symptoms include neck pain and unilateral shoulder and/or arm pain; numbness or tingling in the fingers; and reduced shoulder, arm, and/or finger muscle strength that follows a myotomal pattern. The diagnosis is confirmed if sensation is reduced in a dermatomal pattern and the corresponding muscle stretch reflex is abnormal. Manual muscle testing has higher diagnostic specificity compared with clinical examination of sensoric disturbances and reflexes. Diagnostic accuracy of manual muscle testing averages from between 75% to 80% (figure 5.5). Spurling's maneuver (figure 5.11) may reproduce the symptoms. In terms of differential diagnosis, the practitioner should ask whether the patient has bladder dysfunction and whether walking or balance has deteriorated (an indication of possible myelopathy).
- Diagnosis: The diagnosis is first and foremost clinical. It is based on radiating pain, paresthesias, hyperesthesia and dysesthesia, and motor weakness and reduced reflexes in a nerve root pattern. If the diagnosis is in doubt, MRI of the cervical spine and X rays with oblique views are useful. Ordering an MRI examination depends on accessibility, but it is normally not useful in the early phase. EMG and nerve stimulation studies are often diagnostic but seldom necessary.
- Treatment by physician: The natural history of cervical radiculopathy is generally good without surgery. Oral corticosteroids have the best anti-inflammatory effect and are the first choice for drug therapy. Stronger analgesics are indicated for sleep disturbance caused by pain. A cervical collar limits extension and may bring relief during the first phase. Bladder paresis and progressive weakness of the legs are indications for immediate hospitalization and neurosurgical consulation.
- Treatment by physical therapist: Traction may be indicated if information, drugs, and a cervical collar do not provide sufficient pain relief. Active exercises may counteract stiffness in the neck. Manipulation is contraindicated.
- Self-treatment: The athlete should maintain daily activities and seek alternative training that does not further aggravate the pain.
- Prognosis: The prognosis varies greatly among individuals. Improvement may be marked in the first 14 days; still, the condition may result in chronic symptoms that force the athlete to discontinue participation in competitive sports for several months.

Thoracic Outlet Syndrome

Thoracic outlet syndrome is a condition related to compression of nervous or vascular structures between the neck and the axilla. Contrary to popular belief, symptoms are rarely directly related to a cervical rib. The etiology is more often related to muscular dysfunction that includes tense scalene musculature.

- Symptoms and signs: Symptoms worsen when the arm is elevated, with paresthesias in a distribution corresponding to segments C8-T1, with tenderness over the brachial plexus or above the clavicle, and with a positive Roos test.
- Diagnosis: The diagnosis can be made when at least three of the above symptoms and signs are found.
- Treatment by physician: The outcome of surgery is good in less than 40% of the patients, and some patients suffer disabling complications. Therefore, the physician

must diligently evaluate the patient's symptoms and functional level in order to initiate proper treatment. This includes a thorough differential diagnostic evaluation, measuring range of motion of the neck, evaluating muscle strength in the upper extremities, and watching for evidence of somatization. Hence, a physical medicine and rehabilitation or neurology specialist should evaluate the patient.

- Treatment by physical therapist: Supervised exercise seems to improve the condition in most patients. The purpose of the exercises is to normalize the pattern of movement in the neck and shoulder girdle in order to create more space for the neurovascular structures.
- Prognosis: The prognosis is good with nonsurgical treatment, poor with surgery.

Transient Pain and Paresthesia in the Upper Extremities

The occurrence of transient neck pain with radiation and numbness (burning and stinging) is high in contact sports such as football and rugby. It is believed that repeated hard tackles with lateral flexion of the neck and depression of the ipsilateral shoulder increases the risk of chronic neck pain in this type of collision sport. The symptoms may result from a traction injury of the brachial plexus or to one or more cervical nerve roots. Often, the symptoms last only a few seconds, but some patients have chronic discomfort.

- Symptoms and signs: Symptoms include burning pain and numbness in the upper extremity. These symptoms are localized more regionally than in a dermatomal pattern. The symptoms may be transient, or they may be more persistent and chronic. Physical signs include muscle weakness.
- Diagnosis: The differential diagnosis includes cervical radiculopathy and thoracic outlet syndrome, both of which should be ruled out. If the proportion between the midsagittal diameter of the spinal canal and the diameter of the vertebral joints is <0.7 the patient is at an increased risk of developing chronic discomfort.
- Treatment: To prevent problems, the practitioner should advise an athlete who is at increased risk to wear a cervical collar or to give up contact sports.

Back Pain

Jens Ivar Brox and Roger Sørensen

Definition

Aside from the common cold, back pain is our leading public health problem. Well-defined conditions as well as symptoms for which no specific treatments are available are the focus of this section (see table 5.5).

Occurrence

Acute back pain is common among athletes. The prognosis is favorable, even without comprehensive evaluation and treatment. Most athletes may resume their normal sporting activity within 1 or 2 weeks. Ninety percent of athletes who develop acute lumbago for the first time are asymptomatic within 1 or 2 weeks.

The prevalence of back pain varies from sport to sport. In weightlifting, nearly every elite athlete is affected annually, whereas other athletes, such as runners, rarely have back trouble. It has been reported that 30% to 40% of elite swimmers and more than 60% of elite cross-country skiers have back pain that periodically affects their activity level. Problems among cross-country skiers are more often related to the classical technique than to skating. A Swedish epidemiological study that included soccer and tennis players, wrestlers, and gymnasts revealed that 50% to 85% of the athletes had experienced back pain. Radiographic changes were found in 36% to 55% of the athletes, depending on the sport. The prevalence of spondylolysis among wrestlers was five times higher than in the general population. Former wrestlers have nearly twice the prevalence of back pain as the general

Most common	Less common	Must not be overlooked !
Acute lumbago (p. 121)	Muscle contusion (p. 100)	Tumor (p. 120)
Chronic lumbago (p. 122)	Muscle rupture (p. 114)	Diskitis (p. 116)
Spondylolysis or spondylolisthesis (p. 124)	Ligament damage	
	Acute sciatica (p. 126)	
	Chronic sciatica (p. 127)	
	Scoliosis (p. 129)	
	Scheuermann's disease (p. 129)	
	Ankylosing spondylitis (p. 130)	
	Spinal stenosis (p. 128)	

Table 5.5 Overview of the differential diagnosis of acute and chronic back pain.

population, but lower absence due to illness! The back is the second most common location for injuries in dancers, but there is disagreement about causes of the pain. The prevalence of isthmic spondylolysis or spondylolisthesis is high among dancers–both among those who have back pain and those who do not.

Differential Diagnosis

An overview of the most relevant differential diagnosis of non-specific low back pain is listed in table 5.5. Back pain is usually attributed to a strain of the lumbar muscles, degeneration of the intervertebral disks, or arthritis of the facet joints. Often several structures are involved. Reflex interplay between the structures may make it difficult to make an exact diagnosis during the acute stage. If the pain is chronic, diagnostic imaging using CT or MRI often provides a specific diagnosis (e.g., disc protrusion or prolapse, spinal stenosis, lateral recess stenosis, facet joint arthrosis, degeneration of the intervertebral disk, osteochondritis, or spondylolisthesis). If a corresponding evaluation of people with healthy backs was undertaken, the proportion of radiographic diagnoses would have been nearly as high as in those patients with back pain. Therefore, the physician must relate findings from diagnostic imaging to clinical findings before giving the patient a specific diagnosis. For example, in adults there is no statistical relationship between radiographic spondylolysis or spondylolisthesis and pain. However, spondylolysis or spondylolisthesis should be excluded in young athletes who have back pain.

If the patient has chronic sciatica caused by disk herniation or lateral recess stenosis, a decision must be made about whether or not to perform surgery on the patient and what consequences surgery would have for sporting activity in both the long and short term. In the elderly, pain with ambulation that improves when the patient bends forward may be caused by spinal stenosis (neurogenic claudication). In terms of the differential diagnosis, peripheral vascular disease should be considered. Recent studies also indicate a relationship between degenerative back problems and cardiovascular disease.

In downhill and cross-country skiing, in weightlifting, and in sports that involve throwing (including ball sports), the tendon insertions may become inflamed or may rupture because of sudden or repeated loading. Repeated loading during martial arts, such as judo and karate, may cause muscle and ligament damage. For example, pain referred from the quadratus lumborum muscle projects toward the groin, thigh, and iliac crest and becomes worse with lateral flexion, extension, and rotation.

Diagnostic Thinking

If the patient has chronic pain, the diagnosis should include a functional evaluation relating to the individual sport. In addition to the examination based on patho-anatomy, psychological and social factors should be evaluated.

First, the practitioner should determine whether the pain derives from the back or from some other area or cause (e.g., from the abdomen, genitalia, or systemic disease). The practitioner should then determine whether the condition requires immediate attention or referral (e.g., spinal cord injury or cauda equina lesion), whether the symptoms and signs indicate serious back disease (red flags are noted in table 5.6), nerve root involvement, or non-specific back pain. If red flags are uncovered during the examination, it is the physician's job to communicate this without causing unnecessary anxiety. If a supplemental examination is necessary, the patient should be informed that these examinations are often negative, that the specialist will provide additional advice, and that it may be advisable for the patient to reduce his activity level somewhat until after he has been examined by the specialist.

Pain that does not worsen with activity
Clinical history: doping, cancer, HIV
Impaired general condition, weight loss
Neurological abnormalities without obvious radicular characteristics
Structural deformity

Table 5.6 Red flags for back pain. The patient should be referred within 4 weeks.

Most patients with acute back pain become asymptomatic within 1 or 2 weeks without treatment. Initially, the pain is often severe and accompanied by significant dysfunction. A patient seeks medical assistance because she wants pain relief and advice about what to do. The patient should be informed that the prognosis for acute low back pain is generally good. A complete examination is not always necessary. Because it is difficult to make a specific diagnosis during the acute stage, the patient should be given an opportunity to return for a complete re-examination within 2 weeks. Surgery is indicated during the acute stage if the patient has lost control of bowel or bladder function or if there is evidence of progressive motor deficit. In the latter case, the patient should be referred for appropriate orthopedic or neurosurgical care immediately. The prognosis for acute bladder or rectal paresis is worse if it lasts more than 11 hours. Patients with kyphosis or structural scoliosis should be referred for orthopedic evaluation. If ankylosing spondylitis or another inflammatory disease is present, a rheumatologist should also evaluate the patient.

The diagnosis and clinical course are used to determine when to refer a patient to a specialist in physical medicine and rehabilitation, neurology, orthopedics, or rheumatology. If the condition has lasted less than 2 weeks, the patient may be examined and treated by a primary care physician. If it has lasted more than 8 weeks, a specialist should evaluate the patient.

If the pain is subacute or chronic, the practitioner should take the time to listen to the patient's history and to perform a thorough clinical examination. Diagnostic imaging is usually not a shortcut to the proper diagnosis and treatment, but it can be a useful supplement to the clinical examination.

Patients in different age groups normally develop back pain for different reasons. Table 5.7 indicates the conditions that should be given primary consideration for each age group. Back pain during childhood, puberty, and adolescence is fairly common. Most patients do not seek a physician or physical therapist, nor do they need to do so. The challenge lies in figuring out which patients need regular checkups and/or treatment.

Clinical History

Distinguishing between disk-related (discogenic) and muscular pain is difficult. The practitioner should consider why the patient has chronic pain. Was the underlying pathology undiagnosed during the acute phase? Following a natural course, would the patient be unlikely to recover within 2 weeks? Has treatment been adequate? Did the athlete return to competition too soon after the worst acute pain wore off? Are the athlete's complaints related to their patient's activity level (or lack of activity)? Are other factors contributing to the development of chronic pain?

Athletes are like other patients with back pain—they often feel helpless and afraid that they have a serious diagnosis or that their pain may prevent planned training and

Children

- Congenital (structural) abnormalities, such as hemivertebra or lack of segmentation of the vertbra, accompanied by potentially progressive, unbalanced growth
- By the age of 8 years, the prevalence of spondylolysis is comparable to the prevalence in adults
- In case of strong back pain that does not subside, a tumor/diskitis or juvenile prolapse should be ruled out (primary tumors also occur in patients in other age groups)

Puberty

- Structural abnormalities that manifest during a growth spurt, such as idiopathic scoliosis, Scheuermann's disease, and spondylolysis
- Extreme loading during the growth spurt (e.g., in gymnastics or weightlifting)

Adolescence

- Fractures in high risk sports
- Soft-tissue injuries
- Anorexia or hormone imbalance as the cause of a stress fracture

Adults

- Soft-tissue injuries
- Degeneration of intervertebral disk and facet joints contributing to lumbago or sciatica
- Fractures in high-risk sports
- Anorexia or hormone imbalance as the cause of a stress fracture
- Ankylosing spondylitis or other rheumatic disorder

Elderly

- Degeneration contributing to lumbago, sciatica, or spinal stenosis
- If the patient has nonspecific back pain that begins at a late adult age, a tumor/metastasis should be ruled out, especially if the patient is older than 60 years
- Osteoporosis causing a compression fracture

Table 5.7 Diagnoses of the back for various age groups.

competitive activity, or worse, even end their sporting career. Therefore, the way in which the practitioner handles the patient during the initial consultation is of major importance. The practitioner must instill confidence in the patient and develop a mutual understanding of the condition to create a basis for providing individual treatment advice.

Acute Pain

The origin of the athlete's pain, as well as their main symptoms and functional limitations, must be described in the history. The physician must identify the patient's primary symptom. Is the pain localized in the back or in the lower extremities? Patients with an acute disk herniation and pain in the lower extremities do not always have back pain. Conversely, a patient with pain referring from the deep muscles in the hip may have pain in both the back and in the lower extremities. Is the pain alleviated at rest or does it get worse when the patient coughs or sneezes? If hyperextension increases the pain but flexion does not, the cause may be spondylolysis or spondylolisthesis.

Distinct back pain accompanied by fever may indicate purulent diskitis. In that case, the sedimentation rate, C-reactive protein, and the white blood cell count will be elevated. MRI is positive early in the course of diskitis.

If the patient has intense pain and is bedridden, anxiety and fear often contribute to the dysfunction. Therefore, the practitioner should have the patient explain what she thinks is causing her pain. Rapid exclusion of red flags (table 5.6) is good therapy. If the patient has had similar complaints in the past, the physician must find out what type of treatment she was given and whether it was effective. The patient's expectations about treatment are vital to the outcome of the treatment.

Knowledge of the individual sport may make it easier to understand the injury mechanism. In soccer, the injury mechanism may be extension (throwing), hyperflexion (deflection), compression (falls or collisions), or torsion (dribbling or kicking). In golf, repeated twisting may cause a stress fracture in one or more ribs and trigger pain in the mid- or upper section of the back. Dancers compensate for increased external rotation of the hips by increasing lumbar lordosis. In addition, lifting above the head and large numbers of jumps make them susceptible to injuries. Common injury mechanisms are listed in table 5.8.

Injury mechanism	Sport
Repeated loading	Roller skis, cross-country skiing, rowing, paddling
Repeated loading in contact sports	Soccer, handball, ice hockey, wrestling, judo, karate
Lifting partners	Ballet, dance
Loading during growth period	Weightlifting, gymnastics
Sudden strong muscle contraction	Throwing sports
Hyperextension or torsion	Throwing sports, gymnastics

Table 5.8 Frequently occurring injury mechanisms related to back pain.

Chronic Pain

If the patient has chronic pain, the practitioner must carefully review the entire clinical history. Information is often available from diagnostic imaging or from a specialist when the complaints are chronic. Psychosocial yellow flags should be clarified if the patient does not respond to treatment (table 5.9, p. 123). The patient should be allowed to tell his story in his own words. A tentative diagnosis should be made independent of previous examinations. Allowing enough time for the examination provides a good basis for further treatment.

The clinical history must reveal the nature of the patient's primary complaints. To locate the pain, the patient may point to, or make marks on, a pain drawing of the entire body. Widespread pain suggests somatization. Radiating pain that worsens when the patient sneezes and that follows a dermatomal pattern suggests nerve root involvement. Pain and dysfunction that increase only in connection with sport activity indicate a need to evaluate technique and physical capacity. Weakness or reduced strength in the lower extremities during sport activity suggests mild paresis caused by nerve root involvement. The gradual onset of pain and morning stiffness tends to indicate a rheumatic (inflammatory) disease. If no treatment has helped and the patient dramatizes the irritation verbally and with body language, this more often suggests abnormal illness behavior than a serious back disorder. The physician should determine whether the patient actually wants to return to his sport career.

Clinical Examination

Acute Pain

The purpose of the clinical examination is to determine whether the patient's symptoms are consistent with the clinical signs. Is there an indication for hospitalization or for a quick evaluation by a specialist? Is the patient apprehensive with major dysfunction, even though the clinical findings are otherwise normal? The physician should rule out any red flags (table 5.6). If possible, he should make a tentative diagnosis as to whether the pain originates from the nerve root, the spinal segment, the superficial musculature, the pelvis, the hips, or is referred from other organs. Diagnostic imaging is usually not indicated at the time of the initial evaluation of acute, first episode low back pain. The following points should be evaluated during the initial examination of a patient with acute back pain:

- If the patient has bladder and bowel disturbance, he should be examined for saddle anesthesia and for sphincter function by digital rectal exploration. To confirm good sphincter control, the patient should be asked to squeeze down on the examiner's finger.
- If there is radiating pain or reported muscle weakness in the extremities, the patient should be asked to walk on his toes (S1) and heels (L5) and perform a deep knee bend (L4). The distal sensation of the calves and feet should also be examined. If certain testing is not possible because the patient is bedridden, neuromuscular function can be evaluated with the patient in a supine position.
- If there is radiating pain or reported muscle weakness in the extremities, nerve tension tests should be performed (figure 5.13, a and b). Nerve tension can be tested with the patient in a supine position. For the Lasegue (straight leg raise) test, the patient's lower extremity is lifted with the knee extended. The test is positive if the patient's radiating pain is reproduced distal to the knee at an elevation of less than 45°. The test can be strengthened by passively dorsiflexing the foot. Short hamstring musculature may contribute to a falsely positive test. In case of doubt, the knee may be slightly flexed and the foot flexed dorsally. The Lasegue test is considered "crossed positive" when elevation of the contralateral lower extremity reproduces radiating pain down the symptomatic limb. The test is falsely positive if the radiating pain is not reproduced when the examiner performs a diversionary maneuver (such as testing plantar flexion) while administering the test.
- To develop a differential diagnosis, range of motion in the hip joint and soft tissue structures in the hips and pelvis are examined.

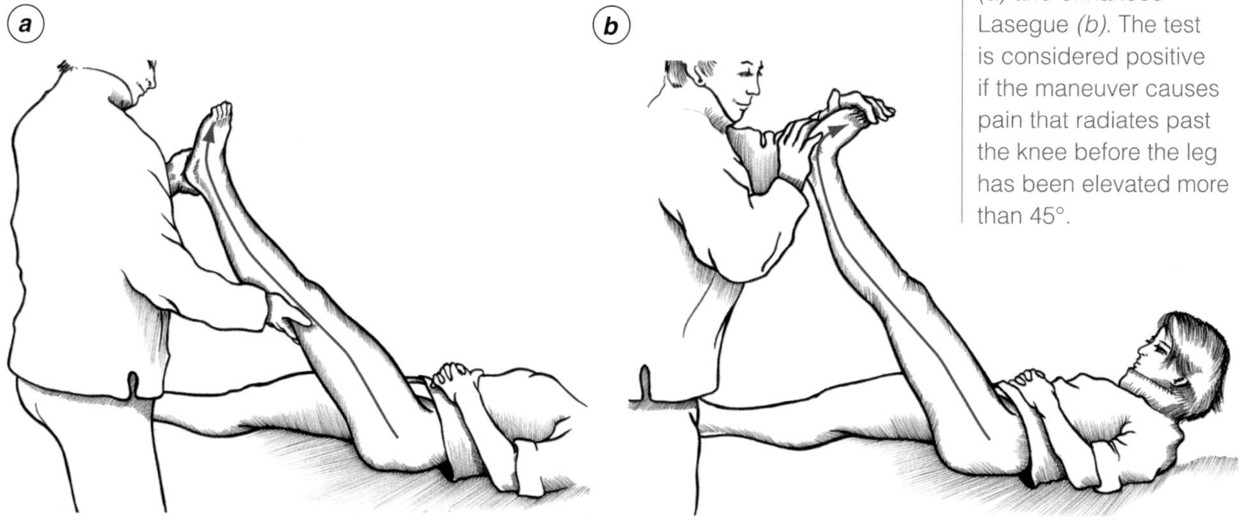

Figure 5.13 Nerve stretch tests: Lasegue *(a)* and enhanced Lasegue *(b)*. The test is considered positive if the maneuver causes pain that radiates past the knee before the leg has been elevated more than 45°.

- Malalignment suggests leg length discrepancy, a divergent posture that affects the intervertebral disks, or idiopathic scoliosis. Reduced active range of motion when bending forward and to the side may be due to pain, shortened musculature, or rheumatic disease. Pain triggered by extending a single leg suggests spondylolysis or spondylolisthesis (figure 5.14), because the motion results in impingement of the posterior elements of the spinal column.

Chronic Pain

Although the main goal of examining patients with acute back pain is to uncover red flags that would by necessity lead to an expanded evaluation, patients with chronic back pain must be thoroughly examined in an effort to make a patho-anatomical diagnosis that explains the clinical history. The examination should be performed with the patient disrobed to their underwear.

- How does the patient walk? Does he roll his hips (hip arthritis)? Does he limp (which could indicate trouble with the back or sciatica)?
- Does the patient walk differently when she is asked to walk than she does when she walks spontaneously? Are there signs of a functional gait pattern?
- Is there paresis when he walks on his heels or toes or when performing a deep knee bend?
- Is there muscle atrophy?

Inspection of the patient from behind
- Determine whether the patient has scoliosis and/or pelvic obliquity. Is the scoliosis structural (figure 5.15)? The best way to observe scoliosis is to have the patient bend forward, because the torsional component in scoliosis makes the costal arch prominent on the convex side. Scoliosis that is caused by leg length discrepancy disappears when the patient uses an orthosis, such as a heel lift or a shoe build-up.
- Can the patient touch the floor with straight legs? If not, what limits movement: tight hamstring muscles or back pain? If the patient needs to push off with his hands when he stands up again, this indicates muscular dysfunction.
- Is lateral flexion symmetrical? Unilaterally reduced lateral flexion may indicate that the facet joint is affected. Pain that is provoked by combined rotation of the upper body and pelvis indicates that the pain does not derive from the back.
- Single leg hyperextension that results in pain (figure 5.14) suggests spondylolysis or spondylolisthesis.

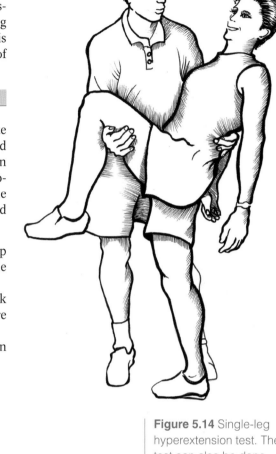

Figure 5.14 Single-leg hyperextension test. The test can also be done with the examiner standing behind the patient and providing support to the shoulders. The goal is to provoke hyperextension of the lumbar portion of the spinal column.

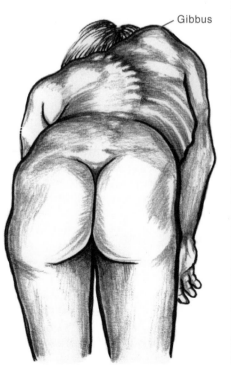

Gibbus

Figure 5.15 Structural scoliosis. The scoliosis is most easily seen when the patient bends forward, because the torsional component in the scoliosis causes the costal arch to become prominent on the convex side. This is also referred to as a gibbus deformity.

Supine position
- In the supine position, the patient should be tested for passive flexion of the hips with flexed knees. Pain during the Patrick test (flexion, abduction, and hip external rotation) could be the result of greater trochanteric bursitis or sacroiliac joint dysfunction.
- The Lasegue test is positive when pain radiates distal to the knee at hip flexion angles of less than 45°. For comparison, the practitioner should examine the contralateral side to rule out a crossed Lasegue sign. The diagnosis may be further tested by repeating aspects of the exam while distracting the patient, thereby guarding against contrived patient reactions.
- The strength of the anterior tibialis, toe extensors, peroneus longus, peroneus brevis, toe flexors, and the triceps surae of the calf should be examined with the knees flexed. Knee extension and hip flexion strength should be tested as well. Is the display of strength jerky (i.e., characterized by non-physiologic "give way" weakness)?
- The patellar, Achilles, and plantar muscle stretch reflexes are tested at 90° of knee flexion.
- If the patient has pain in the hip or gluteal region, the practitioner should assess the flexibility of the piriformis and the hip external rotator muscles through combined hip flexion, internal rotation, and adduction.
- If the quadratus lumborum seems to be affected, the practitioner should palpate the muscle at the same time that the patient is abducting and pulling his hip toward his body.
- The physician should perform an examination of skin sensation in the L4, L5, and S1 dermatomes and, if indicated, rule out "saddle anesthesia."

Prone position
- The patient's hip rotation should be examined in the prone position, and the differences between the sides should be noted.
- The Lasegue test (femoral stretch test) should be "reversed" (e.g., combined hip extension with increasing flexion in the knee causes nerve root pain radiating down the anterior thigh with L4 root affection involvement).
- The practitioner should palpate for pain in the gluteal musculature, over the ischial tuberosity, the greater trochanter, and the external rotators of the hip joint.
- The practitioner should palpate for pain in the paravertebral musculature, and in the midline above and between the spinous processes. Is the pain localized or widespread? Is pain provoked by light touching or by strong, distinct pressure?

Waddell signs (nonorganic tests)
- The five tests described by Waddell include the Lasegue test with distraction, combined rotation of the upper body and pelvis, nonphysiological signs (loss of sensitivity in a stocking distribution and jerky paresis), tenderness caused by palpation of both the skin and of the deeper structures, and exaggerated pain behavior. If at least three of the five tests are positive, the patient may have abnormal illness behavior.

Supplemental Examinations

Ordering diagnostic imaging examinations during the first consultation is usually unnecessary. Skeletal X rays are indicated if a fracture or tumor is suspected or if the patient is elderly and has back pain without radicular characteristics. If the patient has a neurological disorder, a CT is the initial examination of choice. A CT is also indicated if spondylolysis is suspected. This must be specified on the order form so that the image sections can be taken at the proper levels. Scintigraphy is used if the case history and clinical findings indicate spondylolysis but the CT is negative. The primary health care provider normally should not order an MRI during the first consultation for back pain, but it may be indicated preoperatively if the patient is hospitalized. An immediate MRI is also indicated to exclude hematoma that requires quick evacuation if neurological deficit increases postoperatively. Skeletal X rays, scintigraphy, MRI, and biopsy are indicated for differential diagnostic evaluation of malignancy and infection. MRI is the first choice for evaluating infection.

When ordering supplemental examinations, the order form should be carefully completed. The patient's history and main clinical findings can be briefly summarized. If images have been obtained recently, cost considerations and the risk of additional radiation exposure should temper the impulse to request additional imaging studies.

Overview X ray of the lumbosacral spine. A routine X ray provides information about degenerative changes, spondylolisthesis, previous posterior element fractures, or compression fractures. If the primary physician finds structural scoliosis during a clinical examination, standing images of the entire spine can be ordered—or the patient may be referred to the orthopedic department without first obtaining the imaging. If Scheuermann's disease is suspected, lateral images of the thoracolumbar spine should be obtained.

Lumbar CT. If the patient has radicular pain, a lumbar CT is the imaging modality of choice and can be requested by the patient's primary physician. A CT is also useful for examining the facet joints and for ruling out spondylolysis.

MRI. An MRI is best suited for suspected malignancy and diskitis and usually replaces myelography for evaluating spinal stenosis or recess stenosis. The examination is sensitive, revealing early degeneration of the intervertebral disks ("black disks" on water weighted images) or other disk pathology such as protrusions. However, these findings are somewhat nonspecific and should not influence treatment unless well-correlated with the findings on physical examination. Contrast enhanced MRI is better than CT for distinguishing between scar tissue and a new disk herniation.

Skeletal scintigraphy. Scintigraphy is used if a stress fracture or malignancy is suspected. Degeneration, tendinitis, and aseptic necrosis of bone may also generate a positive scan.

Diskography. This procedure is used preoperatively for matters regarding disk-related pain. The patient's description of pain on injection is more important diagnostically than is the morphology of the intervertebral disk (e.g., rupture of the annulus fibrosis). Contrast leakage will almost always occur after prolapse extirpation. To make the diagnosis of discogenic lumbago, the patient's pain must be reproduced on injection of the affected disk while an adjacent disk should be pain free. The actual prognostic value of diskography is questionable, and thus the procedure should be ordered exclusively by spine specialists as part of the diagnostic evaluation of selected patients.

Facet joint anesthesia. The examination must be done using fluoroscopy and must produce at least 50% pain reduction to be positive. In addition, there should be a negative saline injection to permit the diagnosis of facet joint syndrome.

Common Painful Conditions

Acute Lumbago—Acute Low Back Pain

Acute lumbago is most common in the 20- to 55-year age group. The cause may be vertebrogenic, discogenic, or muscular. Often several structures are involved.

Because it may be difficult to make an exact diagnosis, the syndrome is described by the collective term "acute lumbago."

- Symptoms and signs: Pain in the lumbar region may or may not radiate to the hip, groin, or posterior side of the thigh. The patient often has difficulty moving in a normal manner and may have sciatic scoliosis. Often, all movements are painful and limited. The Lasegue test may be positive but is usually negative when the patient is simultaneously distracted.
- Diagnosis: The diagnosis is made clinically, based on the description above and by excluding other potential causes of acute back pain. An X ray is not necessary.
- Treatment by physician: The patient should be informed that the best treatment is to maintain a normal activity level. Restricting the patient's ability to bear weight (e.g., by prescribing crutches) is not recommended. Over-the-counter analgesics or NSAIDs for 3 to 7 days may decrease the duration of the painful period. Stronger (narcotic) analgesics are seldom needed. The athlete should not participate in competition before he can complete a normal training routine.
- Treatment by physical therapist: Although treatment by a physical therapist is unnecessary during the acute phase, the patient may benefit just as much from an initial assessment by a physical therapist as from an examination performed by a physician. There is no purpose in starting abdominal and back muscle exercises during the first painful phase, but alternative training to maintain general endurance and strength in the extremities may be started soon after the injury. It is important to be positive when giving advice and not to place unnecessary restrictions on specific movements. The evidence for manipulation is under debate. It may be indicated if the patient has great expectations for this type of treatment or needs supplemental pain therapy.
- Self-treatment: The patient should be advised to keep their activity level as normal as possible, to remain ambulatory, and to resume training within a few days.
- Prognosis: The prognosis is generally favorable. Most patients are asymptomatic within a week, but nearly half experience a recurrence within the year. Therefore, a "wait and see" attitude toward treatment should be taken. Patients who don't have red flags should be informed that back pain is a common occurrence and not harmful per se but may recur in the future. Recurrent episodes of low back pain should not be considered to result from a new injury each time. The patient should be advised that gradually increasing his level of activity and restricting competitive activity until he is able to train normally may contribute to reducing the frequency of recurrence.

Chronic Lumbago—Chronic Low Back Pain

Low back pain may be caused by multiple potential pain generators, including muscular insufficiency, intervertebral disk degeneration, central disk herniations, or facet joint arthrosis. The diagnosis of segmental dysfunction is also used. There is no specific clinical or diagnostic imaging examination that serves as the basis for this diagnosis. The criteria for discogenic pain or facet joint syndrome are specified in the section on supplemental examinations. Muscular insufficiency or imbalance may also occur in very well-trained athletes. In a study that included elite rowers, increased fatigability in the multifidus musculature (verified by EMG) was associated with chronic lumbago. Degeneration of the intervertebral disks is not necessarily associated with pain, but occurs frequently in young athletes (figure 5.16) in a few sports.

The practitioner should evaluate psychosocial yellow flags if the patient has not responded to treatment (table 5.9). Psychosocial factors, in particular thoughts about the consequences of back pain (fear avoidance beliefs), and "doctor shopping" are more important risk factors than biomedical symptoms or signs.

- Symptoms and signs: Pain that worsens during monotonous activities, for which the patient often changes position while standing or sitting, is a symptom of chronic lumbago. Unilateral pain with morning stiffness that is relieved by NSAIDs points toward arthrosis, whereas more diffuse pain that worsens when working in a stooping position suggests muscular pain. Typical symptoms and signs include reduced range of motion during flexion and lateral bending, intermittent malalignment, and short hamstring and psoas muscles. Waddell signs should be assessed as part of the examination.
- Diagnosis: The diagnosis is clinical, according to the symptoms and signs described above. The criteria for discogenic pain or facet joint syndrome are listed in the section on supplemental examinations. They should be used with caution because of indefinite treatment and prognostic consequences. Diagnostic imaging criteria are described above, in the section on supplemental examinations.
- Treatment by physician: NSAIDs or acetominophen is the first choice. Stronger analgesics are indicated for pain-related sleep dysfunction. Surgery is rarely indicated.
- Treatment by physical therapist: Group exercise is the first choice. The quota principle may apply if it is hard to get started. In some studies, manual therapy has been documented to be effective.
- Prognosis: Patients who learn to live with the pain often function at a high level despite brief bad spells. The athlete may need to change his short- or long-term goals. Psychological and social factors assume greater prognostic significance than

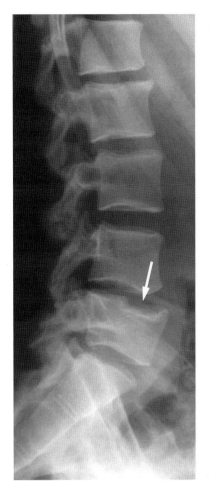

Figure 5.16 Degenerative changes in the lumbar column of a former gymnast. Reduced disk height and mild exostoses at L1-L2. Injury to the upper endplate and deformation of L5.

Previous back pain
Long time away from sports or work
Radicular pain
Reduced muscle strength and endurance in the abdominal and back muscles in relation to the requirements of the individual sports
Reduced range of motion in relation to the requirements of the individual sport
Atypical illness behavior and somatization
Psychological stress and depression, difficulty sleeping, social isolation
Dissatisfaction
Personal problems: alcohol, cohabitation, finances
Insurance claims
Belief that back pain is harmful and may cause disability
Fear avoidance beliefs about physical activity
Anticipates passive treatment modalities like drugs, electrotherapy, and massage

Table 5.9 Yellow flags or risk factors for chronic back pain.

diagnostic imaging and clinical factors. Because the prognosis of chronic low back pain is generally worse than for acute back problems, a comprehensive evaluation is a prerequisite for any surgery.

Spondylolysis and Spondylolisthesis— Stress Fracture of the Pars Interarticularis (possibly with slippage)

In both of these conditions, a defect typically exists in the interartical portion of the vertebral arch. Although this defect may be caused in various ways, among athletes spondylolysis is usually the result of a stress fracture. Its prevalence is about 7% in the adult population of the Western world. A large epidemiological study of elite Spanish athletes revealed an 8% prevalence. The highest prevalence was in throwing sports (27%). In dance sports and acrobatic sports the prevalence ranged from 10% to 30% and in rowing it was 17%. Sport-related spondylolysis is often associated with truncal hyperextension, rotation, and torsion against resistance, such as in throwing sports. The occurrence is due to the specific risk factors inherent to the sport.

It has previously been reported that about 80% of athletes have spondylolisthesis between two vertebrae (usually L5 and S1). However, only 30% of the athletes in the Spanish study had spondylolisthesis. Slippage is usually low grade. Spondylolysis and spondylolisthesis can be graded from I to V (figure 5.17), where grade I is defined as slippage of up to 25% of the sagittal diameter and grade V is defined as one vertebra lying in front of the vertebra beneath it. There is no statistical relationship between radiographic spondylolysis and symptoms in adults. It is estimated that about 10% of the people who have spondylolysis have symptoms. Slippage may increase during the childhood years and in adolescence, but it almost never increases during adulthood (after puberty).

- Symptoms and signs: Pain in the lumbar region that radiates to the gluteal musculature and to the thighs is a symptom of spondylolysis and spondylolisthesis. Patients are often asymptomatic in the morning but get worse with activity throughout the day. Sciatica due to degeneration of the associated intervertebral disk(s), facet joint(s), or hypertrophic tissue in the pseudoarthrosis fissure may occur. The patient may experience distinct pain when one leg is extended while she is standing or lying prone (figure 5.14). If there is a great deal of slippage, it is possible to palpate a depression above the spinous process of the slipped vertebra.
- Diagnosis: The diagnosis is made by clinical examination, a history of appropriate symptoms and by radiographic confirmation of spondylolysis and/or spondylolisthesis. X rays of the lumbosacral column should include frontal and lateral views, which will usually demonstrate spondylolisthesis and the degree of slippage. Flexion and extension views can be used to examine instability. A CT is indicated if the clinical history is positive but the X ray is negative. In case of remission, it should be noted that spondylolysis is suspected so that the sections are obtained through the pars interarticularis. A CT is the best method of demonstrating defects in the vertebral arch. Skeletal scintigraphy with SPECT views is an extremely sensitive means of detecting a recent stress fracture (spondylolysis), but the diagnosis should be confirmed by CT.
- Treatment by physician: It has not been documented whether the use of a brace improves the prognosis and contributes to healing a recent stress fracture of the pars interarticularis. Acetominophen or NSAIDs are the first-line agents if drug therapy is necessary. Surgery is indicated for grade III-V spondylolisthesis, if slippage increases, or if conservative treatment does not help control the patient's pain.
- Treatment by physical therapist: The patient should be provided with instructions to improve activation of the deep trunk musculature. Progress is not made

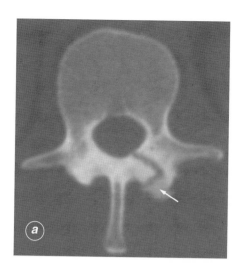

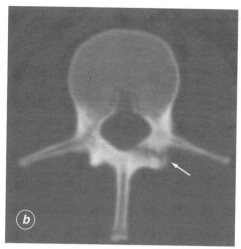

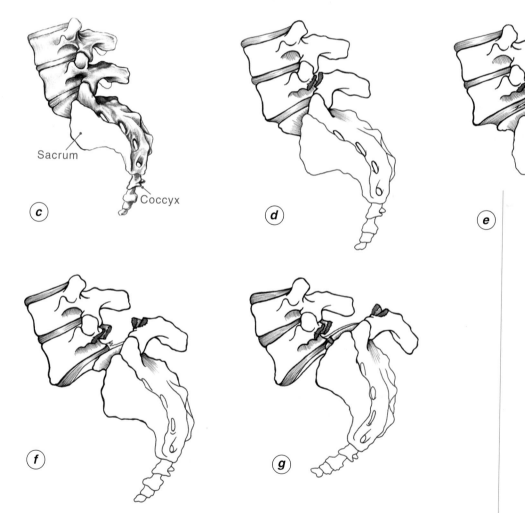

Figure 5.17
Spondylolysis/
spondylolisthesis. CT
images demonstrate
spondylolysis in levels
L1 *(a)* and L2 *(b)* in an
internationally competi-
tive javelin thrower. The
patient achieved normal
throwing function without
surgery. The drawings
show the grading of
spondylolysis *(c)* and
spondylolisthesis, grade
I *(d)*, grade II *(e)*, grade
III *(f)*, and grade IV *(g)*.

NECK AND BACK

by increasing the number of repetitions but by integrating increasingly complex activities into the activity pattern. The effectiveness of this treatment strategy has been documented in a recently published randomized study.
- Self-treatment: The patient should be advised to maintain their normal activity level if possible.

Other Painful Conditions

Acute Sciatica

Disk herniation (figure 5.18) is the most common cause of sciatica. Recent research suggests that immunological factors contribute to the pain. An autoimmune reaction occurs with the formation of antigen-antibody complexes when the nucleus pulposus ruptures out into the spinal canal. Therefore, inflammation from an immunological source may cause sciatica. Neurological deficit is usually related to compression of the nerve root. No clear relationship exists between a positive Lasegue test and pressure around the nerve root. A herniated disk may be asymptomatic or cause back pain with or without radicular symptoms but is not, in itself, an indication for surgery.

- Symptoms and signs: The radiating pain of lumbar radiculopathy is normally worse than the associated low back pain. Radiating pain distal to the knee and pain that worsens when the patient coughs suggest radicular pain. Numbness and paresthesias can also be present. On examination, the athlete may walk with a limp and with a stooped upper body. This is often referred to as "sciatic scoliosis." If the patient has radiating pain and reports muscle weakness in the extremities, muscle function should be tested by having him walk on his toes (S1) and heels (L5) in addition to performing a deep knee bend (L4). The practitioner should also examine the patient for sensory disturbances distally in the calves and in the feet. If this is not possible because the patient is bedridden, motor function may be tested with the patient in a supine position. If the patient's bladder and bowel function are affected, he must be examined for saddle anesthesia. In addition, anal sphincter function must be assessed by digital rectal examination. The Lasegue test is positive when hip flexion in excess of 45° (with the knee extended) causes the patient to experience pain distal to the knee. The test may be falsely positive, so the patient should also be examined while being distracted.
- Diagnosis: The clinical diagnosis is highly reliable if the patient has dermatomal sensory deficit, corresponding myotomal specific weakness, and diminished

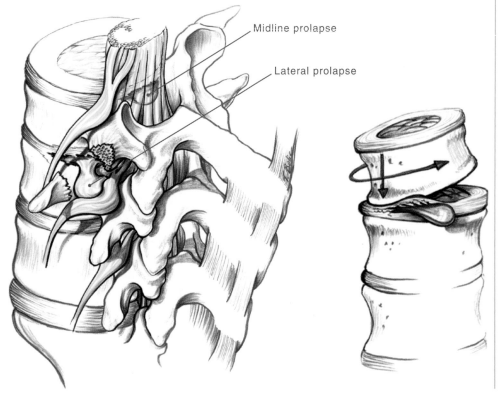

Midline prolapse

Lateral prolapse

Figure 5.18 A midline disk prolapse and a lateral disk prolapse with herniation.

muscle stretch reflexes in a similar nerve root pattern (figure 5.5). The physician must exclude conditions that require immediate treatment (e.g., fractures, bladder paralysis, or progressive paresis in the lower extremities), for which the patient should be referred to a specialist. It may be sufficient to make a referral based on symptoms and findings of a clinical examination. Imaging is unnecessary if primary treatment is effective. An MRI should be obtained if a CT indicates that the root symptoms are not caused by a disk prolapse.

- Treatment by physician: Oral corticosteroids, NSAIDs, or acetominophen are the first-line treatments. Corticosteroids have the best anti-inflammatory effect, and the patient can usually easily tolerate a 40 mg dose of prednisolone for three days. Stronger analgesics are indicated for pain-related sleeping problems. Nerve root pain is usually not a cause for alarm. Inform the patient that most patients recover well without surgery and that normal activity does not delay healing. Referral to a specialist is usually unnecessary unless the athlete remains symptomatic after 4 weeks have passed.
- Treatment by physical therapist: Manipulation is contraindicated. Lifting and repeated twisting should be avoided. The most important step the patient can take is to adjust to alternative training. The effect of lumbar traction is usually temporary and furthermore has not been proven to influence the outcome of lumbar radiculopathy. When the condition improves, exercises for the transverse muscles may be added to the treatment program.
- Self-treatment: The patient should be advised to maintain daily activities rather than staying in bed and to find alternative exercises that do not increase the pain.
- Prognosis: Individual variation is great. Intermittent symptom reduction over the first 14 days should be expected, but the course may be long term, and the athlete typically needs to revise their current goals and prepare for the next season.

Chronic Sciatica

Chronic sciatica is usually due to a prolapse of the 4th or 5th lumbar intervertebral disk or lateral recess stenosis due to facet arthropathy. Intraspinal tumors are rare but may present with nerve root pain as the initial symptom. Peripheral irritation of the sciatic nerve (e.g., as it passes the piriformis muscle in the pelvis or as its peroneal branch passes the head of the fibula) may produce a convincing mimic radiculopathy (pseudosciatica).

- Symptoms and signs: The diagnosis of chronic sciatica is warranted if signs and symptoms of lumbar radiculopathy persist beyond 6 weeks. Lumbar CT is indicated if there has been no clinical improvement after 2-4 weeks despite treatment.
- Treatment by physician: Oral corticosteroids, NSAIDs, or acetominophen are the medications of choice. More potent analgesics may be indicated for pain-related sleep dysfunction. The patient should be informed that most patients recover without surgery and that normal activity does not delay healing. Return to play decisions will depend on the sport in which the athlete is involved, their personality, the degree of pain and paresis, and the treatment plan. Progressive or persistent muscle weakness in the lower extremities, coupled with a history of persistent radiating pain over 3 months, is an indication for surgical intervention. Minimally invasive disectomy, flavectomy, and partial or full laminectomy have all been shown to be effective in the appropriate situation. If the surgeon uses a microscope, it is called microsurgery. Numerous studies have found that more than 80% of patients no longer have radiating pain but that an almost equal number continue to have back pain after surgery. Consequently, the effectiveness of surgery for disk herniation and for non-radicular back pain is uncertain. Percutaneous nucleotomy has no documented effect on disk herniation.
- Treatment by physical therapist: The activity level for those with progressive symptoms should be reduced or changed. Ballet dancers and others (such as ice dancers) who lift a partner may be able to maintain their activity level by wearing

a brace or a weightlifter's belt. There is no consensus opinion regarding the need for rehabilitation after disk surgery. A new study indicates that a normal level of activity should be resumed as soon as the surgical wound is healed.

• Self-treatment: The patient should be advised to find alternative training that does not worsen their radicular pain. Pain is a signal for the athlete to change his activity and should not (by itself) be considered indicative of a relapse. There is no reason for restrictions, with the exception of heavy lifting.

• Prognosis: If sciatica without neurological deficit is likely, the athlete should plan to resume normal sport activity in 6 to 12 weeks. If neurological deficit is present, the course is usually longer, in the range of 12 to 24 weeks. Therefore, the caregiver or care giving team should work with the athlete to create a long-term plan to get him back to his former level of sporting activity. If the patient does not follow the anticipated course, further diagnostic testing may be indicated to better prognosticate the final outcome, so that the athlete can adjust his goals accordingly.

Spinal Stenosis (Spinal Claudication)

Symptoms of spinal stenosis most commonly occur in the elderly (average age at onset is 65 years) because the degeneration of intervertebral disks and facet joints combine to reduce the size of the central spinal canal (figure 5.19). Spondylolysis, previous fractures, and prior back surgery may also contribute to the development of spinal stenosis.

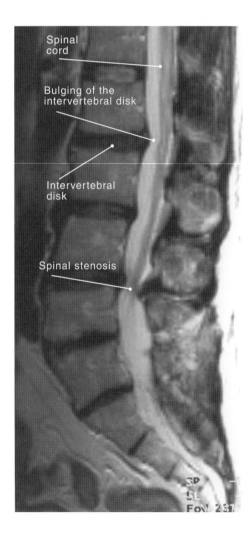
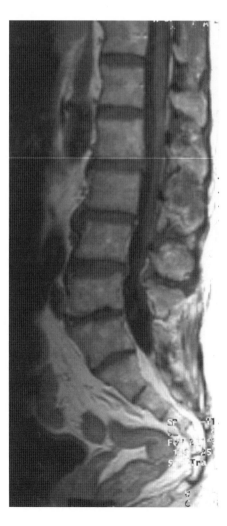

Figure 5.19 Spinal stenosis in levels L4-L5. Moderate degenerative changes with protrusions.

- Symptoms and signs: Symptoms and signs include back pain and morning stiffness, radiating pain, paresthesias, and muscle weakness related to activity. Limited walking tolerance is a key symptom. Bending forward at the waist usually relieves the pain. The Lasegue test is typically negative, while motor disturbance and absence of the patellar muscle stretch reflex are common.
- Diagnosis: The diagnosis is made in patients with characteristic symptoms and a reduced sagittal diameter of the spinal canal. The practitioner must rule out a vascular etiology for the patient's claudicatory symptoms, which may include diminished gait distance, reduced distal pulse, and diffuse sensory disturbance.
- Treatment by physician: NSAIDs or acetaminophen is the treatment of choice. Stronger analgesics are indicated for pain-related sleep dysfunction. Progressive walking intolerance is an indication for surgical referral.
- Treatment by physical therapist: The physical therapist may recommend active individual or group exercises to improve back function.
- Self-treatment: The patient should be advised to maintain daily activities rather than stay in bed.
- Prognosis: Lower extremity pain tends to respond favorably to surgery, but the effect on back pain is less certain.

Scoliosis—Back Curvature

Curvature of the spine in the coronal plane is called scoliosis. Structural scoliosis differs from nonstructural scoliosis in that the latter includes functional or postural scoliosis (which disappears when the patient bends forward) in addition to compensatory scoliosis (which may result from a leg length discrepancy). The five categories of structural scoliosis are idiopathic, neuromuscular, congenital, iatrogenic, and rare syndromes. Collectively, the prevalence of scoliosis in the general population is about 3%. Idiopathic scoliosis occurs about seven times more frequently in girls than in boys. Scoliosis tends to progress as long as the individual is growing. The condition is hereditary, and it is presumed that the inheritance is multifactorial or dominant with reduced penetrance.

- Symptoms and signs: Patients with structural scoliosis generally do not have more back pain than their non-scoliotic peers. Activity of the musculature will be different on the concave and convex side of a scoliosis, and this may explain why patients with scoliosis tend to report muscle fatigue more often than they report pain. Grade school students should undergo an annual screening for scoliosis. The screening involves having the students bend forward at the waist. If a student has structural scoliosis, pronounced asymmetry resembling the keel of a boat is evident, corresponding to the costal arch on the convex side (figure 5.15).
- Diagnosis: The patient should be referred to an orthopedic department for further evaluation. The diagnosis is confirmed and classified by X rays.
- Treatment: The disease may follow its natural course if left untreated. Alternatively, a stiff brace or surgery may be prescribed. The patient must be checked regularly until she is fully grown to rule out interval progression of the spinal curve.
- Self-treatment: The patient should participate in physical activity with her peers. Carrying heavy bags like a backpack is not recommended; therefore, the patient should have two sets of schoolbooks (one for school and one for home).

Scheuermann's Disease

Scheuermann's disease usually occurs during the pubertal growth spurt and is more common in boys than in girls. The prevalence of Scheuermann's disease in adolescents is about 5 %. Repetitive trauma during the growth period may be a significant contributing factor. The most probable cause of the disorder is aseptic bone necrosis, with a reduced blood supply to the growth zone. Necrosis is most pronounced anteriorly and causes the vertebral body to become wedge-shaped (figure 5.20). The changes are localized to the thoracic column in 70% of the patients.

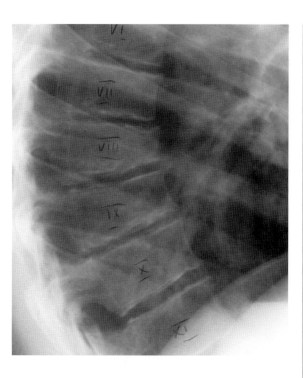

- Symptoms and signs: Increased kyphosis in the thoracic or thoracolumbar column is a common finding. The normal curvature of the thoracic spine in the sagittal plane (kyphosis) is 15° to 30°. Curvatures greater than this are often seen in association with congenital changes, fractures, growth disturbance (e.g., Scheuermann's disease), and systemic diseases (e.g., ankylosing spondylitis). Sometimes it is difficult to distinguish between kyphosis and a normal relaxed posture. Most patients with moderate radiographic changes in the thoracic spine are pain free. Patients with Scheuermann's disease in the thoracolumbar or the lumbar region usually have pain.
- Diagnosis: Scheuermann's disease is diagnosed by X rays demonstrating anterior vertebral body wedging in excess of 5° in three or more vertebrae. If the diagnosis is suspected during the growth period, the athlete should be referred for appropriate pediatric orthopedic care.
- Treatment: Physical therapy to strengthen the back and abdominal muscles is recommended. A brace can be used if the kyphosis is completely rigid. Surgery is rarely indicated.

Figure 5.20 Scheuermann's disease. Lateral X ray shows an athlete with increased thoracic kyphosis, due to wedging of the T7-T10 vertebral bodies of more than 5°.

Ankylosing Spondylitis

Ankylosing spondylitis (AS) occurs more often than Scheuermann's disease and tends to have an earlier onset in men compared to women. In Norway, the prevalence of AS is about 1 or 2 per thousand adults, with 300 to 400 new cases diagnosed annually. The condition is hereditary, and it is assumed that transmission is multifactorial.

- Symptoms and signs: Lumbar pain and stiffness gradually progress over time. The pain is often localized to the entire spine and to the sacroiliac joints. Night pain and morning stiffness predominate. Symptoms often improve throughout the day and with physical activity.
- Diagnosis: The diagnosis is made if reduced range of motion in one or more sections of the back is present, in addition to tenderness to palpation over the spinous processes and the sacroiliac joints. Ankylosing spondylitis affects the ischial tuberosity, the iliac crest, and the tendon insertions in the heel. Recurring eye inflammation (iridocyclitis) may be the first sign of the disorder, which also affects the large joints (shoulders and hips). Chest excursion may be reduced early on, but major limitations are usually present only during the late stages. Thoracic kyphosis and a lack of lumbar lordosis (figure 5.21) produce a characteristic posture and walk. Radiographic examination of the pelvis and vertebral column is diagnostic, but plain film imaging is rarely useful during the early stages. Because ankylosing

spondylitis is relatively rare, and since only 1% to 2% of people who are HLA-B27 positive AS, a positive HLA-B27 test has no real diagnostic value.

• Treatment: Patients who are suspected of having ankylosing spondylitis should be referred to a rheumatologist. Regular exercise and flexibility training is an important part of the treatment program. NSAIDs may be helpful during the most symptomatic periods. Surgical treatment may be indicated if the patient has advanced thoracic kyphosis that makes it impossible to maintain a normal visual angle.

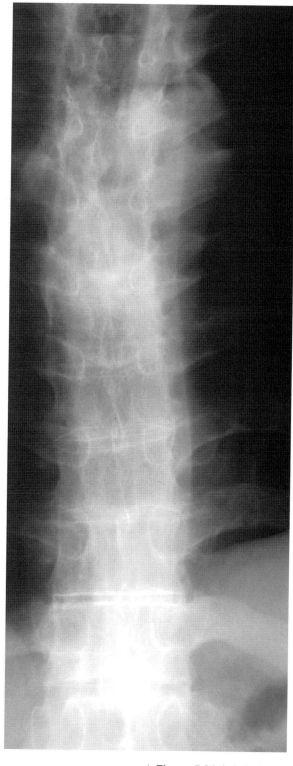

Figure 5.21 Ankylosing spondylitis. The frontal X ray view demonstrates the characteristic ossification of the longitudinal ligaments ("bamboo spine").

Rehabilitation of Neck and Back Injuries

Bjørn Fossan and Jens Ivar Brox

Goals and Principles

Table 5.10 lists the goals of rehabilitation.

Acute phase. The treatment and information given to the patient depends on the diagnosis. In most cases, NSAIDs and acetominophen provide sufficient pain relief. It is often difficult to become completely pain free through activity restrictions and drug therapy. It has not been documented that complete rest will shorten the acute phase. Therefore, the patient must be mobilized as quickly as possible. Short-term relief can be achieved by wearing a support belt. The exercise program should be deferred until after the acute phase.

	Goals	Measures
Acute phase	Create calm and confidence, improve pain management, limit inflammation, invalidate red flags	Information, drug therapy, and eventually PRICE (protection, rest, ice, compression, and elevation), if relevant
Rehabilitation phase	Create a rehabilitation plan Restore normal function Maintain general strength and endurance Prevent recurrence	Create an overview of the diagnosis, prognostic factors, and sports activity, and create a plan in consultation with the athlete and trainer Advice based on the anticipated natural course Individual, specific, and progressive exercise program In case of chronic pain, chart yellow flags and counteract passive pain mastery Individually adjusted alternative training program Counteract the risk factors based on the sport-specific, individual, and general evaluation
Training phase	Lead the athlete back to sport activity	Exercise or training to meet sport-specific requirements Provide athletes with the information necessary to make independent evaluations of their career prospects

Table 5.10 Goals and measures for rehabilitation.

Rehabilitation phase. The documented natural history of acute nonspecific neck and back pain suggests that the athlete should recover well in a short period of time. How long training and competition are interrupted will depend on the diagnosis and the requirements of the athlete's sport. Training to maintain general endurance and strength can often begin within a few days of injury. Function often improves significantly during the first week and makes treatment and rehabilitation unnecessary.

If the patient has recurring or persistent symptoms, a physician and/or a physical therapist must conduct a functional evaluation in consultation with the athlete or trainer to provide a basis for a rehabilitation plan. The functional evaluation should be performed by a physical therapist or a physician who is familiar with the demands of the sport to which the athlete will be returning. For example, because shoulder and hip flexibility is necessary in gymnastics, if the range of motion in these joints is reduced, the athlete may increase their lumbar lordosis to compensate and satisfy the performance requirements–thereby increasing the load on the lumbar spine. As this example demonstrates, treating the back in isolation is often an insufficient means of rehabilitating the patient so that she can return to sports. Simple methods, such as observation during various activities, testing muscle strength, and measuring the extent to which the joints are affected, provide a good basis for a goal-oriented rehabilitation process. If resources allow, video, ultrasound, and EMG can be used to evaluate movement patterns and muscle use.

Rehabilitation Methods

Because of the neuromuscular network in the back, the involvement of various structures in the same segment may well result in a similar physiological reaction (figure 5.5): pain of an identical nature within the same boundaries, increased muscular tension within a specified area, and reduced active (and available) range of motion at the affected level of the back/spine.

Interventions for restoring normal range of motion may be started if reduced range of motion continues beyond the acute phase. Reduced range of motion may contribute to a change in loading patterns throughout the back. Stretching is indicated for restricted range of motion thought to be due to muscular factors. If, however, joint-related causes are suspected, joint mobilization and subsequent muscle stretching may be prescribed (exercises 5.1, 5.2, and 5.11). In both cases, activity with full range of motion and numerous repetitions are recommended (exercises 5.3 and 5.12).

The patient should be instructed to use the thigh and buttocks muscles for heavy lifting. He should otherwise be informed that there is no reason to be overly worried about his back. Positive information and advice may help to instill a sense of confidence coincident with improved range of motion and muscular function.

The deep musculature in the lumbar region and the neck are important for segmental stability and control. The deep-seated muscles (multifidus muscles) work together with the deep abdominal muscles (the diaphragm) and pelvic floor muscles as a functional stabilizing unit. Recent studies indicate that patterns of back muscle activation and fatigability differ between asymptomatic controls and individuals with low back pain. Pain has a reflex effect on muscle activity by inhibiting the deep stabilizing musculature while activating muscles like the iliopsoas and the erector spinae. Therefore, weakness of the deep musculature and increased activation of the superficial musculature can reinforce a dysfunctional pattern of movement. Back pain contributes to an altered activity pattern by affecting both central and peripheral mechanisms. Increasing awareness, practice, and automatic activation of the deep musculature may begin early in the rehabilitation process. This type of training (exercises 5.4, 5.13, and

5.14) has been documented to have a positive effect on patients with spondylolisthesis and on the frequency of recurrence of subacute back pain. Gradual repetition and integration into regular sport activity is necessary to automate the activation pattern. The superficial musculature will also contribute to stiffening the upper body and neck in situations requiring extra stabilization (e.g., when attempting to lift a great load) (exercises 5.5, 5.15, and 5.17). Therefore, training must be specific to the demands of the individual sport (exercise 5.9).

Neuromuscular function training is an optimal form of stabilization training for athletes (exercises 5.6, 5.7, and 5.18). For the lumbar spine, this should take place in a closed kinetic chain on a mobile surface. As shown in exercises 5.8, 5.14, 5.17, and 5.18, sling exercise therapy is an ideal tool to exercise the neck and lumbar spine in a closed kinetic chain, while simultaneously challenging neuromuscular control. At first, the training routine should take place while the athlete is sharp and in good form. It should be repeated as often as possible and for a minimum of 10 minutes a day. As soon as the athlete masters this training, strength and endurance training for the superficial musculature in an open and closed kinetic chain may be integrated (exercises 5.8 and 5.16) into the routine.

For patients with chronic pain, standard medical diagnostic and functional testing should be supplemented with an evaluation of psychological factors influencing the athlete's condition. In doing so, the caregiver may be better able to determine what areas should be emphasized during the rehabilitation process. Even for otherwise robust athletes, pain or fear of pain may be more significant and limiting than, for example, changes in the diagnostic images.

When rehabilitation does not follow the anticipated course and there is no indication for surgery, the practitioner should modify the rehabilitation plan. If it is impossible to begin active treatment, a quota-based exercise program may be attempted. To initiate this program, the therapist first chooses six to ten functional exercises that the patient subsequently attempts to exhaustion or until pain limits further activity. The testing is then repeated in a day or two. The initial training load should be established at 50% of the average result of the two tests, and the series of exercises is completed three times per week. The volume is thereafter increased by one to five repetitions every other training day. The exercise regimen can be gradually adjusted according to normal physiological training principles. The key element of the quota principle is that volume of activity is regulated not by pain but by the athlete's test results. Rest follows training. In case of a relapse, the patient can return to the starting amount but may progress more rapidly if able.

For patients with chronic symptoms, aerobics or various other forms of group training are as effective as individual exercise programs and are more cost effective. Generally, chronic pain weakens cardiovascular function. Improving aerobic capacity may contribute to increasing the body's load tolerance.

Back to Sports

Most athletes will be able to return to their sport after an acute neck or back injury. The athlete needs to participate in normal training activity before participating in competition, but does not need to be completely pain free. Nevertheless, the athlete should only stretch as far as he can, while still performing the movement in a technically correct manner. In certain situations, it may be appropriate to advise an athlete to switch to a different sport or to reduce his activity level so as to limit the risk of reinjury. Young athletes are subject to injuries to the growth zones in the vertebrae, and these injuries may contribute to accelerated degeneration of the intervertebral disks. In addition to a diagnostic and a functional evaluation, young athletes with recurrent back pain should be thoroughly evaluated for correctable risk factors before returning to normal training.

Back Exercise Program

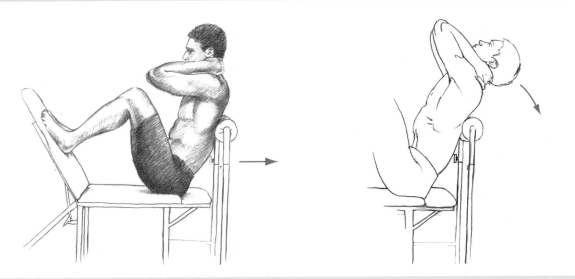

Exercise 5.1 Mobilization/stretching the thoracic spine in extension

- Lock the lumbar region of your back by maximum flexion of your hips.
- Arch your thoracic spine backward over the pole in an extreme position.
- Do range of motion training and stretching.

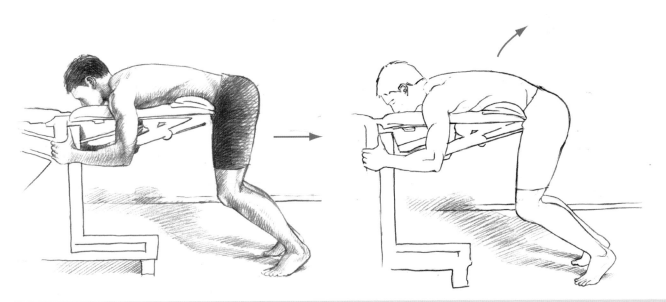

Exercise 5.2 Mobilization/stretching the lower lumbar region in ventral flexion

- Rest your upper body on the bench.
- Lower your pelvis and back toward the floor.
- Help regulate mobilization force by loading your legs.
- Do stretching and range of motion training.

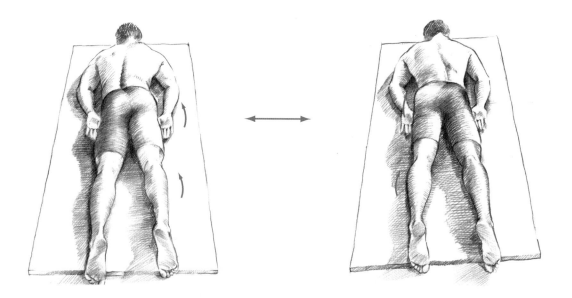

Exercise 5.3 Active mobilization of the lower lumbar region in lateral flexion

- Keep your legs and pelvis on the floor the entire time.
- Keep your legs slightly apart.
- Alternately pull up with one leg and push down with the other, with small swings.
- Do range of motion training.

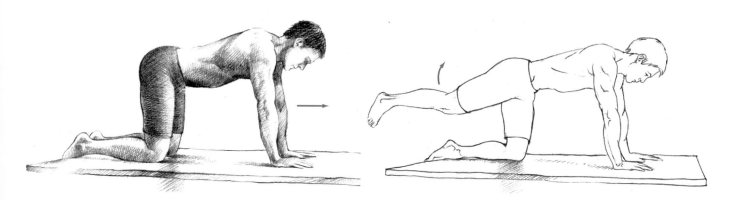

Exercise 5.4 Deep trunk muscle exercises

- Position yourself on your hands and knees and slightly hollow-backed.
- Pull in your abdomen without moving your lumbar region and without holding your breath.
- Alternately extend your right and left leg backward without moving your back.
- Release the tension in your abdomen between repetitions.
- Increase loading by placing your hands farther forward.

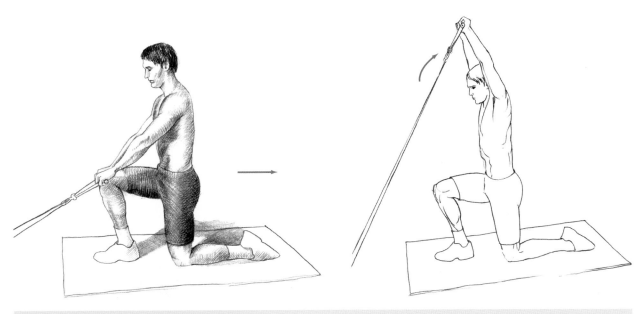

Exercise 5.5 Functional stability training

- Kneel on one or both knees.
- Pull in your abdomen and don't move the lumbar region of your back.
- Focus on stability and quality of movement while gradually increasing loading.

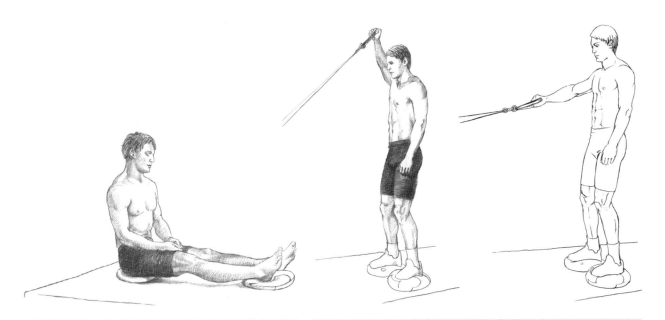

Exercise 5.6 Neuromuscular training

- Keep your balance while sitting on an air pillow, rubber pillow, balance board, or the like.
- Increase the degree of difficulty by placing your legs on a movable surface, by closing your eyes, or by moving your arms or head at the same time.

Exercise 5.7 Neuromuscular training

- Keep your balance with your back stable while doing increasingly difficult movements and more combined movements.
- Increase the degree of difficulty by closing your eyes.
- Gradually adjust the exercises to be more like the sport to which the athlete will return.

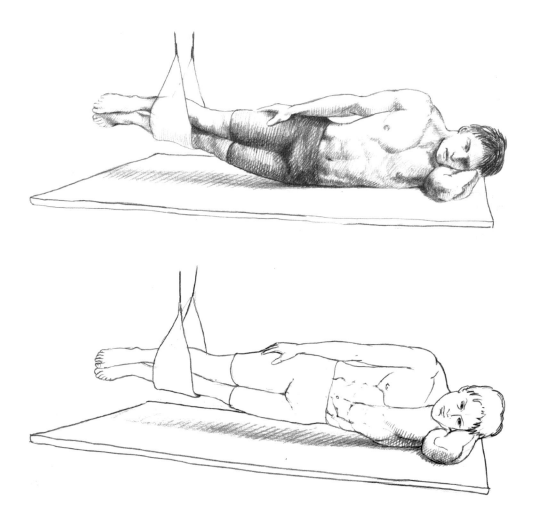

Exercise 5.8 Muscle strength and/or endurance training

- Keep your lower back slightly arched and pull in your abdomen before lifting your pelvis.
- Avoid swinging in the sling.
- Increase loading by moving the sling distally or by spreading your legs in the air.
- Repeat exercise while lying on your back or on the other side.

Exercise 5.9 Functionally oriented stability training (for preparing to return to sport)

- Jump with a Telemark landing, throw a medicine ball, pass a soccer ball.
- Focus on stability during the exercise.
- Vary throwing, kicking, and receiving positions.
- If pain is provoked, preactivate the local muscles by pulling in your abdomen.
- Increase loading with longer jumps, throws, kicks.

Neck Exercise Program

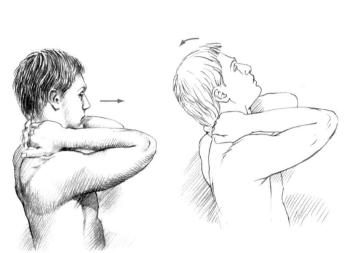

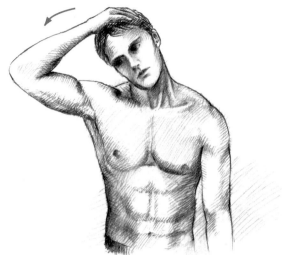

Exercise 5.10 Mobilization and stretching of the neck in extension

- Lace your little fingers on the lowest vertebra of the segment you want to mobilize, stabilize the lower portion of your neck, move your head and neck backward over your hands.
- Do range of motion training or stretching.
- Mobilize and stretch in the same manner in ventral and lateral flexion.

Exercise 5.11 Stretching the lateral flexors of the neck

- Actively press the shoulder girdle down during all stretching.
- Use your hand to strengthen the pull.
- Use minimal strength and a long stretching time.
- Alternate ventral flexion and rotation to the right when you bend to the right, and to the left when you bend to the left.

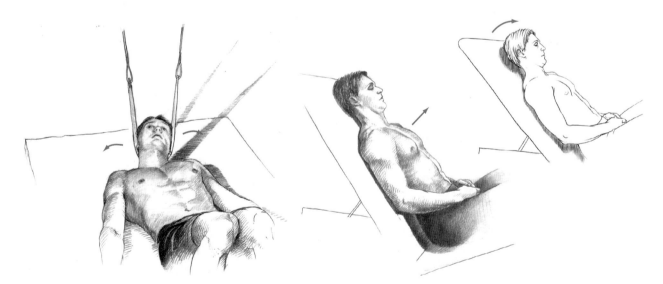

Exercise 5.12 Active mobilization of the neck in lateral flexion

- Move your head gently between extreme positions in lateral flexion.
- Mobilize and stretch in the same manner in ventral flexion and extension (lying on your side) or in rotation.
- Do range of motion training.

Exercise 5.13 Deep neck muscle training

- Pull in your chin, relax your jaw, and lift your head as high off the bench as possible without activating the superficial flexors (use a mirror to check) and without holding your breath.
- Increase holding time before loading.
- Increase loading by decreasing the angle of the bench.

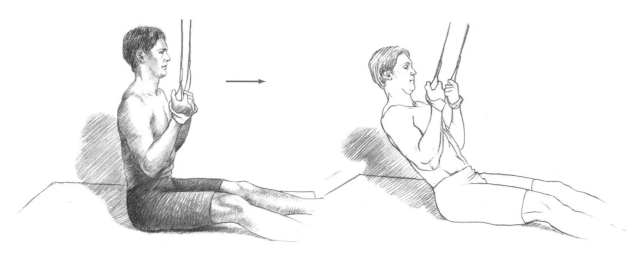

Exercise 5.14 Stability training for the neck

- Pull in your chin, stabilize your head and neck, relax your jaw, and gradually lean as far back as you can without activating the superficial flexors (look in the mirror to see when the other muscles start to kick in).
- Increase holding time before loading.

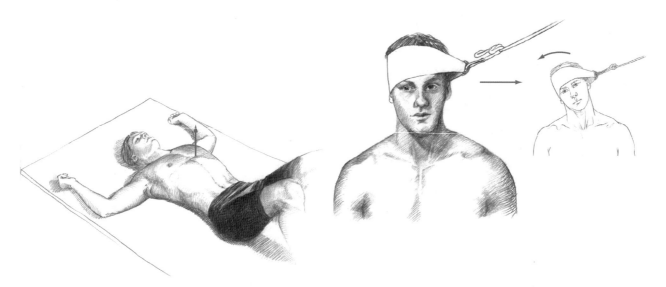

Exercise 5.15 Functional stability training

- Stabilize your neck before pulling your shoulder blades together, and lift your chest.
- Do not make any undesired movements with your neck or head.
- Increase loading by gradually increasing holding time.

Exercise 5.16 Training for muscular strength or endurance

- Assume a weight-bearing position, with resistance from the pulley apparatus; note the direction of the pull.
- Stabilize your neck using the deep flexors before movement.
- In the same manner, train the flexors, extensors, and rotators.
- Vary loading with the help of weights.

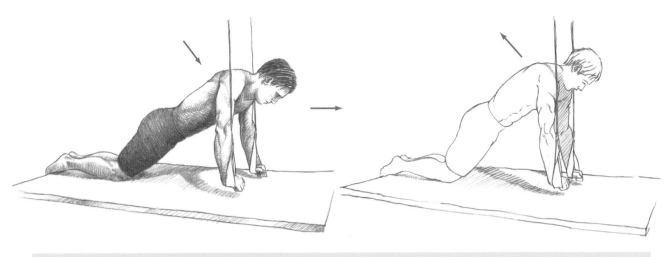

Exercise 5.17 Functional stability training

- Allow your body to "fall through" your shoulders with your arms extended, and push up again.
- Increase loading by moving the contact point from your knees toward your toes.
- Avoid jerky movements of your neck and head.

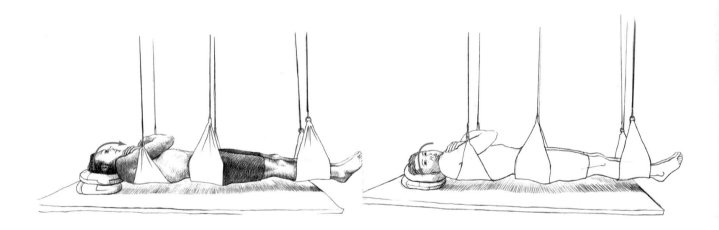

Exercise 5.18 Neuromuscular training

- Lie freely suspended with your head as the only contact point with the floor.
- Make controlled movements of the head in flexion, extension, or rotation.
- Increase the degree of difficulty by closing your eyes.

Chest Injuries

Arne Kristian Aune

Occurrence

Uncomplicated chest injuries, such as broken ribs, are common in sport (table 6.1). More severe chest injuries are less common but may occur in high-energy sports. If a high-energy trauma occurs, it is always necessary to quickly exclude severe chest injury first, because such injuries may be life threatening to the athlete. In most cases, a clinical examination is all that is needed to make this determination. Simple first aid measures are usually lifesaving. On-site caregivers are responsible for providing this care.

Diagnostic Thinking

Every athlete who sustains an injury as the result of a high-energy sport trauma should be given a rapid prioritized examination. The patient may have life-threatening injuries to the head, chest, and abdomen, and the importance of immediately establishing an open airway and reestablishing and maintaining effective ventilation cannot be overemphasized. Health care practitioners covering sporting events during which this type of trauma may occur should have ready access to medical supplies that permit the administration of intravenous fluids and oxygen supplementation during ventilation. When an open airway and adequate ventilation have been established, the athlete's uniform or clothing should be removed so that a good clinical examination can be performed. Both the abdomen and the chest need to be examined.

Clinical Examination

Examination. The examination is principally intended to rule out life threatening or other serious injury to the thorax. If the injured athlete becomes anxious, restless or panicked, hypoxia or hypotension should be considered to be the cause until there

Most common	Less common	Must not be overlooked !
Costal fractures (p. 146)	Diaphragmatic rupture (p. 148)	All thoracic injuries with the exception of broken ribs (p. 148)
Pneumothorax (p. 146)	Cardiac injuries (p. 148)	Lung contusion (p. 148)
	Major vascular injury (p. 148)	

Table 6.1 Overview of the differential diagnosis of thoracic injuries.

is proof to the contrary. Cyanosis of the skin and lips may indicate a blocked airway or a severe chest injury. Enlarged neck veins may indicate severe intrathoracic injury, such as hemopericardium, or increased intrathoracic pressure, such as that caused by blood in the mediastinum, pneumothorax or hemothorax, mediastinal emphysema, or tension pneumothorax. An asymmetrical chest wall may be a sign of subcutaneous emphysema, pneumothorax, multiple displaced rib fractures, sternal fractures, or bleeding in the chest wall. Asymmetrical movement of the thorax may indicate an injury to the side that moves the least. Multiple rib fractures may make the chest wall unstable, causing a paradoxical movement of the chest wall (e.g., retraction with inspiration and expansion with expiration).

Palpation. Palpation and visual inspection should permit the examiner to detect the abnormalities mentioned above. If the patient has subcutaneous emphysema, a leakage of air is present, as is a feeling of crepitice on palpation. The physician should palpate both the patient's carotid pulse and the peripheral pulses in the upper and lower extremities. Percussion will result in hyperresonance if the patient has tension pneumothorax. Conversely, dullness to percussion will result from an intrathoracic accumulation of blood or fluid.

Other examinations. Breath sounds (and other intracavitary sounds) can best be appreciated through auscultation. The practitioner should check the patient's pulse and measure her blood pressure at regular intervals to watch for signs of circulatory failure.

Common Injuries

Costal Fractures

- Symptoms and signs: The area above a single fractured rib will be tender to palpation, and respiration will be painful. Multiple rib fractures may be immediately life threatening. The patient may have significant respiratory problems and possibly an unstable chest wall.
- Diagnosis: The diagnosis is based on the mechanism of injury and the physical examination, including palpation and auscultation. The examiner must be attentive so as not to overlook signs of lung parenchymal injury or of pleural injury, including pneumothorax. If it is suspected that only one rib is fractured, an X ray is unnecessary. An X ray of the chest should be obtained, however, if multiple rib fractures are suspected or if the patient has other injuries to the chest.
- Treatment: A single fractured rib may be extremely painful but will heal by itself. It may take as long as six weeks before the patient can return to full activity. Primary care physicians are quite capable of treating this type of injury. The only treatment required is analgesic drugs and rest. If there are signs of more severe injuries such as multiple rib fractures or an unstable chest wall, the chest wall is stabilized by laying the patient on the injured side and applying pressure with a flat hand or by a tight wrap or bandage. The patient's airway should be secured, oxygen administered, and the patient transferred to the hospital immediately.

Pneumothorax

Trauma or a single fractured rib may puncture the lungs and pleura so that the negative pressure disappears and the lung collapses (figure 6.1). Subcutaneous emphysema or air leakage may also occur. If air leakage is minimal and the lung seals itself up quickly, the lung collapse is only partial, and the lung continues to conduct air. If the air leak is substantial, a total lung collapse may occur. Circulation and ventila-

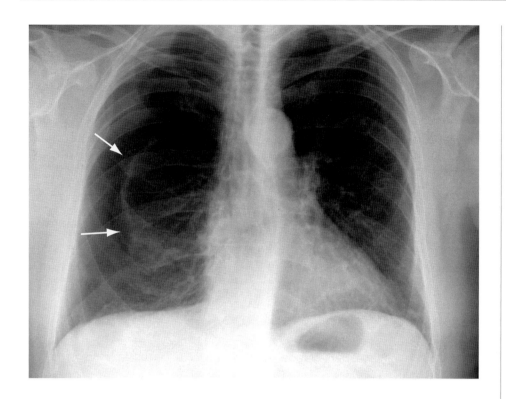

Figure 6.1 Pneumothorax after a rib fracture. The rib fracture is not visible on the X ray, but the pleural edge is visible (marked by the arrows).

tion both decrease as the degree of collapse increases. The contralateral lung takes care of ventilation in case of a total unilateral collapse. However, if the injury creates a one-way valve that allows air to enter into the pleural space but prevents it from exiting, hemithoracic pressure builds, in turn displacing the mediastinum toward the opposite side and compressing the uninjured lung. Such a "tension" pneumothorax can rapidly result in significant cardiopulmonary impairment and should be considered a medical emergency.

- Symptoms and signs: Early on, respiratory symptoms may be minimal. Dyspnea will worsen as the degree of lung collapse increases. Tension pneumothorax increases respiratory problems and can also result in anxiety, dyspnea, tachycardia, and cyanosis. The neck veins become distended and the mediastinum is gradually displaced.
- Diagnosis: The diagnosis is made if percussion of the chest wall produces a hyper-resonant sound with decreased respiratory sounds on the affected side. Chest X ray reveals free air in the pleural cavity, the degree of lung collapse, and any mediastinal displacement.
- Treatment: Treatment consists of establishing an open airway, giving morphine for pain relief, administering oxygen through a mask, and transporting the patient to the hospital. Morphine reduces anxiety and pain, thereby improving spontaneous ventilation. It is seldom necessary to provide further on-site treatment, unless the athlete has a probable tension pneumothorax and the hospital is more than half an hour away. If this is the case, insertion of a needle drain with a valve (Heimlich valve) into the pleura can be a lifesaving procedure. If a chest X ray reveals a small accumulation of air, the physician should attempt conservative treatment with bed rest and daily radiographic checkups. If the air leak closes itself, the air is resorbed within a few days and the lung expands. If the air jacket in the pleura is more than 2 cm wide and covers the entire convexity of the lung, a chest drain with suction is inserted to pull the lung into the chest wall.

Lung Contusions !

If the athlete sustains blunt trauma to the thorax, the lung tissue may be injured even if there is no evidence of superficial trauma or injury. The resulting parenchymal edema and bleeding will compromise ventilation and result in hypoxia.

- Symptoms and signs: Depending on the degree of injury, the patient may exhibit dyspnea, anxiety, tachycardia, bloody sputum, and other signs of oxygen debt.
- Diagnosis: This diagnosis is difficult to make, but it is always necessary to rule out lung trauma if the patient has multiple rib fractures and simultaneous pneumothorax. If the patient is bleeding into the pleural cavity (hemothorax) as well, the symptoms will also include circulatory failure. Hemothorax causes dullness to percussion and decreased respiratory sounds on auscultation.
- Treatment: Morphine is used as an analgesic, and other interventions include maintaining the airway, providing oxygen via a mask, establishing intravenous access for infusion of fluids and medications, and rapid transport to the hospital.

Other Injuries

Injuries to the trachea or bronchus often cause tension pneumothorax, with subcutaneous emphysema, bloody sputum, and eventually severe dyspnea. Treatment includes intubation and a chest tube. A tracheostomy is typically performed in such major injuries. An injury to the lower portion of the chest and abdomen may cause the diaphragm to rupture. Dyspnea and shock are common clinical signs of this type of injury. Cardiac injuries may be caused by blunt trauma or by the penetration of a thin, sharp object (such as a ski pole) into the upper abdominal region or the chest. If there is no pericardial rupture, the patient will be able to survive for a while. However, cardiac tamponade may occur very suddenly, requiring rapid intervention. If the hospital is more than half an hour away, a catheter should be inserted via the xiphoid region, slanting upward toward the precordial area. Cardiac contusion may cause the same symptoms as acute myocardial infarction, including both chest pain and arrhythmia. Injuries to the large vessels in the thorax are relatively rare, and most patients will die before treatment can be started, even with surgical intervention.

Abdominal Injuries

Arne Kristian Aune

Occurrence

High-energy sport trauma may result in abdominal injury, but even minor trauma may cause severe intra-abdominal bleeding that could be life threatening. Consequently, medical preparations to handle this type of trauma during high-risk sporting activities should be adequate.

Differential Diagnoses

The intra-abdominal organs may be injured as a result of external trauma to the abdomen or to the lower chest wall (table 6.2). Splenic injuries occur most commonly, but in principle, all of the abdominal organs are vulnerable to injury.

Diagnostic Thinking

In addition to thoracic injuries, serious injuries to intra-abdominal organs that may result in bleeding or significant tissue damage must be considered and ruled out when high-speed or high-energy trauma is the cause of the injury. If this type of injury is suspected, an open airway must be established and maintained, oxygen and intravenous fluids must be provided, and the patient must be immediately transported to the hospital.

Case History

The energy of the trauma may indicate an abdominal injury, but minor trauma (such as a blow or kick under the left costal arch or a fall over bicycle handlebars) may also cause severe splenic bleeding. The main symptom is abdominal pain, but the

Most common	Less common	Must not be overlooked !
Splenic rupture (p. 150)	Liver injury	Any intra-abdominal organ injuries
	Pancreatic injury	
	Gastric injury	
	Intestinal injury	
	Vascular injury	
	Urinary tract injury	
	Renal injury	

Table 6.2 Overview of the differential diagnosis of abdominal injuries.

patient may have additional symptoms and signs, such as hypovolemic shock with anxiety, tachycardia, and hypotension.

Clinical Examination

The patient should be given a full clinical examination of the chest and abdomen. When the abdomen is affected, the physician should examine the patient for evidence of peritoneal irritation and evaluate the patient's circulatory condition. He should explore and inspect the natural orifices and obtain either a clean-catch or straight-catheterized urine sample for urinalysis.

Common Injuries

Ruptured Spleen !

- **Symptoms and signs:** The spleen is the abdominal organ that is most frequently injured as a result of blunt abdominal trauma. Generally, blood loss and pain are present, as is left-upper-quadrant tenderness that radiates, off and on, to the left shoulder. If minor bleeding or hematoma under the splenic capsule occurs, symptoms and signs may be sparse.
- **Diagnosis:** The diagnosis may be difficult to make before the patient is hospitalized and given supplemental examinations, but the patient should always be hospitalized for observation if a splenic injury is suspected. It is not uncommon for a patient with abdominal trauma to feel fairly well, until entering hypovolemic shock as the result of gradual but persistent bleeding. Therefore, the patient should be under medical observation.
- **Treatment:** On-site treatment consists of securing the airway and establishing the infusion of intravenous fluids, instituting pain-relieving measures, and transporting the injured athlete to the hospital.

Other Injuries

Liver injuries present with symptoms similar to those caused by injury to the other abdominal organs. If the patient has suffered a major injury, bleeding symptoms will predominate. If the patient has sustained only minor injuries, his symptoms may be sparse. On-site treatment is the same as for other abdominal injuries. Signs of a minor pancreatic injury may often appear sometime after the accident occurs, and the patient may have a retroperitoneal hematoma that could eventually rupture, causing symptoms and signs of shock and peritonitis. In most patients, gastric and intestinal injuries will cause notable peritoneal signs, including a rigid abdomen. Blunt trauma may cause sheer injury to the mesenteric arteries or other blood vessels, resulting in hypovolemic shock. Injuries caused by an impact or blow to the kidneys or to the upper urinary tract will routinely cause hematuria. Such bleeding is rarely severe, and conservative treatment usually suffices. However, the patient should be referred to a urology or nephrology department for further evaluation of the injury.

Acute Shoulder Injuries

Arne Kristian Aune

Occurrence

Acute shoulder injuries frequently occur in sports in which falls and collisions are common. Shoulder dislocations constitute 4% of the injuries in the 20- to 30-year-old age group, with most dislocations occuring during sporting activity. Dislocations are three times more common among men than among women, and the vast majority of shoulder dislocations occur anteriorly. In ice hockey, shoulder trauma accounts for 20% of all injuries, with 8% of shoulder injuries due to dislocation. Eleven percent of all injuries sustained by skiers are shoulder injuries, with dislocations, acromioclavicular (AC) joint injuries, and rotator cuff injuries representing the leading diagnoses. Twenty percent of all shoulder injuries are fractures, with fractures of the clavicle and of the greater tubercle of the humerus predominating.

Differential Diagnosis

Shoulder pathology and injuries affect people in all age groups. When preparing a differential diagnosis for shoulder pain, the clinician should consider the influence of age on the incidence of specific conditions. For example, in children, falls that result in direct trauma to the shoulder are the predominant cause of clavicular fractures. In young adults, the population traditionally most active in sport, AC injuries and dislocations are the most common type of shoulder injury. In middle-aged patients, painful subacromial conditions and rotator cuff pathology occur most often. In the elderly, particularly among women, osteoporotic fractures of the proximal humerus predominate. Osteoarthritis of the shoulder joint is relatively rare as a primary disease; it usually occurs as a delayed consequence of intra-articular injuries or chronic rotator cuff dysfunction. This chapter describes the acute and chronic shoulder injuries that are most common in sport (see table 7.1).

Diagnostic Thinking

It is essential to distinguish between a fracture and a dislocated joint or a soft tissue injury. The injury mechanism and the clinical examination are the determining

Most common	Less common	Must not be overlooked !
AC joint injury (p. 157)	Rotator cuff tears (p. 162)	Posterior shoulder dislocation (p. 162)
Anterior shoulder dislocation (p. 159)	Fractures (p. 162)	Brachial plexopathy (p. 163)
Clavicular fractures (p. 156)	Sternoclavicular joint dislocation (p. 163)	Vascular injury

Table 7.1 Overview of the differential diagnosis of acute shoulder injuries.

factors. Vascular and peripheral nerve or brachial plexus injuries must be excluded. After assessing the athlete, the physician should make a tentative diagnosis, so that appropriate radiographs can be ordered. An acute shoulder injury should be evaluated at the primary-care level if radiography is available. Because it is easy to overlook posterior dislocation, the practitioner must ensure that axillary or lateral images are taken, in addition to frontal images. No other examinations are necessary during the acute phase. The need for subspecialty level referral depends on the expertise and experience available during the initial care and on access to radiography.

Clinical History

It is important to determine the injury mechanism, the direction of the energy that caused the injury, and the amount of force involved. If an athlete is injured by falling directly on her shoulder or on an outstretched arm, a fractured clavicle or a dislocated shoulder would be the diagnoses most likely to result from the mechanism of injury (figure 7.1, a and b). Direct trauma to the lateral side of the shoulder often causes AC joint injury (figure 7.2, a and b). Powerful external rotation-abduction, such as that caused by overturning in motocross or falling while downhill skiing, increases the likelihood of neurovascular damage with an anterior shoulder dislocation. It is important to ask the patient if he has a history of previous shoulder injury or chronic shoulder problems. Middle-aged or older patients with degenerative changes of the rotator cuff more commonly sustain rotator cuff ruptures than do younger athletes.

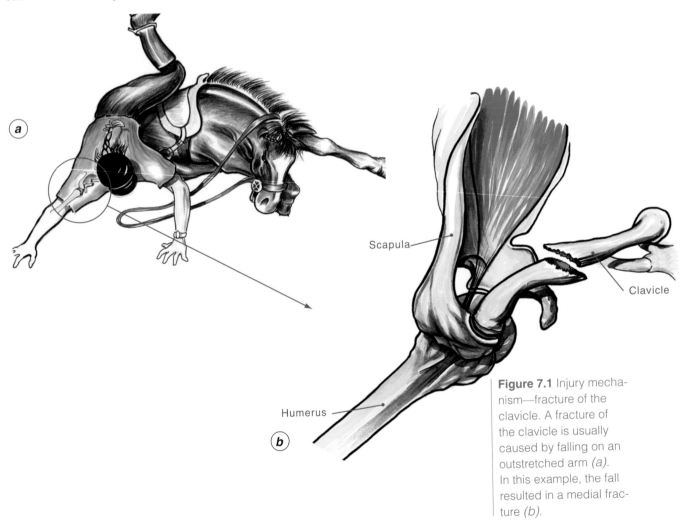

Scapula

Clavicle

Humerus

b

a

Figure 7.1 Injury mechanism—fracture of the clavicle. A fracture of the clavicle is usually caused by falling on an outstretched arm *(a)*. In this example, the fall resulted in a medial fracture *(b)*.

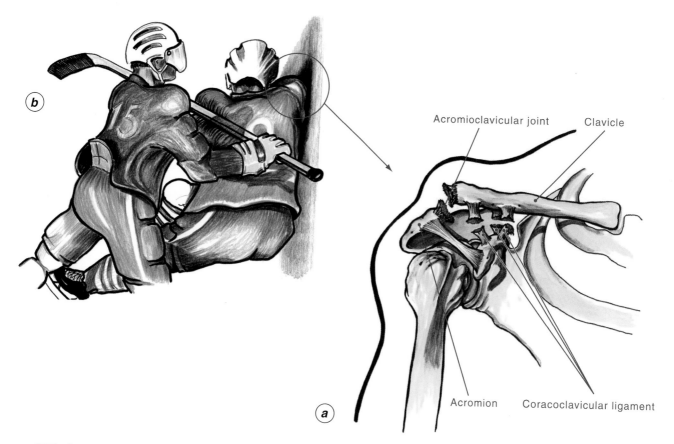

Clinical Examination

Inspection. Changes in the contour of the shoulder beneath the deltoid and an arm fixed in slight external rotation and abduction are typical signs of an anterior dislocation. A dislocated AC joint or a fractured clavicle is easily detected upon examining the patient. Bruising or hematoma formation and superior dislocation of the lateral end of the clavicle with "tangent phenomena" are typical of AC joint injuries, but the patient may also have a lateral clavicular fracture. Hematoma above the clavicular metaphysis indicates a medial clavicular fracture. Swelling and subcutaneous bleeding must also be noted if present.

Palpation. The physician should palpate all the important anatomic structures. The distal pulses should be palpated, and the athlete's appreciation of cutaneous stimulation should be assessed, particularly laterally over the deltoid muscle, to rule out damage to the axillary nerve.

Functional tests. The examiner should assess both active and passive joint range of motion. Generally, during the acute phase, it is neither possible nor necessary to perform functional tests, stability tests, or specific tests. However, these examinations are an extremely important tool in the evaluation of a chronic shoulder injury. Patients with acute rotator cuff injuries may have "pseudoparalysis" of shoulder abduction and extension. Instead, individuals with acute rotator cuff pathology may attempt to compensate by elevating and rotating the scapula, effectively "shrugging her shoulders" (the shrug sign).

Supplemental Examinations

Radiographic examination. X rays should be taken of all acutely injured shoulders. Radiographic studies are ordered specifically on the basis of the clinical diagnosis.

Figure 7.2 Injury mechanism—direct trauma to the shoulder. An acromioclavicular joint dislocation *(a)* is usually caused by direct trauma to the shoulder, such as being tackled into a side-board *(b)*.

If a clavicular fracture is suspected, two X rays of the clavicle are obtained to get inferior and superior views. Both the sternoclavicular joint and the AC joint must also be examined. For pediatric patients, it may be helpful to image the opposite side for comparison, so that it is possible to distinguish between fractures and a normal apophysis, if, for example, an acromial fracture is suspected. If the patient has an AC joint injury, images of the opposite side are taken for comparison. Images with and without handheld weights may be taken to gauge any instability. Images with superior angling must be included. If the patient has a glenohumeral joint injury, such as a dislocation or suspected juxta-articular fracture, a trauma series is obtained (that is, frontal, axillary, and lateral X rays). The axillary projection may be difficult to take if the patient is in a great deal of pain and has difficulty with abduction. It is always possible to take a lateral projection. Posterior dislocations are easily overlooked if no lateral or axillary views are taken. A control X ray must always be taken to check the position of the shoulder after a dislocation has been reduced.

Computerized tomography (CT). CT scans may be useful to distinguish between juxta-articular fractures and fracture/dislocations when determining the need for surgical intervention. However, CT is rarely advisable as an initial examination and is never indicated for care at the primary level.

Magnetic resonance imaging (MRI). MRI is seldom necessary for acute injuries but can be indicated in specialty-level care in order to evaluate potential brachial plexus or rotator cuff injuries.

Angiography. If vascular damage is suspected, angiography should be performed.

Common Injuries

Clavicular Fracture

Clavicular fractures (figure 7.3, a and b) are extremely common in children and adolescents who fall directly on their shoulder or on an outstretched arm. Such injuries may also occur as a result of a direct blow to the clavicle. In lateral clavicular fractures, the trauma is usually directly over the lateral aspect of the shoulder, as happens with injuries to the AC joint. Clavicular fractures are typically divided into medial and lateral fractures, depending on whether they occur medially or laterally to the coracoclavicular ligaments.

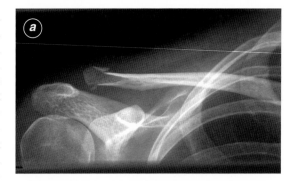

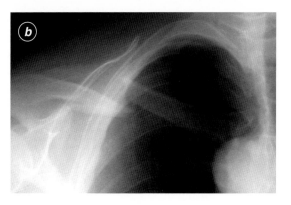

• Symptoms and signs: Swelling and structural malalignment of the clavicle are easy to detect. If the patient has a lateral fracture, swelling, pain, and possibly malalignment are localized toward the AC joint.

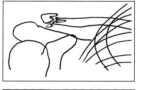

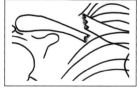

Figure 7.3 Fracture of the clavicle. The X rays demonstrate a lateral clavicle fracture *(a)* and a medial clavicle fracture *(b)*.

- Diagnosis: Diagnosis is made on the basis of two plain film radiographs that must include the AC joint and the sternoclavicular joint.
- Treatment of medial clavicular fractures: Most clavicle fractures are relatively easy to treat, and tend to heal within a few weeks. A figure-eight bandage or collar 'n cuff should be used only for the purpose of pain relief and not to reduce the fracture. All displaced fractures heal with shortening and a bump above the fracture site. This seldom causes functional problems. Surgery is rarely indicated for acute fractures, except in cases involving an open (compound) fracture, or a concomitant scapular fracture (resulting in a "floating shoulder"), or in cases of multiple trauma. Range of motion exercises and functional use of the arm may begin as soon as the patient can tolerate such activity. Physical therapy is not usually necessary. Treatment may take place at the primary-care level. In high-energy and comminuted fractures the patient may have subclavicular vascular damage. A vascular surgeon may treat these types of injuries by means of simultaneous open reduction and fixation of the fracture using a plate osteosynthesis. Healing problems and pseudoarthrosis after fractures of the medial clavicle are rare and occur in less than 1% of patients. Shortening and deformity (e.g., a bump above the healed fracture) may be cosmetically disfiguring but should not be treated surgically. There may be a great deal of callus formation in children, but the callus should decrease in size over time. Patients should be advised to accept the consequences.
- Treatment of lateral clavicular fractures: Stable fractures are treated conservatively at the primary-care level, in the same manner as medial fractures. If the fracture is displaced, surgery may be necessary because this type of fracture often proves difficult to heal and carries an increased risk of pseudoarthrosis. Therefore, lateral fractures with malalignment should be referred to an orthopedic surgeon for evaluation.
- Prognosis: The prognosis is favorable, and the athlete should anticipate returning to their original level of activity without problem. However, lateral injuries may have sequelae of pain and reduced function, making resection of the lateral end of the clavicle necessary. In these cases the patient should be referred to an orthopedic surgeon for evaluation. Shoulder function is generally good after such operative intervention.

Acromioclavicular (AC) Joint Injuries

The AC joint is often injured during sporting activity, usually as a result of falling on the shoulder. If the trauma comes directly from outside the shoulder (i.e., laterally), the AC joint is compressed, and the articular surface and the intra-articular disk can be injured. If the energy comes at an angle from above, the shoulder, including the scapula, is depressed while the clavicle remains in place. This mechanism injures the coracoclavicular ligaments, increasing the degree of dislocation of the AC joint. AC joint injuries are graded according to the degree and direction of the malalignment (figure 7.4, a-d).

- Diagnosis: The diagnosis of AC joint injury is made based on the presence of swelling and pain above the AC joint. Superior, posterior, or inferior dislocation of the lateral clavicle (in relation to the acromion) may also be present. The injury is graded by comparing the results of weight-bearing and nonweight-bearing radiographs, using the healthy side for comparison.
- Treatment: Grade 1 to 3 AC joint injuries can be treated conservatively at a primary-care level. The few patients who have delayed late symptoms may be surgically treated at a later time. The natural history of mild AC joint injury is generally good. Most of the time, malalignment and instability create only cosmetic problems. If the injury is difficult to classify, the patient should be referred to an orthopedic surgeon for evaluation. Injuries marked by significant dislocation

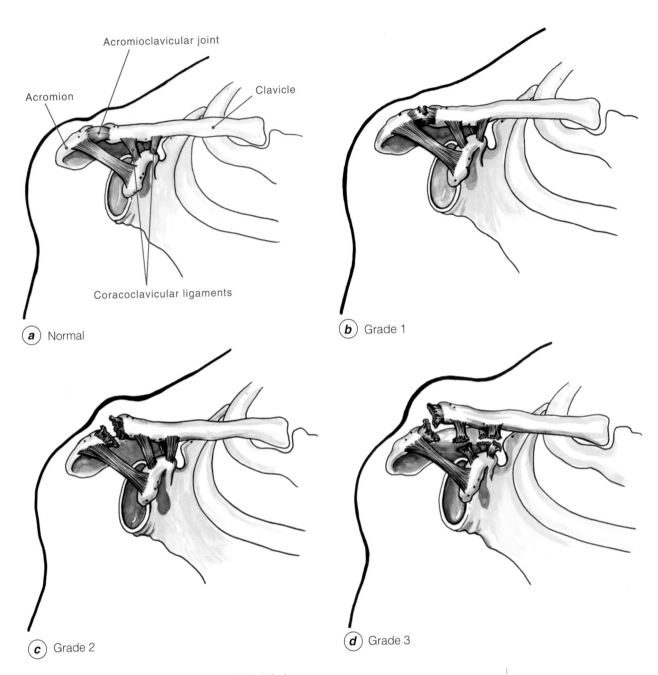

Acromioclavicular joint

Acromion

Clavicle

Coracoclavicular ligaments

(a) Normal

(b) Grade 1

(c) Grade 2

(d) Grade 3

Figure 7.4 Grading of acromioclavicular joint injuries.

Grade	Injury
1	Injury of the AC joint capsule without dislocation
2	Like 1, but with superior subluxation or increased joint distance compared to the healthy side
3	Total dislocation where the AC joint capsule and the coracoclavicular ligaments are torn off
4	Like 3, but with posterior dislocation where the clavicle penetrates the upper arc of the trapezius muscle because of tearing of the deltoid muscle's insertion into the deltoid tuberosity
5	Pronounced superior dislocation due to a tear of the deltoid muscle's insertion on the humerus at the deltoid tuberosity
6	Inferior dislocation—the lateral clavicle is locked under the coracoid process

(grades 4 to 6) should be treated surgically. Otherwise, treatment options include short-term pain relief and brief immobilization with a triangular bandage (or the like). Then, in accordance with the patient's level of tolerance, the patient should be instructed to resume shoulder use incrementally, first emphasizing range of motion, and then progressing to resistance training. The patient may return to sporting activity when her range of motion and strength have returned to normal, and she can do sport-specific exercises without pain. Persistent pain and restricted function may make surgery necessary for some patients.

Anterior Shoulder Dislocation

Most shoulder dislocations (95%) occur anteriorly (figure 7.5, a-c) and are frequently caused by sport-related shoulder trauma. Posterior dislocations are much less common. The most common cause of an anterior shoulder dislocation is a fall on an outstretched arm or forceful external rotation of an abducted arm (such as when a team handball player is tackled while shooting the ball).

• Symptoms and signs: When the shoulder (i.e., the humeral head) is dislocated anteriorly, the patient will tend to hold her arm in a slightly externally rotated and abducted position. Voluntary or passive range of motion of the joint will be

Figure 7.5 Anterior shoulder dislocation. The X ray views demonstrate anterior dislocation of the humeral head with a Hill-Sachs lesion (a) and reduction of the dislocation (b). The drawing (c) shows how the labrum-ligament complex is torn loose from the glenoid fossa by the anterior translation of the humeral head, resulting in what is known as a Bankart lesion.

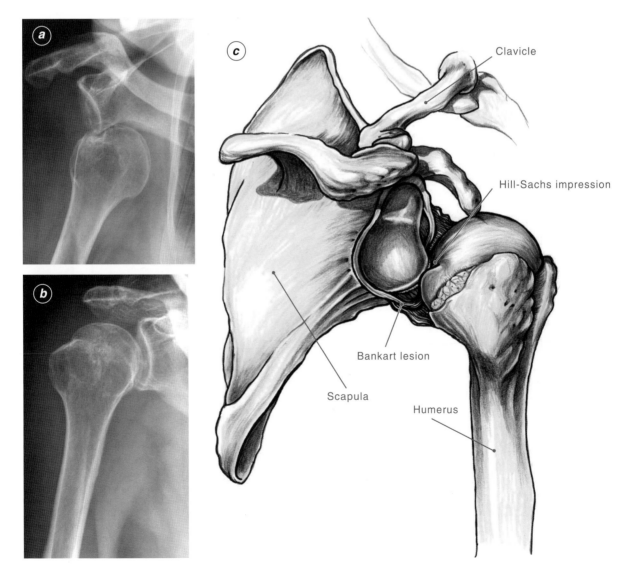

Clavicle

Hill-Sachs impression

Bankart lesion

Scapula

Humerus

SHOULDER

severely restricted. The contour of the shoulder above the deltoid may be altered. The physician should examine innervation, especially cutaneous sensibility laterally over the middle deltoid (axillary nerve distribution). An injury to the brachial plexus resulting from pressure produced by the dislocated humeral head may have serious functional consequences. In addition, the distal circulation should also be examined bilaterally.

• Diagnosis: A radiographic examination (trauma series) is necessary to determine in which direction the humeral head is dislocated and to rule out any concomitant fractures. Frontal and lateral images are taken, and if the patient can tolerate it, axillary projections are obtained. A simultaneous fracture of the greater tubercle is involved in 5% to 13% of anterior shoulder dislocations. The incidence increases with age. Even if these fractures are displaced, they will usually be reduced at the same time the dislocated glenohumeral joint is reduced. In the case of an anterior dislocation, the inferior glenohumeral ligament complex, including the labrum, is usually torn loose from the glenoid (Bankart injury). In 3% to 10% of these cases, the patient also sustains an intra-articular fracture/avulsion off the anterior glenoid. This injury is usually minor and does not affect the initial treatment. Occasionally, the fracture involves a major portion of the glenoid, making surgical fixation to stabilize the shoulder necessary. All patients with a first-time dislocation sustain a compression fracture of the humeral head posteriorly when the humeral head, in its dislocated position, is pressed posteriorly toward the glenoid margin (Hill-Sachs lesion). This may be a cartilaginous injury, and therefore may not be visible on an X ray. The presence of a Hill-Sachs injury should not affect the initial treatment. Posterior dislocation causes a reverse Hill-Sachs lesion.

• Treatment: The level of treatment depends on the experience and competence of the caregiver, whether the athlete has sustained a first-time dislocation or whether this is a recurring phenomena, and on access to radiography. The physician must reduce the dislocation as soon as the diagnosis is made. Dislocations that remain untreated for a long period of time increase the risk of neurovascular damage. Early reduction is easier because there is less muscle spasm. However, first-time dislocations must be documented radiographically. In case of a recurrent dislocation, a radiographic examination may well be unnecessary. Before reduction, the patient should be given either 20 ml of 1% lidocaine intra-articularly via a direct lateral injection 1 cm below the acromion, or morphine and diazepam. Of the various methods of reduction, this author prefers the Stimson method (figure 7.6). The patient is placed in a prone position with her arm hanging down from the side of the examination table. The arm

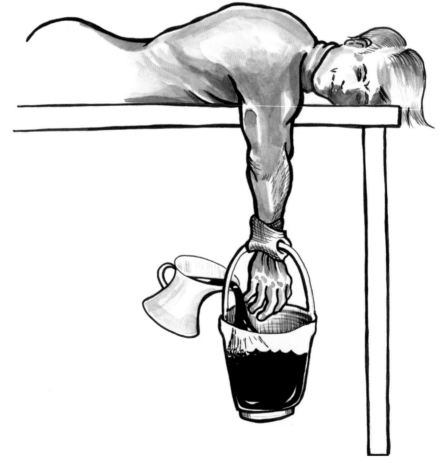

Figure 7.6 Reduction of a dislocated shoulder—Stimson's method. Traction of the arm with the patient in a prone position on the bench.

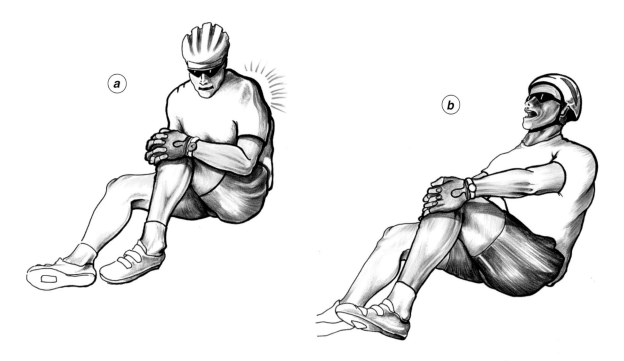

Figure 7.7 Reduction of a dislocated shoulder—self-reduction. The patient wraps his hands around his knee *(a)* and extends his hip while leaning backward *(b)*.

is distracted longitudinally; the key to successful reduction is to get the patient to relax the shoulder girdle musculature. Alternatively, one may tape a bucket to the athlete's ipsilateral wrist and gradually increase traction by slowly filling the bucket with water. Reduction must be done slowly (it often takes 5 to 10 minutes before the shoulder is in place). In contrast to the "foot in the axilla" Hippocratic method, this method is complication free. It may also be used for posterior dislocations. Another method of self-reduction, equally complication-free (figure 7.7, a and b), may be taught to patients who have a tendency to dislocation or for whom transport to the hospital will be delayed. In this method, after the shoulder is reduced, innervation and circulation are reexamined and the reduction is documented by an X ray. For pain relief (until the patient can comfortably move her shoulder) the shoulder is immobilized in an arm sling (or something like it) for as short a time as possible. The immobilization period is usually 3 to 4 days. Increasing the period of immobilization does not further reduce the risk of recurrent dislocation.

- Treatment by physical therapist: After a brief period of immobilization, exercises for range of motion, muscular balance, and strength begin.
- Return to sport: Before returning to sport, the patient must have achieved the same range of motion and strength in the injured shoulder as in the contralateral shoulder, and the apprehension test must be negative. Returning to sport too quickly has been proven to increase the risk of recurrent dislocation. Therefore, a rehabilitation period of at least 3 months is recommended before return to sport.
- Prognosis: Various studies report a high frequency of recurrence (46% to 95%) in young, active athletes. However, there is no routine indication for surgery after the first dislocation; otherwise, numerous athletes would have surgery unnecessarily. Nevertheless, young patients who participate in throwing or other "overhead" sports and who have dislocated their dominant shoulder should be offered surgery after their initial dislocation because of the extremely high frequency of recurrence. Between 5% and 60% of patients with anterior shoulder dislocations sustain nerve damage. Nerve damage, however, is more common in older patients. Most nerve damage goes into spontaneous regression after 3 to 12 months. If axillary nerve function has not returned after 4 months, the patient is referred for consideration of surgical nerve grafting. Rotator cuff ruptures occur in 40% to 90% of the middle-aged and elderly patients after the first dislocation. If this type of injury

causes persistent pain and reduces strength, and if the athlete does not respond favorably to exercise therapy, he should be referred for surgical evaluation.

Other Injuries

Rotator Cuff Tears

Acute rotator cuff tears are rare among younger athletes, but a fall (e.g., while skiing) may result in a tear in active older athletes with pre-existing degenerative tendinopathy. Rotator cuff tears are usually the end result of a multifactorial degenerative condition that is precipitated by an age-related reduction in circulation to the tendon, chronic tendinosis, and persistent impingement. A fall may trigger a complete tear of the weakened tendons. Athletes in throwing sports may also sustain partial tears as a result of repeated eccentric loading of the tendinous tissue. The evaluation and treatment of rotator cuff injuries are discussed in the section on painful shoulder disorders.

Fractures

The most common juxta-articular fractures are avulsion of the greater tubercle of the humerus and intra-articular scapular fractures. These are discussed in connection with shoulder dislocation (see page 159). A fracture of the greater tubercle that has been dislocated should be surgically reduced and fixed. Fractures without dislocation are treated conservatively by short-term immobilization in an arm sling for pain relief, followed by range-of-motion exercises and strength training. The patient may be treated at the primary-care level and occur typically in elderly osteoporotic people. Fractures of the proximal humerus are less common in younger individuals. The rule is conservative treatment, as mentioned previously, but open reduction and internal fixation may be indicated for displaced or comminuted fractures and major dislocations. Therefore, fractures of this type should be referred to an orthopedic surgeon for further evaluation and management. Fractures of the body of the scapula heal well. Treatment is conservative, with immobilization for pain relief, followed by range-of-motion exercises and strength training by a physical therapist at the primary-care level. Fractures that extend into the scapular notch may lead to entrapment of the suprascapular nerve. In such cases, surgery may be necessary. Suprascapular nerve lesions can cause paresis of the supraspinatus and/or the infraspinatus muscles, depending on the site of entrapment. Should suprascapular neuropathy be suspected, the athlete should be referred for evaluation.

Posterior Shoulder Dislocation !

Posterior shoulder dislocations represent less than 5% of all dislocations. The injury is often caused by a fall on an outstretched arm or by an epileptic seizure. Posterior dislocations may be overlooked, primarily because the initial radiographic evaluation of the injured shoulder is inadequate. Inspection from behind reveals an obvious change in the contour of the shoulder. The diagnosis is made using radiographic examinations with axillary and/or lateral views. The Stimson reduction method (figure 7.6) may be used to reduce the dislocation. The injury may be treated at the primary-care level in the same manner that anterior dislocations are treated—that is, depending on access to radiography and personnel with the proper expertise.

Brachial Plexus Injuries !

Brachial plexus injuries may be divided into root avulsion injuries and more distal injuries. Root avulsion injuries result in myotomal-specific paresis on the affected side. If MRI or CT myelography demonstrate evidence of avulsion, the prognosis for recovery is poor. The prognosis is better for more distal brachial plexus injuries. Electrodiagnostic testing can facilitate localization of the lesion and provides an estimate as to the severity of the injury. Brachial plexopathies should be followed expectantly to gauge spontaneous improvement. If after 3 months there is no evidence of clinical recovery, surgery must be considered. Sural nerve graft surgery may improve elbow and hand function to some extent, but the effect on shoulder function is minimal. If a plexus injury is suspected, the patient should be referred to a neurologist or to a neurosurgeon.

Sternoclavicular Joint Dislocation

Sternoclavicular joint dislocations (figure 7.8, a-c) are rare. They may be serious and difficult to treat if the clavicle dislocates posteriorly and threatens the large thoracic vessels behind it. Therefore, the patient should be evaluated and treated in the hospital.

A radiographic examination may be completely negative, and a CT scan is recommended. Anterior dislocations may remain untreated with satisfactory functional results. The prominence of the clavicle is only of cosmetic significance. It is not reduced because it rarely becomes stable. Children and adolescents may suffer a growth plate injury, in which case the dislocation will not be capable of remodeling. Posterior dislocation may threaten the mediastinal structures, and therefore the recommended treatment is reduction (with preparedness for emergent vascular surgery if necessary). Posterior dislocations are usually stable following reduction.

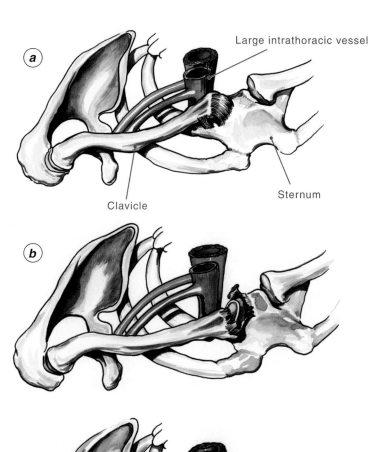

Large intrathoracic vessel

Clavicle

Sternum

Figure 7.8 Sternoclavicular joint dislocation. Normal anatomy *(a)*, anterior dislocation *(b)*, and posterior dislocation *(c)* are shown. Posterior dislocation may be life threatening if the large intrathoracic vessels are affected.

SHOULDER

163

Chronic Shoulder Disorders

Arne Kristian Aune

Occurrence

Painful conditions caused by overuse, muscular imbalance, and instability are the predominant shoulder injuries that occur in throwing sports and in sports such as swimming and tennis. The incidence of chronic shoulder disorders in these sports is between 17% and 26%. Overuse injuries to the shoulders of volleyball players and athletes in other throwing and racket sports are increasing, with a disproportionate share occuring among female athletes. In fitness sports, shoulder overuse injuries are twice as common among older athletes as they are among younger athletes.

Differential Diagnosis

The differential diagnosis for chronic shoulder pain depends on the age, activity level, and injury history of the athlete (table 7.2). For example, recurrent dislocations after a primary traumatic, anterior shoulder dislocation are common in younger athletes. Chronic shoulder pain is a problem in all age groups. In throwers, swimmers, and athletes who play racket sports, shoulder pain is usually caused by multidirectional instability resulting from muscular imbalance and overstretching of the anterior joint capsule due to unilateral activity and repetitive microtrauma. Tendinitis, tendinosis, and impingement of the rotator cuff in these athletes are usually secondary phenomena caused by the underlying instability. Injuries to the glenoid labrum may cause pain and a feeling of instability. In middle-aged and elderly athletes, tendinosis, degenerative conditions, and rotator cuff tears are the most common causes of pain. Even if the clinical course after AC joint dislocation is usually benign, joint pain and osteoarthritis may occur as late sequelae. Weightlifters may have pain in the lateral clavicle caused by increased stress that may result in osteoarthritis and

Most common	Less common	Must not be overlooked (!)
Posttraumatic shoulder instability (p. 170)	Labral injury/SLAP lesion (p. 171)	Cervical radicular pain (p. 111)
Multidirectional instability (p. 172)	Rotator cuff tears (p. 176)	Adhesive capsulitis (p. 180)
Subacromial pain syndrome (p. 174)	Recurrent posterior dislocation (p. 178)	
	AC joint osteoarthritis (p. 178)	
	Entrapment of the suprascapular nerve (p. 179)	

Table 7.2 Overview of the differential diagnosis of chronic shoulder disorders in athletes.

distal clavicular osteolysis. Entrapment of the suprascapular nerve is a relatively rare cause of posterolateral shoulder pain and muscle atrophy that should be entertained in the appropriate clinical setting.

Diagnostic Thinking

Typically, most painful shoulder conditions, whether due to instability or tendinosis in the rotator cuff, should be treated conservatively with a rehabilitation program. However, it is important to make an accurate diagnosis so that the rehabilitation program can be tailored to the situation. The treatment of recurrent shoulder dislocation is often surgical. The goal of the evaluation is to determine what pathoanatomical changes have occurred to the joint so that proper surgical treatment may be planned.

Clinical History

The patient's history is an extremely important tool to understanding chronic shoulder disorders. A thorough history may facilitate narrowing the differential diagnosis so that further evaluation can proceed more efficiently.

First, it should be determined how and when the athlete's symptoms started. Were they post-traumatic in etiology? In what type of activity was the patient engaged when their symptoms first appeared? If the athlete has a history of shoulder dislocation, the problem is likely to be caused by glenohumeral instability. Does the patient hear or feel a click, clunk, or crunching sound in the affected shoulder? If so, the symptoms may be the sequelae from a cuff or a labral injury. Did the pain begin gradually, or did it arise suddenly? Acute pain is typical of inflammatory conditions, whereas chronic pain is indicative of tendinosis or multidirectional instability. The practitioner should determine whether the athlete was able to continue his activity in whole or in part once the symptoms began.

The practitioner should record the medical history and symptoms and should also indicate what therapy was attempted and the subsequent response (e.g., physical therapy, drugs, surgery, or steroid injections). The patient should be asked specifically whether she has a history of neck pain or problems.

The specific symptoms and the degree to which the symptoms affect sport activity, work, or daily life must be determined. Even if there is no history of shoulder dislocation, the patient should be asked whether his shoulder feels unstable. If it was dislocated, he should be asked how many times, under what circumstances, and whether he needed to go to the hospital to have it reduced. If the patient has pain that may be caused by instability, the practitioner must determine whether the shoulder locks up and whether it clicks in certain positions. These findings point toward labral pathology. During the interview, the patient should be asked about any restricted movements–for example, does reaching behind his back or combing his hair provoke symptoms?

Finally, the patient's history should be as specific as possible with respect to pain. Pain is often the main reason that the patient seeks medical care. The practitioner must distinguish between pain at rest and pain from loading and identify which activities cause pain. Pain at rest or pain that is associated with severely restricted shoulder range of motion suggests adhesive capsulitis. Patients with tendinosis or a rotator cuff rupture suffer from pain when lying on their affected arm and when lifting their arm or doing activities at shoulder level or above. Pain during activities requiring external rotation and abduction indicates anterior instability.

Clinical Examination

Inspection. Abnormal positioning of the shoulder at rest may reflect underlying spinal deformity, a muscle injury, or even occult neurological disease. Changes in positioning may also occur in an effort to compensate for the sequelae of chronic pain. Muscular atrophy (e.g., of the supraspinatus and the infraspinatus muscles) may indicate a rotator cuff rupture or entrapment of the suprascapular nerve. Injury to the axillary nerve affects the deltoid muscle.

Range of motion. When examining the active range of motion, the physician should note the scapulohumeral rhythm (i.e., the rotation of the scapula when the arm is abducted). He should stand behind the patient and observe the scapulolohumeral rhythm bilaterally, using the uninvolved side as a control. Active range of motion is not always the same as passive range of motion. Disrupted scapulohumeral rhythm in the plane of the scapula indicates subacromial pain or weakness, or it may indicate muscle imbalance (which is relatively common in the presence of instability). Normal shoulder range of motion is commonly accepted to be 180° flexion, 30° extension, 180° abduction, 30° adduction, 70° internal rotation in the neutral position, and 60° external rotation in the neutral position.

Palpation. Tenderness can often be elicited by palpation at several sites throughout the shoulder girdle. Subacromial tenderness along the humeral head at the insertion of the rotator cuff is a sign of rotator cuff degeneration or tendinosis. The radiographic presence of calcium deposits at the tendon insertion suggests calcific tendinitis. Pain around the coracoid process is rare but may occur in the case of subscapular tendinosis or coracoacromial impingement, which frequently causes shoulder pain in swimmers. Pain corresponding to the tendon of the long head of the biceps brachii is common in impingement syndrome, rotator cuff tendinosis, or in the case of a complete rotator cuff tear. However, if the patient has a history of remote rupture of the bicipital tendon, the biceps sulcus is usually pain free. Pain and thickening over the AC joint are signs of degenerative arthropathy as AC joint stability may be assessed by depressing the clavicle inferiorly while the humerus is being pressed superiorly. Pain above the clavicle is rare but may occur if the patient has a late healing fracture or pseudoarthrosis. Tenderness to palpation above the sternoclavicular joint may be a sign of chronic instability. Sometimes the patient may spontaneously dislocate and reduce this joint. The shoulder girdle muscles and their respective insertions should be palpated. Frequently, tender points or trigger points will be identified that do not reflect specific injury but which may occur secondary to other pathology in the neck or shoulder.

Neuromuscular function. A general neurological examination of the upper extremity should be performed, in particular to look for accompanying injuries to the peripheral nerves, including injuries to the suprascapular nerve and the axillary nerve (e.g., after shoulder dislocations). If the patient has injured the long thoracic nerve, the serratus anterior muscle will be paretic, resulting in "winging" of the ipsilateral scapula. Winging can be demonstrated by having the patient perform push-ups against the wall. On the paretic side, the relatively unopposed action of the trapezius against a paretic serratus anterior will result in prominence of the medial border of the scapula. The cervical spine should be examined for range of motion and evidence of nerve root irritation to rule out a referred cervical etiology of the patient's shoulder pain.

If the clinical history suggests recurrent dislocations or instability, the practitioner should assess shoulder stability by using specific tests.

Drawer test (translation test) (figure 7.9). Normally, the humeral head can only be moved a few millimeters anteriorly and posteriorly. If translation increases when the patient hangs his arm at his side, it is a sign of increased capsular laxity (figure 7.7).

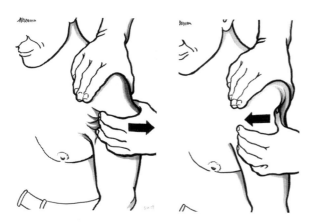

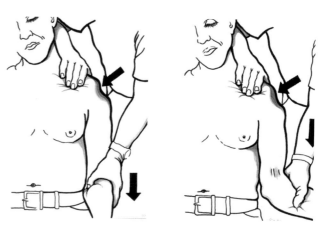

Figure 7.9 Drawer test (translation test). The patient's arm hangs by his side. One hand fixes the shoulder blade while the other grasps the upper arm and pushes it anteriorly and posteriorly.

Figure 7.10 Sulcus sign. The patient's elbow, hanging by his side, is distracted distally. The test is considered positive when a depression is visible beneath the acromion.

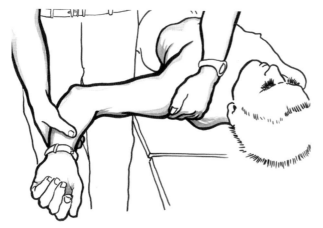

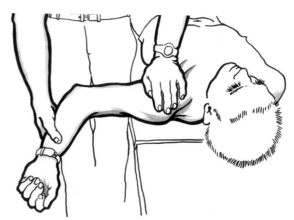

Figure 7.11 Apprehension test. With the arm in 90° abduction and 90° flexion, the limb is externally rotated at the shoulder. This test for anterior instability is positive if the patient indicates discomfort, pain, or the fear that the shoulder is going to dislocate.

Figure 7.12 Relocation test. The examiner follows the same procedure as for the apprehension test but, in addition, applies counterpressure to the humerus from the front. If this brings pain relief when compared with the apprehension test, the test is positive and indicates anterior instability.

Sulcus sign (figure 7.10). Inferior translation, resulting in the so-called sulcus sign, is achieved by pulling the elbow distally. The presence of a depression inferior to the acromion is indicative of significant laxity. This is particularly common in patients with multidirectional instability, where shoulder pain is caused by increased laxity.

Apprehension test (figure 7.11). The test is performed with the patient in a supine position or sitting with her arm at 90° abduction, the elbow flexed to 90°, and externally rotated at the shoulder. The examiner attempts to force external rotation further, and if the patient complains of discomfort, pain, and becomes fearful that her shoulder will dislocate anteriorly, the test is considered positive.

Relocation test (figure 7.12). With the patient in the supine position, the examiner repeats the procedure for the apprehension test but applies even posteriorly directed pressure on the humerus so that the humeral head is held in place in the glenoid cavity. If this brings pain relief following a provocative anterior apprehension test, the relocation test is considered positive and suggests that the athlete's pain may be the result of anterior instability.

Jobe relocation test. If the patient complains of posterior shoulder pain during the apprehension test, it is a sign of posterior instability. The Jobe relocation test is administered by pressing against the proximal humerus in a posterior-anterior direction. If the patient's symptoms are relieved, this test for posterior instability is considered positive.

Test for posterior instability. This test is conducted by having the patient sit or stand in a forward-leaning position, elevating his arm at the shoulder to about 45° and internally rotating the upper limb while the humeral head is being pushed from behind in the longitudinal direction of the humerus. The test is positive if there is posterior subluxation or frank dislocation of the humeral head.

Generalized joint laxity. Generalized joint laxity may be the result of connective tissue that is more flexible or distensible than normal. The patient should be examined in five areas: hyperextension of the knees and elbows (in excess of 10°), hyperextension of the fingers (of more than 90°), dorsal extension of the ankle (to more than 45°), and the Steinberg thumb sign (positive if the patient's thumb can be passively bent to touch the volar portion of the forearm). If the patient meets three of these five criteria, there is generalized joint laxity that makes the patient vulnerable to multidirectional shoulder instability.

Tests for labral injury and SLAP lesions. The O'Brien test is generally considered to be a useful means of evaluating the integrity of the glenoid labrum and for the presence of AC joint pathology (figure 7.13, a and b). The test is conducted with the patient standing with his arm at 90° flexion at the shoulder, 10° to 15° adduction in relation to the sagittal plane, and with maximal internal rotation, so that the thumb points downward. The examiner stands beside the patient and applies even pressure downward against resistance. The maneuver is repeated with the patient in the same position, only this time the palm of the patient's hand points up and the upper limb is maximally externally rotated. The O'Brien test is described as positive if the patient feels pain during the first part of the test and then experiences significantly reduced symptoms (or no pain at all) during the second part. Pain or clicking in the shoulder joint suggests an injury to the fibrocartilaginous labrum. Pain on top of the shoulder indicates damage to the AC joint.

Another test for a labral pathology is the crank test (figure 7.14, a and b). The patient lies supine with his arm abducted 160°, and the examiner stands behind the patient and applies compression and rotation internally and externally. The test is considered positive if the patient experiences pain or a clicking sensation.

Impingement tests. Specific examination techniques can be used to provoke pain due to degeneration of the rotator cuff or if the rotator cuff is persistently entrapped under the acromion. Pain that occurs when the arm is abducted,

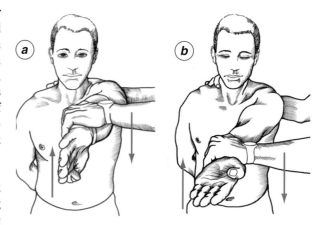

Figure 7.13 O'Brien test. The examiner applies even pressure downward on the affected upper limb, which has been positioned in 90° flexion and 10° to 15° adduction and internal rotation (a). Pain in the shoulder joint and/or a click indicates an injury to the glenoid labrum. Pain over the acromioclavicular joint indicates AC joint pathology. External rotation of the arm relieves the symptoms (b).

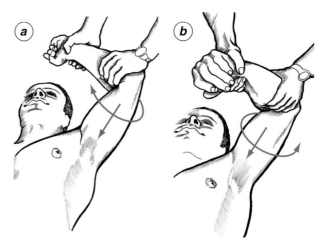

Figure 7.14 Crank test. With the arm abducted to about 160°, compression is applied and the humerus rotated. If the patient feels pain or a clicking sensation, the test is considered indicative of a labral injury.

particularly between 70° and 130°, is defined as a positive painful arc. The examiner demonstrates the Neer sign by stabilizing the acromion and pressing somewhat inferiorly, while internally rotating the humerus and raising the arm in full flexion to 180° (figure 7.15, a and b). The patient usually reacts with pain between 120° and 180°, as he does with a positive sign when the rotator cuff is trapped below the acromion. The Hawkins impingement sign is somewhat simpler to test than the Neer sign, particularly for patients with reduced range of motion (figure 7.15, a and b). The shoulder is flexed to 90° in the horizontal plane, and in this position it is internally rotated. If the patient reacts with pain, the sign is positive. To complete the impingement test, the patient is given a subacromial injection of 5 ml to 10 ml of local anesthetic, and the examination is repeated. Pain relief is a positive sign of impingement. This test can be used to distinguish between primary impingement and secondary impingement caused by instability. The outcome of the impingement tests will be positive in a patient with instability and secondary impingement problems, but the relocation sign is often positive, indicating that the pain is caused by instability.

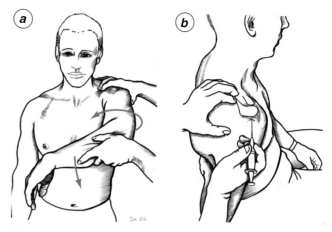

Figure 7.15 Impingement tests and injection technique. The Hawkins impingement test is performed with the upper arm at 90° flexion in the horizontal plane, with a flexed elbow. If the test is positive, the patient has pain under the acromion *(a)*. After a subacromial injection of local anesthetic *(b)*, the test is repeated. If the injection brings pain relief, impingement is indicated.

Testing of the AC joint (cross body test). The test (figure 7.16) is conducted by having the patient raise his arm in the horizontal plane to 90° and compressing the upper arm axially toward the shoulder with simultaneous maximum adduction of the arm. The test is positive if there is pain in the AC joint, which occurs if the patient has osteoarthritis or sequelae after an AC joint dislocation. To complete the test, inject a local anesthetic into the joint and repeat the test. The previously mentioned O'Brien test, if positive, indicates AC joint pathology.

Muscle strength. Motor weakness is most often the result of pain limiting voluntary muscle function (e.g., tendinosis or inflammation can result in arthrogenic inhibition of the muscles acting upon a joint). Pain triggered by isometric activation of a specific muscle group is a sign of tendinosis. If strength is significantly reduced with a lesser element of pain, the patient may possibly have a ruptured tendon. All muscles in the rotator cuff must be tested as part of a thorough shoulder examination. The supraspinatus muscle is tested by having the patient abduct and internally rotate her arm in the plane of the scapula. The infraspinatus is tested by external rotation with the arm at the patient's side. The teres minor is tested by external rotation with the arm at 90° abduction. The subscapularis is tested by having the patient place her hand back on her lumbar spine and pressing her palm outward. The long head of the biceps brachii, although not one of the rotator cuff muscles, may be tested by elbow flexion and supination.

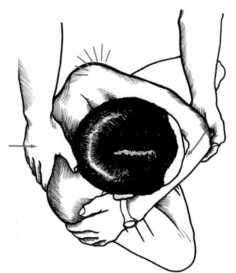

Figure 7.16 Cross body test. The examiner applies compression on an arm that is adducted maximally in the horizontal plane. If the test triggers pain in the acromioclavicular joint, it is considered positive for AC joint pathology.

Supplemental Examinations

Radiographic examinations. Plain radiography provides important supplemental information to the clinical examination. The routine radiographic examination of the shoulder should always consist of at least two views: a frontal image and a lateral or axillary image. In addition, views of the AC joint can be obtained, as can special views to assess the configuration of the acromion (e.g., if the patient has subacromial pain).

MRI. Magnetic resonance arthrography is the best supplemental examination to the usual radiographic images for diagnosing shoulder pathology. However, indications for MRI should be limited, since the examination is expensive. MRI is not indicated for manifest instability in the shoulder, except in patients older than 40 years, more than half of whom also have a torn rotator cuff. If the patient has a painful condition of uncertain etiology but where instability is suspected, MRI is indicated. MRI is not indicated for subacromial pain syndrome but is useful as a preoperative examination if it is suspected that the patient has a rotator cuff tear that requires surgical treatment.

CT. A CT scan with double contrast (in the form of contrast medium and air) is a good test for Bankart lesions and additional osseous injuries due to dislocation. Because this information is seldom of any practical value to treatment (as a supplement to information obtained about clinical symptoms and from plain radiographic imaging), CT scans are not routinely performed during the evaluation of an unstable shoulder or of other chronic painful shoulder conditions.

Ultrasound. Ultrasound is a good method of screening for rotator cuff disease, but it is highly operator-dependent and should be performed only by an experienced operator.

Common Injuries

Posttraumatic Shoulder Instability

After the first dislocation, it is quite common for active young athletes to repeatedly dislocate the same shoulder, whether as a result of trauma or by placing the shoulder in a vulnerable position of external rotation and abduction. The frequency of dislocation may vary from a few times a year to several times a day. More than 80% of the patients have a Bankart injury (defined as tearing of the glenoid labrum and the associated glenohumeral ligaments away from the anterior-inferior portion of the glenoid). A Bankart lesion results in an unstable glenohumeral joint, and as a result the humeral head may sublux or dislocate. In addition to a Bankart injury, overstretching of the capsular ligaments is probably of greater clinical significance in regard to repeat dislocations than previously believed. Indications of instability may vary; some affected individuals experience only a feeling of uncertainty or perhaps pain when the arm is in an externally rotated position.

• Diagnosis: The diagnosis is based on the information in the clinical history (that is, recurrent anterior shoulder dislocation or pain). Typical examination findings include increased anterior translation, a positive apprehension test, and a positive relocation test. Generally no sulcus sign is present. If pain is the only symptom, the diagnosis may be somewhat more difficult to make. However, in these cases the apprehension and relocation tests are usually also positive. Frontal (AP) and axillary view X rays should be obtained. The best way to demonstrate an osseous Bankart injury or Hill-Sachs lesion is by means of an axillary X ray or a CT scan. The finding of a supplemental osseous injury should not determine whether the patient requires surgery or not, but it will reveal the direction of the dislocation and thus may be of significance for the choice of surgical method. MRI is seldom necessary in evaluating recurrent shoulder dislocations.
• Treatment: Recurrent shoulder dislocation is a benign condition. Recurrent dislocations are unpleasant for many younger and active older individuals, but gener-

ally dislocations will occur only infrequently, and the condition can be completely compatible with both work and leisure-time activities. Primary caregivers do not need to refer the patient for surgery unless the patient is unable to tolerate the subjective difficulty caused by the shoulder instability. Surgery to repair the Bankart injury consists of repairing the labrum ligament complex back to the glenoid rim (Bankart operation). It is usually also necessary to tighten up the joint capsule and the glenohumeral ligaments.

- Treatment by physical therapist: For the first 6 weeks, external rotation of more than 0° and abduction of more than 90° are restricted to protect the repaired structures during initial healing. Subsequently, the patient retrains range of motion, balanced neuromuscular function and control, and strength. Sport-specific exercises and drills prepare the athlete for return to play. The patient may return to full activity after 3 to 6 months, depending on the type of activity and sport.
- Prognosis: The Bankart operation is a safe method of providing freedom from recurrence of dislocations in more than 90% of the cases.

Labral Injury—SLAP lesion

In addition to Bankart injuries, trauma often results in other injuries to the glenoid labrum. If the patient falls on an outstretched arm or is subject to strong eccentric contraction involving the long head of the biceps brachii muscle, the labrum-biceps tendon complex may be torn from the upper portion of the glenoid, resulting in a superior labral anterior to posterior (SLAP) lesion (figure 7.17).

- Symptoms and signs: Patients with a SLAP lesion often have pain in the upper or posterior part of the shoulder, especially when they externally rotate or abduct their shoulder. They also have a feeling of instability, sliding, or clicking in the joint.
- Diagnosis: The diagnosis is based on the clinical history and on positive provocative testing on physical examination, which may include O'Brien's test and the crank test. The patient often has clinical signs of anterior instability. However, the diagnosis may be difficult to make on clinical grounds alone. Arthroscopy or MR arthrography are useful imaging adjuncts when the diagnosis is uncertain in cases of chronic post-traumatic shoulder pain.

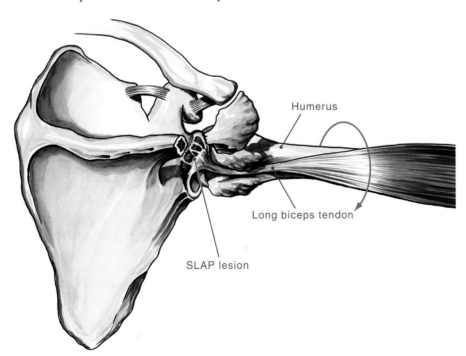

Humerus

Long biceps tendon

SLAP lesion

Figure 7.17 SLAP lesion. Tearing the labrum-biceps tendon complex away from the upper portion of the glenoid.

- Treatment: Patients who are suspected of having a SLAP lesion should be referred for arthroscopy of the shoulder and possible surgical repair of the lesion.
- Treatment by physical therapist: Rehabilitation follows the same principles as discussed for surgical repair of a Bankart injury, but it is also necessary to restrict eccentric loading of the long biceps tendon for 6 to 8 weeks after the operation.
- Prognosis: In most cases the prognosis is good.

Multidirectional Instability

Multidirectional instability never results from a single injury but rather is caused by a longer process in which repeated minor injuries stretch out the joint capsule and the associated ligaments. Congenital generalized joint laxity is a predisposing factor. Multidirectional instability is common in younger athletes, especially girls. Symptoms first appear after persistent excessive loading or repeated trauma—for example, if an athlete trains more for throwing than her tissue can tolerate. Throwers often have increased external rotation and reduced internal rotation, which also predisposes them to stress on the anterior-inferior capsule and ligaments. Therefore, the condition occurs most often in sports with skills that demand particularly extreme movement of the shoulder joint (often to the end of range), such as throwing overhead or selected swimming strokes. When loading exceeds the tissue's intrinsic ability to tolerate and adapt to it, the capsule and ligaments gradually become overstretched (figure 7.18, a-c). Initially, the dynamic shoulder stabilizers can compensate through increased muscular activity, but continued activity results in rotator cuff fatigue, making it impossible to stabilize the humeral head in the glenoid fossa. The situation generally worsens because the scapulothoracic muscles cannot stabilize the scapula in an optimal position with respect to the humerus.

This may result in rotator cuff injury. Direct contact may be made between the rotator cuff, the acromion, and the coracoacromial ligament at the end of a throwing motion, which may cause inflammation in the subacromial space and damage to the bursal side of the rotator cuff. This condition is called secondary impingement. At the beginning of the throwing motion, when the arm is abducted and externally rotated, the humeral head may slide forward due to capsular laxity, thereby creating irritation between the medial aspect of the supraspinatus and the superior posterior portion of the glenoid. This mechanism can result in both a labral injury and supraspinatus tendinopathy, and has been referred to as internal impingement (figure 7.18).

- Symptoms and signs: Multidirectional instability in active young patients with secondary rotator cuff injuries is often quite a challenging problem to diagnose. The shoulder has usually never been dislocated before, and the primary presenting complaint is that of pain. Therefore, this condition may be thought to be simply subacromial pain, and it is as a result easy to treat incorrectly. An accurate clinical history is important. The clinical examination usually produces a positive translation test both anteriorly and posteriorly. A positive sulcus sign is often present, and the apprehension and relocation tests are positive. Signs of inflammation, tendinosis, and impingement of the rotator cuff, with positive isometric tests and impingement tests, are often present. These are distinguished from primary subacromial impingement because they have a positive relocation sign (unlike in patients with subacromial impingement), and they generally affect young patients.
- Diagnosis: Diagnosis is made on the basis of the clinical examination. Radiographic evaluation is recommended to rule out other skeletal injuries, but plain imaging is usually unremarkable. Magnetic resonance arthrography may demonstrate increased joint volume, and secondary impingement may result in abnormal signal intensity in both the posterior portion of the glenoid labrum and the supraspinatus tendon. However, laxity testing comparing both shoul-

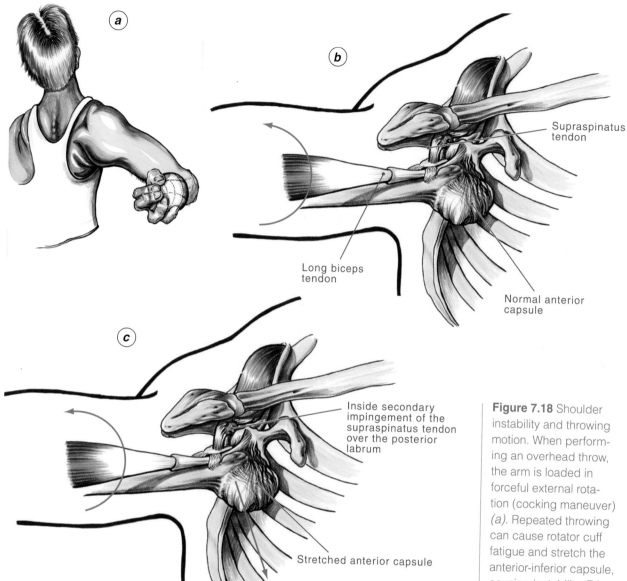

Figure 7.18 Shoulder instability and throwing motion. When performing an overhead throw, the arm is loaded in forceful external rotation (cocking maneuver) *(a)*. Repeated throwing can cause rotator cuff fatigue and stretch the anterior-inferior capsule, causing instability. Friction between the supraspinatus tendon and the posterior labrum may injure these structures *(b and c)*.

ders under general anesthesia and arthroscopy is the best method of making the proper diagnosis.

- Treatment by physical therapist: The main therapy for multidirectional instability and secondary rotator cuff pain is a long-term, goal-oriented rehabilitation program. The patient should be removed from the activity or sport that caused the condition and allowed to rest. Good communication is necessary between the caregiver, the athlete, and the trainer or coach, because a standardized rehabilitation program takes a minimum of 20 weeks before the patient may return to sport training. Therefore, everyone involved in the rehabilitation process (including the athlete and the physical therapist), needs to be highly motivated. Treatment should be provided by a physical therapist with a special interest in shoulder rehabilitation. The rehabilitation program is based on stretching the posterior structures, on strengthening the rotator cuff and the scapular stabilizing musculature, and on improving the neuromuscular control of the shoulder complex. After 20 weeks, progressive training for throwing or other sport-specific training may begin.

- Treatment by physician: If symptoms are still present despite a well-coordinated rehabilitation program, surgery may be indicated. If surgery is required, it will be necessary to tighten the joint capsule. Rehabilitation follows the same general guidelines outlined for the primary conservative treatment. Throwers must not throw at full speed until 1 year after the operation.
- Prognosis: The prognosis is worse after surgical intervention for multidirectional instability than after operative treatment of posttraumatic instability, as only 50% of throwers return to their original level of activity.

Subacromial Pain Syndrome—Impingement Syndrome

In the subacromial pain syndrome, the pain is related to the tendons of the rotator cuff muscles, including the supraspinatus tendon, the infraspinatus tendon, the biceps tendon, and the associated subacromial bursa (figure 7.19, a-c). Pain in this syndrome is thought to occur when these soft-tissue structures become inflamed or undergo degeneration—in either case resulting in an increase in the volume occupied in the subacromial space. This, in turn, may cause impingement of the tendinous structures as they pass underneath the acromion and the coracoacromial ligament, particularly when the shoulder is abducted. Repeated injuries and degeneration of the supraspinatus tendon are a typical cause of the impingement syndrome. The diagnosis may be difficult to make in athletes. It is especially difficult to diagnose against multidirectional instability, which may cause secondary impingement in young athletes. Subacromial pain syndrome compromises the function of the rotator cuff (which is to stabilize the humeral head in the glenoid fossa). Without the rotator cuff functioning as an effective depressor of the humeral head, the deltoid muscle pulls the humerus even further superiorly, resulting in progressive worsening of the subacromial impingement syndrome. It also reduces shoulder function, limits voluntary range of motion even further, and alters the scapulohumeral rhythm. The natural history of the condition begins with tendinitis or tendinosis and may progress to severe rotator cuff degeneration and may potentially lead to a rotator cuff tear. Three stages of rotator cuff dysfunction have been described: stage 1 is acute inflammation, with swelling and edema in the rotator cuff, stage 2 is scar formation and a chronic irreversible change in the rotator cuff. Stage 3 represents the final stage, with increasing degeneration and rupture.

- Symptoms and signs: The patient is usually more than 40 years of age. However, if the patient is an 18-year-old swimmer or athletic thrower with subacromial pain syndrome, the clinician should strongly suspect the diagnosis of multidirectional instability with secondary impingement. The onset of symptoms is often related to minor or to repeated trauma, to a long career in sport, or to a job that demands repetitive overload of the shoulder. Pain is often nonspecific at first but later localizes to the anterio-lateral surface of the acromion and the AC joint. Night pain is typical for this condition, and the patient often has difficulty lying on the affected shoulder. It is painful to carry, and especially to lift, objects with the elbow extended above shoulder level. The typical painful arc is between roughly 70° and 130° of abduction, at which point the affected soft-tissue structures are trapped between the acromion and the humeral head. Both active and passive shoulder motion are often reduced because of pain and weakness. Scapulohumeral rhythm is generally compromised on the affected side, and there is often contracture of the posterior glenohumeral joint capsule. The patient with impingement syndrome may also demonstrate mild weakness of upper limb flexion, abduction, and external rotation at the shoulder.
- Diagnosis: The diagnosis is made after a physical examination of the shoulder, including an assessment of glenohumeral joint stability. Atrophy of the supraspinatus muscle may be present, particularly if the patient has chronic pain. Findings on

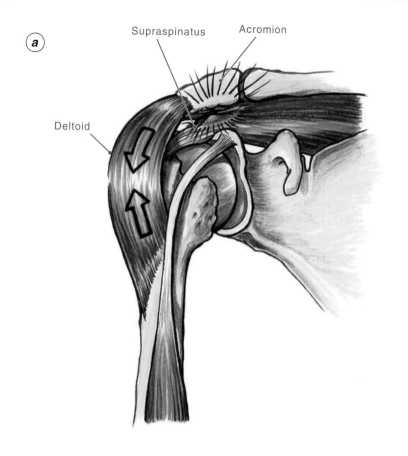

(a) Supraspinatus Acromion

Deltoid

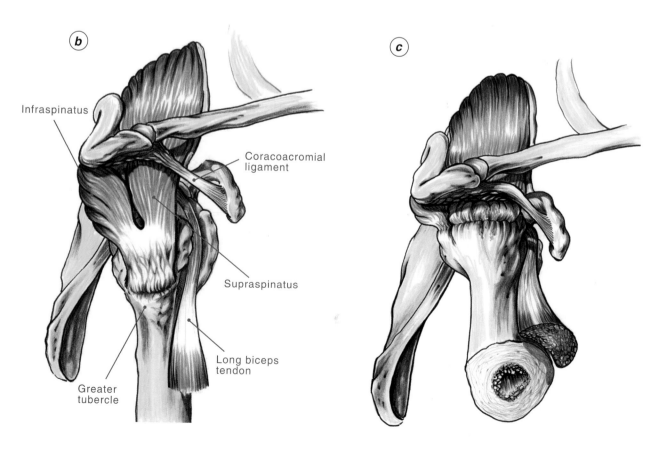

(b) Infraspinatus

Coracoacromial ligament

Supraspinatus

Long biceps tendon

Greater tubercle

(c)

Figure 7.19 Subacromial impingement of the rotator cuff. Impingement impairs the ability of the supraspinatus and the infraspinatus to depress the humeral head. Relatively unopposed, the deltoid pulls the head up toward the acromion and makes subacromial impingement *(a)* worse. When the arm is at the patient's side, the insertion of the supraspinatus and infraspinatus tendons onto the greater tubercle occurs laterally to the acromion *(b)*. When the arm is abducted, the tendons will come into contact with the anterior underside of the acromion and the coracoacromial ligament and impingement occurs *(c)*.

palpation may be variable, but generally tenderness is present over the site where the supraspinatus tendon inserts onto the greater tubercle of the humerus (beneath the anterolateral corner of the acromion). Shoulder range of motion is generally limited, especially abduction, internal rotation, and flexion. The scapulohumeral rhythm is also altered. Muscle strength is generally reduced, especially when the supraspinatus is tested. Pain provoked by isometric activation is diagnostic for tendinosis. The Neer and Hawkins signs are diagnostic for impingement. To confirm the diagnosis, the impingement tests can be repeated after the patient is given a subacromial injection of local anesthesic. Reduction of symptoms following the injection is considered diagnostic of impingement syndrome. Some patients with chronic subacromial pain may develop osteophytes beneath the acromion. These osteophytes represent ossification of the coracoacromial ligament at its insertion. If inflammation is long-standing, calcium deposition may also occur at the tendon's insertion. The osteophytes and calcium deposits are visible as shadows on X rays. Special radiographic views, including the supraspinatus outlet view, may help determine the shape of the acromion. A type 1 acromion is very flat, allowing for satisfactory subacromial space. The type 2 acromion has a curved shape, and a type 3 acromion has a hooked shape that tends to reduce the amount of subacromial space. Type 2 and 3 acromions are commonly associated with rotator cuff pathology. It is possible to distinguish between impingement and degenerative tears of the rotator cuff by using ultrasonography or magnetic resonance arthrography.

- Treatment: Treatment is mainly conservative, with a program that aims to improve the function of the rotator cuff and the musculature that stabilizes the scapula. Nonsteroidal anti-inflammatory drugs (NSAIDs) may be used to ease pain and enhance tolerance for rehabilitation activities. The subacromial injection of cortisone is controversial but may be useful during stage 1. Repeated injections increase the risk of degenerative rotator cuff partial or full-thickness tears. If conservative treatment does not produce a satisfactory result within 3 months, the patient is referred to a specialist for surgical evaluation. Operative intervention may include removal of the subacromial bursa and remodeling of the anterolateral underside of the acromion to make it flatter. At the same time the coracoacromial ligament insertion is released. Subsequent treatment follows the same principles as primary conservative treatment, with an emphasis on retraining range of motion and muscular control. The rehabilitation period generally lasts between 6 to 12 weeks, depending on the type of work or activity to which the patient is going to return.
- Prognosis: The results are good in about 80% of the patients, but it is not possible to predict whether the patient will return to work or sport activity that requires the full, unrestricted use of the shoulder, particularly if the patient is in stage 3.

Rotator Cuff Tears

Injuries to the supraspinatus tendon (figure 7.20, a and b) are a common cause of subacromial pain and limited shoulder function in middle-aged athletes and among individuals whose employment requires repetitive overhead or shoulder level work. The blood supply to the supraspinatus tendon is relatively poor, and repeated trauma can result in a spectrum of pathology, from rotator cuff degeneration to microtears to full-thickness tears. Tendon pathology usually begins anteriorly in the supraspinatus tendon in the area where the bicipital tendon penetrates the sulcus. Tendon degeneration and tearing may gradually spread proximally and involve the infraspinatus tendon over time. In the case of a massive rotator cuff tear, the biceps tendon will also be affected—either ruptured or dislocated out of the sulcus. There may be a concomitant tear of the upper portion of the subscapularis tendon as well. The size of the injury is often directly proportional to the clinical symptoms and functional deficit. Athletes in throwing sports may also sustain partial tears of the supraspinatus tendon as a result of eccentric overloading of the tendon during the

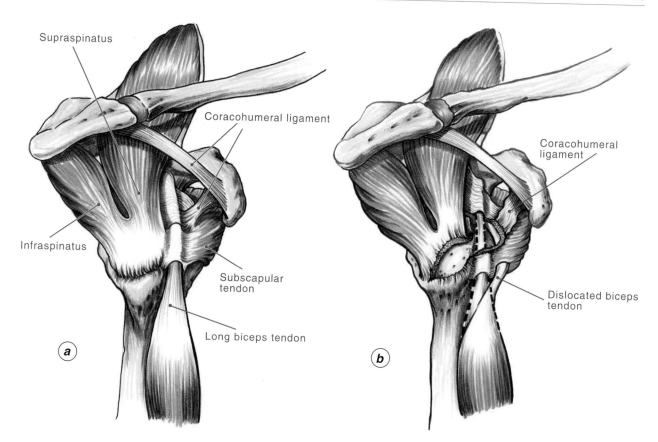

throwing motion. Such trauma to the tendon is frequently associated with rotator cuff tears and usually occurs on the undersurface of the tendon close to the shoulder joint.

- **Symptoms and signs:** The typical patient with a rotator cuff tear is older than 40 and has a history marked by repetitive loading of trauma to the glenohumeral joint. The patient may have had several episodes of acute shoulder pain and "inflammation" and have even received local corticosteroid injections. Physical examination findings are often the same as for patients with subacromial pain syndrome or impingement. The muscles of the rotator cuff may be weak, depending on the size of the tear. An ultrasound examination may be useful if performed by an experienced examiner. The patient should be given a dynamic examination; then both partial and complete tears may be found. Radiographic evaluation is carried out in the same manner as was discussed for subacromial impingement. If a significant tear is present, leakage through the rotator cuff into the subacromial space may be visible on CT arthrography scan, while an MRI examination is sensitive to both partial and complete rotator cuff tears. The disadvantage of MRI is its high cost.
- **Treatment:** The treatment of rotator cuff ruptures is controversial. The primary treatment of a rotator cuff tear is conservative and follows the same guidelines as treatment for subacromial pain syndrome, whether the patient is an athlete or not. Treatment is provided at the primary-care level. For long-term symptoms that do not respond to exercise therapy, the patient is referred for evaluation to consider surgery. Surgical treatment typically consists of acromial resection and possibly repair of the rotator cuff.
- **Prognosis:** A rotator cuff tear does not necessarily signal the end of the athlete's sporting career. Most athletes who have rotator cuff problems have only minor partial ruptures. The outcome of treatment, whether conservative or surgical, is usually good in these patients. Total rotator cuff tears are degenerative disorders

Figure 7.20 Rotator cuff tears. Normal anatomy of the rotator cuff, seen from the side, is shown (a). A complete rotator cuff tear usually begins anteriorly in the supraspinatus tendon and may expand posteriorly into the infraspinatus tendon. If the rupture goes anteriorly through the biceps tendon sheath, the coracohumeral ligament, and down into the subscapularis tendon, dislocation of the biceps tendon often follows (b).

that generally occur in the elderly and rarely happen in connection with sport activity. The functional outcome of rotator cuff repair is generally satisfactory. However, the results depend on how extensive the injury is, how many tendons are involved, and how far advanced the tendon and muscle degeneration has become. Patients may have to modify their routine activities or change their jobs.

Other Conditions

Recurrent Posterior Shoulder Dislocation

Sport-related recurrent posterior shoulder dislocation or subluxation are rare. The patient suspected of a posterior dislocation usually demonstrates clinical signs of posterior instability. Radiographic examinations and magnetic resonance arthrography may demonstrate a reverse Bankart injury. Clinically, the affected individual often complains of moderate discomfort. Treatment is conservative at first, employing exercises to correct muscular imbalance, and may be administered at the primary-level care. If the patient has persistent, disabling pain, surgery may be indicated. However, the frequency of recurrence and the risk of surgical complications are higher for posterior dislocation than they are for surgically corrected anterior dislocation.

Acromioclavicular (AC) Joint Osteoarthritis

Although the short-term outcome following an AC joint injury is generally good, some athletes proceed to develop painful arthrosis of the joint due to instability or intra-articular disk injury (figure 7.21, a and b). Weightlifting, particularly bench pressing, often leads to degenerative conditions in the joint, with resultant pain and development of osteoarthritis or distal clavicular osteolysis.

- Symptoms and signs: The clinical history is generally remarkable for a previous AC joint injury or a history of chronic repetitive overload, as in the case of weightlifters. Patients usually localize their pain and tenderness directly to the joint.
- Diagnosis: The diagnosis is based on tenderness to palpation directly over the joint, positive provocation tests, and pain relief upon local injection of anesthetic. In addition, there may be instability of the joint similar to that which may have occurred after a previous dislocation. The diagnosis is confirmed by X ray of the AC joint, which may demonstrate instability or the development of osteoarthritis.

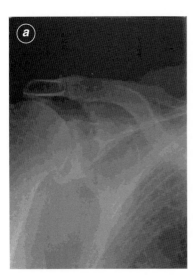 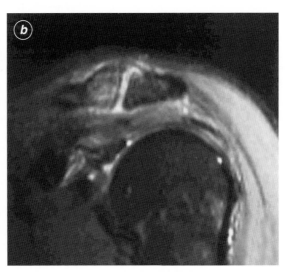

Figure 7.21 Acromioclavicular joint arthrosis. The X ray shows a narrow and uneven joint space *(a)*. MRI demonstrates reactive changes in the soft tissue and signals changes in the distal clavicle *(b)*.

- Treatment: Initial treatment is conservative. The patient is cared for at the primary care level with activity modification and local cortisone injections for pain relief. If this strategy does not succeed in providing relief from symptoms, the patient is referred for possible surgery.

Entrapment of the Suprascapular Nerve

The suprascapular nerve originates off the upper trunk of the brachial plexus and passes through the scapular notch and the spinoglenoid notch (figure 7.22). The nerve is vulnerable to injury in either passage, due to traction of the nerve from repeated activity with the arm abducted above shoulder level. Volleyball players are especially prone to developing suprascapular neuropathy, as are throwers, tennis players, and swimmers. Another potential cause of entrapment is direct compression by a ganglion cyst, which may develop in connection with a SLAP lesion.

- Symptoms and signs: The clinical signs and symptoms include atrophy (figure 7.23, a and b) and weakness of the infraspinatus muscle and possibly of the supraspinatus muscle, depending on the site of nerve entrapment. In addition the athlete may complain of pain posteriorly in the shoulder.
- Diagnosis: If the nerve is entrapped at the suprascapular notch, proximal to the origin of the motor branch to the supraspinatus, testing of both the supraspinatus muscle and the infraspinatus muscle will reveal atrophy and weakness, and resisted external rotation and abduction may cause pain. If the infraspinatus is affected in isolation, the nerve is affected more distally in the spinoglenoid notch. EMG may be used to confirm the diagnosis. An MRI should be performed to exclude a ganglion cyst.

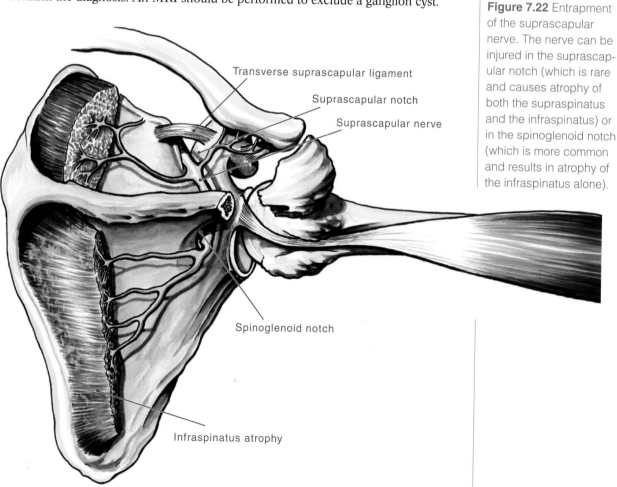

Transverse suprascapular ligament

Suprascapular notch

Suprascapular nerve

Spinoglenoid notch

Infraspinatus atrophy

Figure 7.22 Entrapment of the suprascapular nerve. The nerve can be injured in the suprascapular notch (which is rare and causes atrophy of both the supraspinatus and the infraspinatus) or in the spinoglenoid notch (which is more common and results in atrophy of the infraspinatus alone).

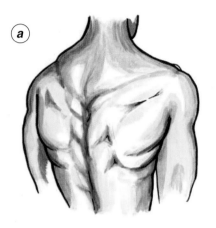
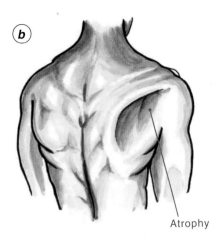

Atrophy

Figure 7.23 Infraspinatus atrophy. Normal muscle volume *(a)*; atrophy of the infraspinatus *(b)*.

• Treatment: If the patient has a ganglion cyst, surgery is indicated. In other situations, initial treatment is conservative and consists of interruption in or modification of activity and a rehabilitation program for the rotator cuff. If satisfactory function has not been achieved after 6 to 12 months, surgery should be considered. Surgical release of the nerve often relieves pain and sometimes atrophy as well.

Adhesive Capsulitis (Frozen Shoulder) !

Adhesive capsulitis, or frozen shoulder, is a relatively rare condition. The joint capsule becomes inflamed, resulting in formation of intra-articular adhesions that in turn lead to increasing stiffness of the joint capsule, eventually causing typical joint contracture. The fact that both surgical and conservative treatment will worsen the course must not be overlooked. The reason why treatment is ineffective is unknown. The condition is best described as painful, restricted shoulder movement.

• Symptoms and signs: The patient has significant pain, and both active and passive range of motion are severely restricted. Motion that does exist generally follows a capsular pattern where abduction takes place almost exclusively between the scapula and the chest wall. External rotation is usually quite limited. The natural history of adhesive capsulitis can be divided into three stages, each of which may last up to half a year. The first stage is the stiffening stage, during which there is pain and restricted motion. In the second stage the condition is static, and in the third stage the pain ceases and the shoulder "thaws out." Taken together, these three stages often last from 1 to 2 years.
• Diagnosis: Typical clinical examination findings are limited range of motion and a capsular movement pattern. It is necessary to distinguish between idiopathic adhesive capsulitis and a rotator cuff rupture with secondary shoulder stiffness. Supplemental radiographic and MRI examinations are of limited value, but magnetic resonance arthrography may demonstrate reduced capsular volume or a rotator cuff rupture.
• Treatment: The natural history of the condition is typically benign, and attempted interventions are generally ineffective and may worsen the condition. Active rehabilitation usually has a negative effect and will restrict movement even further. Manipulation and surgery are contraindicated. Postural and relaxation exercises for the neck musculature may be helpful and provide some pain relief. As mentioned previously, the condition will eventually resolve spontaneously. The practitioner should inform the patient that the expected outcome of the condition is in most cases favorable.

Rehabilitation of Shoulder Injuries

Hilde Fredriksen and Arne Kristian Aune

Goals and Principles

Table 7.3 lists the goals of shoulder injury rehabilitation.

Acute injuries almost always result in dysfunction of the affected body part, and this is especially true for the shoulder, where the pain and swelling of an injury easily alters the scapulohumeral rhythm. To prevent this from changing the athlete's movement pattern (which in turn could predispose the athlete to new injuries), the athlete must be prescribed an individualized rehabilitation training program developed to restore the athlete to their prior functional status.

Important Factors in Shoulder Injury Rehabilitation

Rotator cuff training. The rotator cuff balances the humeral head in the glenoid fossa, so that the joint rotates on physiological axes. For example, the subscapularis

	Goals	Measures
Phase 1	Reduce swelling	PRICE principle
Phase 2	Reduce pain	Possibly short-term immobilization
	Improve the movement pattern in the shoulder girdle as a whole:	Exercise within the limits of pain, with emphasis on scapulohumeral rhythm, range-of-motion training, and sensory motor training
	• Strengthen the rotator cuff	
	• Stabilize the scapula	
Phase 3	Restore the normal movement pattern in the shoulder girdle as a whole:	Functional exercises
	• Strengthen the rotator cuff	Sport-specific training
	• Stabilize the scapula	Recover completely before engaging in maximum activity
	• Improve range of motion	
	• At a minimum, reach the same neuromuscular function, strength, and range of motion as before the injury	
	Reduce the risk of reinjury	

Table 7.3 Goals and measures for rehabilitation of shoulder injuries.

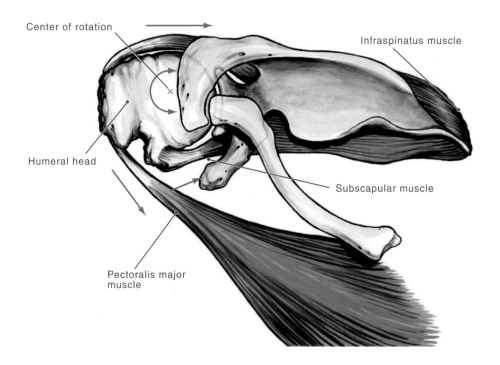

Center of rotation

Infraspinatus muscle

Humeral head

Subscapular muscle

Pectoralis major
muscle

Figure 7.24 Role of internal rotation. The pectoralis major muscle has an anterior force component that contributes to anterior translation of the humeral head. Thus, activation of the pectoralis major muscle causes anterior translation of the humeral head.

muscle and the pectoral muscles are both internal rotators in the shoulder. If their insertions and action angles on the humerus were examined, it would be obvious that in their function as internal rotators they have very different functions in the glenohumeral joint (figure 7.24).

The subscapularis muscle, by contrast, helps to center the humeral head in the glenoid fossa. Like the subscapularis muscle, the posterior muscles of the rotator cuff also play an important role in centering and stabilizing the humeral head in the glenoid fossa. Conversely, larger muscles, such as the pectoralis major, the deltoid, and the latissimus dorsi, may potentially develop into major destabilizing elements in the shoulder. Hence, the role of the rotator cuff as a juxta-articular, stabilizing group of muscles is extremely important to shoulder girdle function. The best way to train the rotator cuff is by low loading (<30% of one repetition maximum), with numerous repetitions throughout the entire rehabilitation period. Early in the rehabilitation period it may also be necessary to train the rotator cuff in isolation, while supporting the arm, to isolate movement to the extent possible. However, as soon as possible, the rotator cuff should be trained in large movement patterns that also require scapular stabilization. When throwing athletes approach the end of their rehabilitation program, eccentric training of the posterior portion of the rotator cuff is particularly important. The quality of and the manner in which the exercises are done is crucial because it controls the progression of rehabilitation.

Restoring normal coordinated scapular movement. It is of limited help to center the humeral head in the glenoid fossa if the ability to stabilize the scapula is also limited. Good scapular control is necessary to provide a stable base for arm movement, both to maintain the glenoid fossa in a position that provides the greatest possible congruence with the humeral head and to ensure proper positioning of the scapula. The ability to stabilize the scapula is often reduced after the injury sequence because of pain-based inhibition of the serratus anterior muscle and the trapezius muscle. The initial goal of scapular stabilization exercises is not necessarily to increase strength and range of motion but to develop good coordination between movements in the humerus and scapula. As shown in exercises 7.7 and 7.8, sling exercise therapy is an ideal closed kinetic chain exercise for the shoulder, as it simultaneously challenges both proprioceptive and neuromuscular control. At the beginning of the rehabilitation process it may be helpful to do exercises in the plane of the scapula–that is, with the humerus in abduction at about 30° flexion anteriorly. In this plane, conditions are optimal for stabilizing the humeral head in the glenoid fossa. With more than 90° abduction, there will be more space under the acromion if exercises are done in the plane of the scapula rather than at full abduction, thus reducing the possibility of impingement and inflammation.

Satisfactory range of motion in the spine. Increased thoracic kyphosis and restricted thoracic extension reduce arm movement as a whole and worsen the working conditions for the scapular musculature, thus increasing the risk of poor glenohumeral joint function. If poor spinal mechanics are detected, the physical therapist should perform both mobilization and exercise therapy.

Satisfactory internal rotation and horizontal adduction in the glenohumeral joint. Throwing sports often result in increased external rotation and decreased internal rotation of the shoulder. Reduced internal rotation is caused by posterior capsular contracture and muscle tightness, and may increase anterior translation of the humeral head and thereby contribute to anterior instability. The patient often needs help stretching out this type of posterior contracture.

Dosage. The manner in which the exercises are done depends on the goal:

- Circulation and movement: Light loading and numerous repetitions are performed.
- Maximum strength: Up to six repetitions with maximum loading are performed.
- Increased range of motion: Patient relaxes in the extreme position to allow for stretching.
- Stabilization: Patient holds contraction in the extreme position to control movement.
- Eventually, the main emphasis of the rehabilitation program for athletes should be on plyometric exercises, in which rapid shifting from eccentric to concentric muscle action occurs.

During the last stage of rehabilitation, the practitioner should place increasing emphasis on sport-specific training, incorporating more plyometric exercises.

Return to Sport

It is advisable to compare the strength, neuromuscular function, and flexibility of the injured side with the healthy side before the player is considered to be fully rehabilitated. Athletes in throwing sports need to realize that the throwing arm normally has increased external rotation and reduced internal rotation and is typically stronger than the contralateral (uninjured) arm. In throwing sports, before the athlete returns to play he must have completed a throwing training program (throwing and catching) of progressive intensity and must have trained at maximal intensity without pain before being allowed to compete. Athletes in team sports also should train in practice games before being allowed to compete. Specific functional tests must be adjusted according to the requirements of the individual sport.

Preventing Reinjury

It is possible to reduce the risk of reinjury by means of optimal rehabilitation, and by paying as much attention as possible to the factors mentioned. By definition, optimal rehabilitation consists of healing all the involved structures and ensuring that the patient has normal scapulohumeral rhythm and neuromuscular function, strength, and range of motion. Posttraumatic and multidirectional instability offer the greatest rehabilitation challenges in connection with sport-related shoulder injuries. Athletes often have very strong muscles for gross arm movements, including the pectoralis major and latissimus dorsi muscles. Therefore, the physician must make sure that the rotator cuff functions correspondingly well. This will ensure that the glenohumeral joint moves on physiological axes, so that every throw or swimming stroke does not increase translation. Training for stability involves holding the inner musculature in its path of motion to allow controlled eccentric movement as far out in the path of motion as possible. It is absolutely essential to train the shoulder in the portion of the path where stability is worst and the chance of subluxation or repeat dislocation is greatest.

Exercise Program

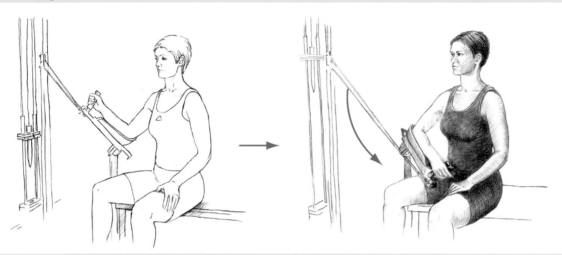

Exercise 7.1 Sitting shoulder rotation (with support)

- Internal rotation: Attach rope at the hand (as shown in the figure).
- External rotation: Attach rope at the elbow.
- In the final position the rope needs to be almost parallel to the forearm.
- Progression: Increase degree of abduction (in the plane of the scapula) in the shoulder joint.

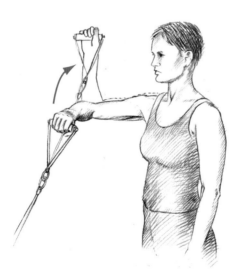

Exercise 7.2 Standing shoulder rotation (without support)

- This exercise requires a great ability to stabilize the scapula.
- External rotation: Stand facing the pulley apparatus (as in the figure).
- Internal rotation: Stand with your back to the pulley apparatus.
- In the final position, the rope must be almost parallel to your forearm.
- Progression: Increase degree of abduction (in the plane of the scapula) in the shoulder joint.

SHOULDER

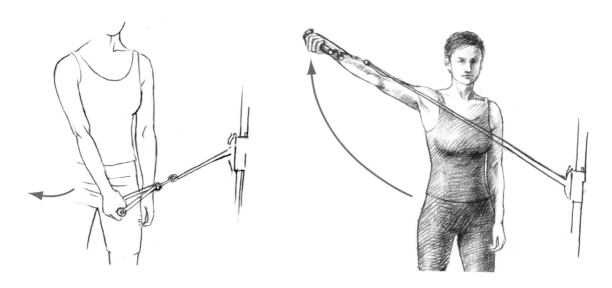

Exercise 7.3 Abduction in the plane of the scapula

- Stand with your side to the pulley apparatus.
- Push down your shoulder and pull out to the side in the plane of the scapula with your thumb on top.
- In the extreme position, the rope must be parallel to your arm.
- Progression: Increase degree of abduction.

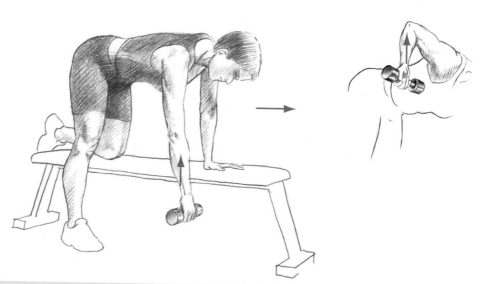

Exercise 7.4 Single-handed rowing motion

- Position yourself with your left hand and knee on the bench.
- Pull your right scapula backward and downward; lift your elbow while your forearm is externally rotated. Hold in the upper position, and restrain your scapula on the way down.
- Include rotation in the thorax at the end of the movement.
- If anterior instability is present, make sure that you don't lift your elbow too high.

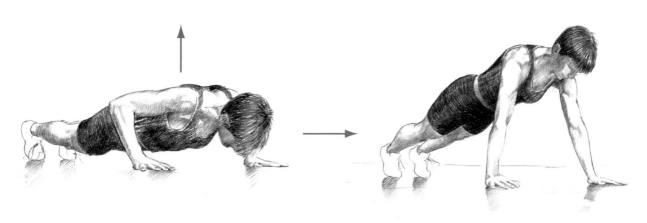

Exercise 7.5 Push-ups with a plus

- Lie on your abdomen with your palms on the floor, shoulder-width apart.
- Keep your back straight, extend your arms, and push up between your scapulae.
- Easier: Do exercise with your hands against the wall or on a step, or with your knees on the floor.
- Progression: Place feet on a step or hang in a sling.

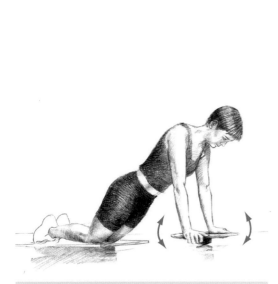

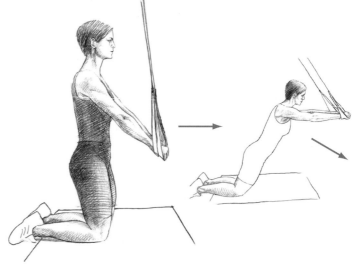

Exercise 7.6 Neuromuscular training

- Stand in the push-up position with your hands on a balance board or in a sling.
- Progression: Keep knees on the floor, feet on the floor.
- Stand at rest and do "small" push-ups, then regular push-ups.
- Use two hands, then use one hand.
- Lean on one hand, and throw a ball or similar object with the other hand.

Exercise 7.7 Shoulder flexion and extension in slings

- Focus on control in the extreme position.
- Kneel with your arms stretched forward.
- Tense your abdominal and back muscles and lean forward. Hold in extreme position.
- Then pull your body back again by pressing your arms downward.
- Progression: Gradually lean farther and farther forward.
- Position yourself farther back from the plumb line of the rope.
- Keep less distance between the sling and the floor.

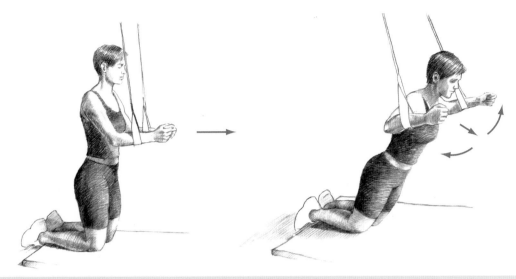

Exercise 7.8 Horizontal abduction and adduction in slings

- Kneel, with the body leaning forward over the elbows bent at 90°.
- Tense your abdominal and back muscles, gently extend your arms out to the sides and lean your body forward. Focus on control in the extreme position; hold. Pull your body back again by pressing your arms together.
- Progression: Gradually extend your arms farther out to the sides.
- Position yourself farther back from the plumb line of the rope.
- Keep less distance between the sling and the floor.

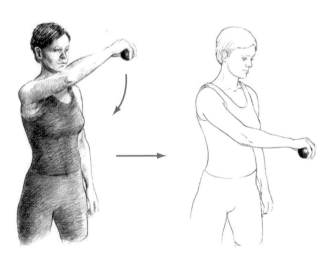

Exercise 7.9 Eccentric training of the internal rotator musculature

- Catch a ball in front of your body.
- Stabilize the scapula and release and catch the ball again or stop it on the way down.
- Progression: Use heavier balls.

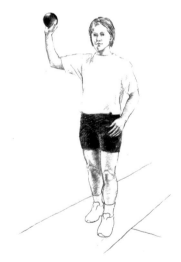

Exercise 7.10 Plyometric training of the internal rotator musculature

- Throw and catch a ball, emphasizing the transitional stage.
- Abduct the shoulder and flex the elbow.
- Progression: Abduct or elevate the shoulder more.
- Progression: Receive harder throws or use greater speed during the transitional stage.

Elbow and Arm 8

Acute Elbow Injuries

Stein Tyrdal

Occurrence

Acute elbow injuries constitute a small portion (3% to 6%) of all sports injuries. Although most athletes with acute elbow injuries are able to continue their activity (sometimes at a reduced level of performance), these injuries can occasionally be career-ending. The elbow joint is the joint most frequently dislocated among children. Among adults, the elbow is the second most commonly dislocated joint (after the shoulder), with an annual incidence of six to eight injuries per 100,000 inhabitants.

Differential Diagnosis

Table 8.1 provides an overview of the most common acute elbow injury diagnoses. Fractures near the elbow are serious but very seldom result from sport-related activity. In children, falls often cause supracondylar fractures of the humerus. Ten to twenty percent of elbow dislocations are accompanied by fractures. In a few sports, particularly throwing sports like javelin and baseball, elbow injuries are common. However, most of the elbow injuries in these sports are related to overuse. The young athlete who sustains an elbow injury as a result of a fall should be carefully examined to rule out ligament damage and/or dislocation. The practitioner should know that this type of trauma in older athletes can cause a wrist fracture. Cartilaginous injuries sometimes occur alone or in combination with ligament injuries or fractures. In children, the growth plates may be injured as well.

Most common	Less common	Must not be overlooked (!)
Sprain (p. 194)	Elbow dislocation (p. 195)	Apophyseal fracture (p. 198)
	Medial collateral ligament rupture (p. 197)	Monteggia fracture (p. 201)
	Antebrachial fracture (p. 200)	Galeazzi fracture (p. 202)
	Supracondylar fracture of the humerus (p. 199)	Radius fracture (p. 231)
	Olecranon fracture (p. 199)	Vascular damage (p. 204)
	Acute olecranon bursitis (p. 204)	Nerve injury (p. 204)
	Distal biceps tendon rupture (p. 202)	Posttraumatic stiffness (p. 204)
	Triceps tendon rupture (p. 203)	

Table 8.1 Overview of the differential diagnosis of acute elbow injuries.

ELBOW AND ARM

In the narrow elbow region there are many structures that can impinge on the nerves that pass through, and nerve irritation is therefore not uncommon. Even if tumors rarely occur, they should be considered within the differential diagnosis.

Diagnostic Thinking

Most elbow injuries can be treated at the primary-care level. The practitioner rarely has a problem distinguishing between sprains (such as partial ligament tears) and dislocations or major fractures. The challenge is to determine which injuries may cause problems later on; these should be immediately referred to an orthopedic surgeon for timely evaluation. It is often difficult to arrive at a prognosis, and over-looked injuries or rehabilitation that is too vigorous can result in range of motion deficits, particularly in extension. Limited range of motion and hemarthrosis are signs of severe intra-articular injuries. Therefore, patients with limited range of motion or intra-articular fluid must be x-rayed. A precise clinical examination, during which the osseous protrusions and landmarks are palpated, is also necessary to determine whether the patient should be x-rayed to exclude fractures.

Most elbow trauma causes only minor injuries, such as capsular injuries, partial ligament injuries, minor cartilaginous injuries, or small osteochondral fractures. However, since advanced cross-sectional imaging is rarely indicated, sprain is often used as a diagnosis of exclusion following plain radiography.

Therefore, the goals of the clinical examination during the acute phase should be (1) to determine that the elbow is not dislocated, (2) to rule out damage to the regional vasculature and peripheral nerves, and (3) to exclude significant fractures. If the most threatening diagnoses can be excluded by means of a clinical examination, further examinations are unnecessary during the acute phase. A minor fracture may be over-looked on a plain X ray during the primary examination, but such an injury does not require immobilization or surgery.

The practitioner must avoid unnecessary or long-term immobilization. The elbow joint of an adult cannot be immobilized for longer than 3 weeks without a significant risk of permanent joint contracture.

Clinical History

The most common injury mechanism in sport is a fall on an outstretched arm, with simultaneous valgus stress and forearm supi-nation (figure 8.1). Other common injury mecha-nisms include traffic acci-dents and direct trauma. Falls directly on the elbow and blunt injuries to the olecranon may cause an olecranon fracture.

In case of a fall on an out-stretched (or nearly out-stretched) arm, the radius and the ulna twist away

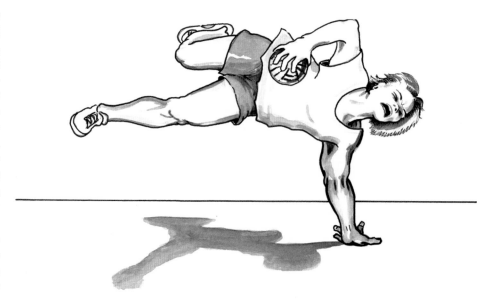

Figure 8.1 Injury mecha-nism. Falling on a nearly outstretched arm is the most common cause of elbow dislocations.

from the humerus laterally by means of combined supination and valgus stress. Most often this type of trauma causes only a sprain. If greater force is involved, total ligament ruptures with dislocation may occur, sometimes combined with fractures. In the case of dislocations, the lateral ligament complex is almost always torn first, while the medial collateral ligament may remain intact. Compression will cause most dislocations to occur posteriorly. Compression may also cause accompanying fractures in the lateral column (the capitulum humeri and the head of the radius) and in the coronoid process. When falling on an outstretched arm, the athlete often lands on the wrist first. Therefore, the physician should also check for accompanying injuries near the wrist and in the shoulder area, first clinically and then possibly radiographically.

Acute trauma may also cause tendon ruptures. Athletes who sustain tendon ruptures have often had tendon pain in the past. Anabolic steroid abuse increases the risk of tendon rupture.

Clinical Examination

When faced with an acute injury, the practitioner must determine whether the patient has a severe injury–that is, a dislocation or fracture. Hemarthrosis and limited range of motion are signs of severe intra-articular injury that necessitate radiographic examination.

Inspection. Dislocated elbows and major elbow fractures will cause diffuse swelling around the elbow, malalignment, significant pain, and limited function with reduced active and passive range of motion. Occasionally, the vascular supply and nerve function may be affected. Active first aid may slightly reduce the pain. The diagnosis is often made by inspection.

Palpation. Palpation is usually painful, so it may be difficult to do an adequate examination. An effort should be made to palpate the osseous prominences and edges to determine whether these are smooth (as they are when there is a dislocation), or sharp (as they are when there is a fracture). Intra-articular fluid is relatively easy to detect by palpating the "soft spot," which is located in the middle of the lateral triangle (the three corners of this triangle are the lateral epicondyle, the anterior margin of the radial head, and the tip of the olecranon) (figure 8.2). Demonstrating fluctuance in the "soft spot" indicates that there is intra-articular fluid.

Neuromuscular function. It is seldom possible to evaluate neuromuscular function completely during the acute phase, because restriction due to pain is often significant. However, the practitioner must demonstrate any nerve injury as early as possible, because later it may be important to know when nerve injury actually started. Normally, hand movements can be examined to help determine whether muscles and nerves near the elbow are likely to be intact. Nerve function is examined as described in Chapter 9 (see figure 9.2, page 229).

Circulation. The physician must also evaluate circulation, because this can easily be overlooked in an acute situation. The capillary nail refill test is used to evaluate circulation. It is easiest to assess the pulse by palpating the radial artery or the ulnar artery, just

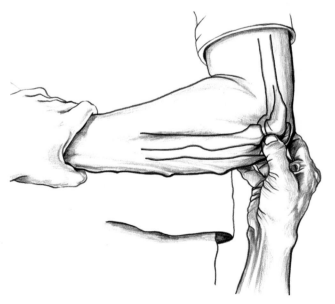

Figure 8.2 Palpation of the elbow to detect intra-articular fluid in the elbow. Fluctuation in the soft spot is a definite sign of joint effusion. The easiest way to find this point is to allow the thumb to slide anteriorly from the tip of the ulna along the lateral edge of the ulna.

ELBOW AND ARM

proximal to the wrist. Because of pain and swelling, it can be far more difficult to palpate the brachial artery in the elbow region.

Movement. The normal range of motion in the elbow joint is from full extension (0°) to 140° to 150° flexion, 75° pronation, and 85° supination. The best way to evaluate the available range of motion is by comparing one side with the opposite side and by using a goniometer. If the range of motion is reduced with a hard "end feel", a mechanical cause is indicated. If the "end feel" is soft or absent, it indicates pseudo-locking (i.e., joint range of motion is being limited by pain). The practitioner must remember to examine pronation and supination by twisting the forearm while the patient is holding something in his hand (like a pencil). Note that the elbow has to be fixed against the body; otherwise, it is difficult to evaluate the patient's ability to rotate the elbow because the patient often "cheats" by using the shoulder.

Stability Tests. During the acute phase, it is often difficult to assess stability because of pain. Pathological movement can usually be established, but more sophisticated tests should be delayed until the patient is under anesthesia.

Supplemental Examinations

Radiographic Examinations. Patients with intra-articular fluid or reduced range of motion after an acute injury should always be examined using frontal and lateral X rays. The physician must make sure that the forearm and the wrist are also examined if a combined injury is suspected, since these are often overlooked. Even if an elbow injury is found, this does not exclude a forearm or wrist injury (and vice versa).

Other X rays may be indicated:
- Oblique views will increase the accuracy of demonstrating minor accompanying fractures and can be helpful if the regular frontal and lateral views are difficult to interpret.
- Frontal and lateral X rays of the forearm are necessary if a fracture/dislocation injury is suspected.

Other diagnostic imaging methods:
- Examination of the elbow under fluoroscopy may be useful in evaluating additional fractures and interpositioned fragments, particularly if reduction is difficult.
- Scintigraphy, ultrasound, computed tomography (CT), and magnetic resonance imaging (MRI) are not normally indicated during the acute phase.

Common Injuries

Sprains

Elbow injuries in young athletes are usually caused by falling on an outstretched arm, throwing, or blows (direct and indirect) to the elbow. Most athletes do not seek medical assistance because the subjective symptoms are usually moderate and temporary. Most elbow trauma results in only minor injuries such as capsular injuries, partial ligament tears, minor cartilaginous injuries, or small osteochondral fractures. These types of small fractures are often not visible on the primary radiographic examination. Because treatment will be early mobilization in any case, it is rarely helpful to evaluate these fractures by using additional diagnostic imaging techniques. The swelling and pain that accompanies such injuries usually subside after a few days.

Elbow sprains are a diagnosis of exclusion in cases where the primary radiographic examination shows no direct signs of skeletal injury or indirect signs of ligament injury (dislocation of intact skeletal parts). The severity of pain caused by these types of injuries varies from person to person.

- Symptoms and signs: Pain, tenderness, swelling, and limited range of motion.
- Diagnosis: If there is intra-articular fluid or reduced range of motion, the patient *must* be referred for a radiographic examination. If the physician does not find objective signs of skeletal or ligament injury during the clinical examination, but the patient indicates that she is in a great deal of pain, she *should* be given a radiographic examination. If pain and swelling do not improve within a week, the patient *must* be referred for a radiographic examination and possibly for supplemental examinations. The clinical examination may demonstrate swelling and limited range of motion, but a sprain will often be a diagnosis of exclusion after supplemental examination(s) have excluded fractures or dislocations.
- Treatment by physician: PRICE treatment is indicated during the acute phase, possibly including nonsteroidal anti-inflammatory drugs (NSAIDs). Immobilization is not mandatory but may be necessary for a few days for pain relief. Sprains are treated using active range of motion exercises within the limits of pain, muscle strengthening, and protection against new trauma until activity is pain free.
- Treatment by physical therapist: The patient should be instructed in self-exercises that are tolerated within the limits of pain. All types of passive stretching should be avoided. When full range of motion (or a range of motion acceptable to the athlete) is achieved, strength training may begin.
- Prognosis: The prognosis is good; most athletes are able to resume full training in less than 3 weeks.

Other Injuries

Lateral Ligament Injury—Elbow Dislocation

In young athletes, injuries to the ligament structures on the outside of the elbow are usually the result of a fall on an outstretched arm. Ligament sprains may be classified according to how significant the associated joint instability is (figure 8.3, a-d). In grade I and II injuries, there is no significant instability, and most athletes will be diagnosed with a sprain injury without actually recognizing the extent of the injury to the lateral ligaments. Grade III injuries carry a risk of simultaneous medial ligament injury. Partial ruptures are probably the cause of many painful conditions on the lateral side of the elbow following minor trauma, such as a hyperextension injury. Lateral instability may also be a complication of a dislocated elbow or a result of excess detachment of the lateral ligament complex after surgery.

The practitioner must be aware that dislocations are often accompanied by fractures, such as fractures of the radial head (5% to 10%), avulsion injuries involving one of the condyles (medial or lateral, about 12%), and fractures of the coronoid process (10%). Major fractures predispose the athlete to recurrent dislocations. Osteochondral injuries, including fractures of the capitulum humeri, apparently occur with greater frequency than standard X rays would seem to indicate.

- Symptoms and signs: Grade I and II injuries cause swelling, tenderness, and occasional ecchymosis above the lateral epicondyle. Grade III injuries cause malalignment and severely limit range of motion. If the patient has a grade III injury, it is impossible to exclude accompanying fractures clinically. Note that in some cases, patients with dislocated elbows can still have a 90° range of motion with relatively

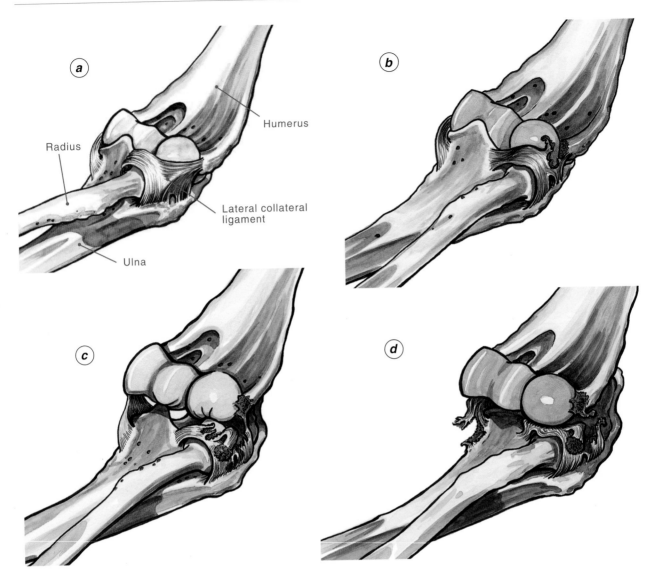

Radius

Humerus

Lateral collateral ligament

Ulna

little pain. The practitioner must remember to check the distal pulse and assess peripheral nerve function.

- Diagnosis: The diagnosis is made clinically, but standard frontal and lateral X rays are necessary to exclude fractures and dislocations of the radial head. Stability tests are of little value during the acute phase.
- Treatment by physician: Grade I and II injuries do not need to be immobilized and are treated with active range of motion exercises within the limits of pain, strength training, and protection against new trauma until pain-free activity is achieved. The ligament must be given time to heal before it is subjected to situations in which a risk of new trauma exists; otherwise, the injury can easily become chronic, resulting in pain that impairs function. A dislocated elbow (grade III) must be reduced immediately, but an X ray should be taken, if possible, before reduction. Rapid reduction is excellent pain therapy and decreases the inflammatory reaction. Dislocated elbows that cannot be reduced require surgery. After reduction, stability is tested, and the elbow is immobilized in accordance with table 8.2. Early movement prevents posttraumatic stiffness. Adults can tolerate a maximum of 3 weeks of immobilization; children can achieve full mobility even after 6 weeks of immobilization. Retraining should be pain-free; otherwise, minor bleeding, which leads to capsule shrinkage and reduced range of motion, may ensue. If full range of motion has not been achieved in 6 to 8 weeks, more aggressive therapy should be started (see the section on Posttraumatic Stiffness).

Figure 8.3 Spectrum of instability. Lateral ligament complex injuries are classified according to the degree of instability: Grade I *(a)*: distortion, partial ruptures without instability; Grade II *(b)*: posterolateral rotation instability—i.e., subluxation of the head of the radius with supination, axial compression, and valgus stress; Grade III: dislocated elbow. In Grade IIIa *(c)*, the humerus "rests" on the top of the coronoid process; in Grade IIIb *(d)*, the entire elbow is dislocated.

Stability after reduction	Treatment	Duration
Stable in all directions	Immediate active exercises	
Stable with pronation	Orthosis that prevents supination but allows flexion and extension	3 weeks maximum
Unstable with pronation	Orthosis (or possibly a cast) that prevents extension in the direction of instability	3 weeks maximum

Table 8.2 Guidelines for immobilization of dislocated elbows.

- Treatment by physical therapist: The patient should be instructed in a home program of exercises that are within the limits of pain. All types of passive stretching must be avoided. When full range of motion (or range of motion acceptable to the athlete) is achieved, strength training may begin.
- Prognosis: Up to 50% of all dislocations (with and without fractures) will result in late symptoms, such as reduced range of motion and strength, pain, or instability. The symptoms are related to the extent of the primary injury or accompanying injuries. It is possible to tolerate a slight limitation of extension in most sports. The prognosis is good for posterior dislocations without accompanying fractures that have been immobilized for 2 to 3 weeks.

Medial Collateral Ligament Rupture

The most common cause of medial collateral ligament ruptures (figure 8.4) is valgus stress—for example, from throwing (the javelin, baseball, or handball), from hyperextension (as in the case of handball goalie's elbow), or from falls. In most instances the ligament is only partially torn. Medial ligament injuries may also occur in combination with dislocations or fractures.

- Symptoms and signs: The primary symptom is medial elbow pain during activity. The principal finding on exam is focal tenderness to palpation and pain with valgus stress. If a total rupture has occurred, acute pain will be accompanied by swelling, ecchymosis, and a feeling of instability. Some patients also experience tingling in the two ulnar fingers, which is a sign of ulnar nerve irritation.
- Diagnosis: The diagnosis is made clinically using a valgus stress test, but a radiographic examination with standard elbow views is indicated to exclude fracture.

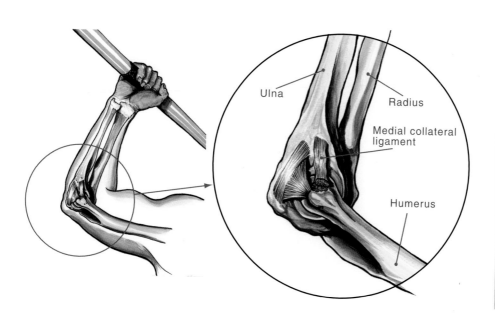

Ulna

Radius

Medial collateral ligament

Humerus

Figure 8.4 Medial ligament injury. Javelin throwing is a classic injury mechanism for tearing the medial collateral ligament in the elbow. Tearing usually occurs at the insertion to the humerus with repeated valgus stress and rotation.

- Treatment: Isolated medial ligament injuries are treated using PRICE treatment and the same functional treatment as for lateral ligament injuries.
- Prognosis: The prognosis is good, but it may take up to a year for the patient to become asymptomatic. Chronic pain will result if the injury is neglected and the athlete returns to play without adequate rehabilitation.

Fractures With Dislocations

In dislocations, the most common accompanying fractures involve the coronoid process, the radial head, and the capitulum humeri. Fractures may occur individually or in various combinations with and without dislocations.

- Symptoms and signs: Typical symptoms include pain, swelling, and reduced range of motion.
- Diagnosis: The diagnosis is made using standard and oblique X rays, with CT or MRI if necessary. Small fractures are often overlooked. If the primary X ray is negative and there is no clinical improvement, it is recommended that a follow-up X ray be obtained after a week.
- Treatment: The only treatment required for minor avulsion fractures is active exercises that are within the limits of pain. Larger fragments may require immobilization for up to 3 weeks, and surgery may be needed to treat dislocations.

Apophyseal Fracture—Little Leaguer's Elbow !

When a child falls on an outstretched arm, he may sustain an avulsion fracture at the site of insertion of the elbow flexor or extensor tendons (figure 8.5). Children may also sustain partial avulsion injuries with growth zone disturbance from intensive periods of repeated throwing (Little Leaguer's Elbow). The incidence is unknown, but about 12% of all growth zone injuries occur in the elbow, usually to individuals between the ages of 2 and 15 years. Unlike other growth plate injuries, boys are more vulnerable than girls.

- Symptoms and signs: The primary finding is distinct tenderness above one of the epicondyles.
- Diagnosis: The diagnosis is based on lateral and frontal X rays of the elbow.
- Treatment by physician: The elbow should be immobilized in a cast (usually for 3 weeks) to prevent painful pseudoarthrosis, followed by mobilization and rehabilitation as soon as pain allows it. If the fragment is displaced by more than 2 mm or is rotated, surgery is recommended.
- Prognosis: The prognosis is good, with normal function usually returning within 6 weeks. Growth disturbances are rare, because the epicondyles do not affect longitudinal growth nor do they articulate with the elbow joint. However, it is necessary to be aware of the possibility of intra-articular fragments since these may precipitate future osteoarthritis.

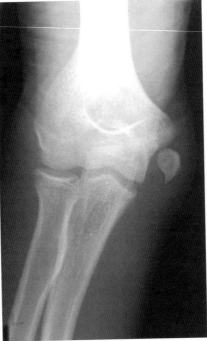

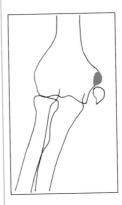

Figure 8.5 Apophysis fractures. When a child falls on an outstretched arm, an avulsion fracture may occur through the growth zone.

Supracondylar Fracture of the Humerus

In children, supracondylar (figure 8.6), diacondylar, transcondylar, and intercondylar fractures of the humerus total 50% to 60% of all fractures in the elbow area. Among boys, the left elbow is fractured more frequently, indicating that the left arm is used more often than the right arm to protect against falls. Because vessels and nerves lie in close proximity to the humerus, it is necessary to carefully examine the patient for vascular nerve injuries.

- Symptoms and signs: Symptoms include significant swelling and, if the fracture is displaced, obvious malalignment. To reduce the risk of skin damage, it is important to reduce and stabilize displaced supracondylar fractures immediately, before the patient is sent to the hospital for an X ray or before other measures are taken.
- Diagnosis: The diagnosis is made by X ray, using standard elbow views. Extra oblique views may be helpful if the standard views are difficult to interpret. The physician should also check skin color, distal capillary refill, the radial arterial pulse, and distal skin sensation.
- Treatment principles: The main goal of treatment is to restore the normal alignment and achieve anatomic healing with normal function. Treatment should take place at a hospital with the patient anesthetized. If there is no palpable pulse distally, the fracture must be reduced (by pulling the forearm in a longitudinal direction) and stabilized before the patient is transported to the hospital.

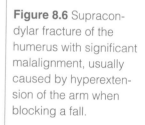

Figure 8.6 Supracondylar fracture of the humerus with significant malalignment, usually caused by hyperextension of the arm when blocking a fall.

Olecranon Fracture

Because of its superficial location, the olecranon is vulnerable to injury from direct trauma, such as falling on the elbow. Olecranon fractures are divided into three types, according to the Mayo classification system (figure 8.7). Type I fractures are nondisplaced, with minimal to no associated crush injury. Type II fractures are stable with displacement, with or without associated crush injury. Type III fractures (the least common) are unstable, with or without associated crush injury, and may have accompanying radial head fractures. If this is the case, it can be difficult to distinguish between a type III olecranon fracture and a Monteggia fracture.

- Symptoms and signs: If no dislocation has occurred, swelling is usually moderate. If a dislocation has occurred, more swelling is usually present because of bleeding from the fracture and the displaced olecranon fragment. Elbow extension is limited. Maximum tenderness is experienced at the level of the fracture. Because the olecranon is superficial, a defect is often palpable.
- Diagnosis: The diagnosis is made clinically, but a standard X ray series of the elbow is necessary. The practitioner must evaluate the need for X rays of the entire forearm.
- Treatment by physician: The goals of treatment are to (1) reconstruct the articular surface, (2) maintain muscle strength, (3) reestablish joint stability, (4) avoid joint stiffness, and (5) avoid complications. To achieve these goals, most olecranon fractures must be treated surgically at a hospital. Simple, nondisplaced, stable fractures

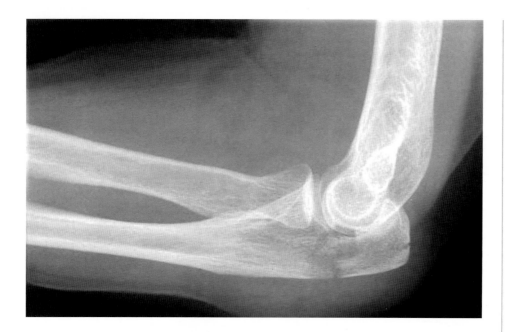

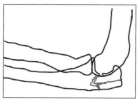

Figure 8.7 Olecranon fracture, usually caused by falling on the tip of the elbow and often requiring surgery.

(type I), which can be immobilized for 2 to 3 weeks represent exceptions to this rule. Repeat X rays should be taken after about 1 week to make sure that the fracture does not become displaced.

• Treatment by physical therapist: The exercise program emphasizes instruction in an independent exercise program within the patient's limits of pain. After the fracture is healed, exercises to improve range of motion are emphasized. However, it is important to be aware that osteosynthetic material may prevent full extension. Strengthening exercises begin after satisfactory range of motion is achieved.

• Prognosis: The prognosis is good but depends on the alignment achieved and on the location of osteosynthetic materials, because this will often affect the extension function of the triceps over the long term. Other complications include ulnar neuropathy, posttraumatic arthritis, instability, pseudoarthrosis, and local irritation of osteosynthetic materials.

Antebrachial Fracture

Antebrachial fractures involve simultaneous fractures of both the radial and the ulnar shafts (figure 8.8, a-c). Most commonly, children sustain these injuries as the result of a fall. Direct trauma (e.g., blows and kicks) may also result in a fracture of one or both forearm bones. A fracture in the ulnar shaft alone may indicate that there is a Monteggia fracture, particularly if the fracture is located proximally in the ulna.

• Symptoms and signs: Symptoms and signs include moderate swelling, obvious malalignment, total motor dysfunction, and significant pain. If the circulation or the skin is threatened by the severity of the injury, the fracture should be reduced and stabilized immediately before the patient is sent to the hospital.

• Diagnosis: The diagnosis is based on the apparent malalignment, but it may be difficult to distinguish this fracture from a Monteggia fracture. An X ray is necessary to confirm the diagnosis and to demonstrate the injuries. The practitioner must check skin color, distal capillary filling, and the radial arterial pulse, as well as distal skin sensation.

• Treatment by physician: The patient is referred to the hospital for immediate evaluation and possible surgery. Usually, however, reduction and immobilization in a high cast are the preferred interventions.

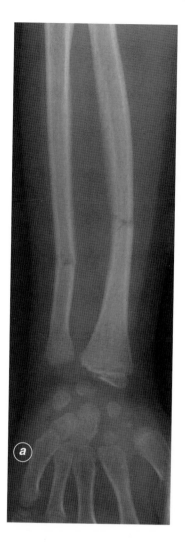

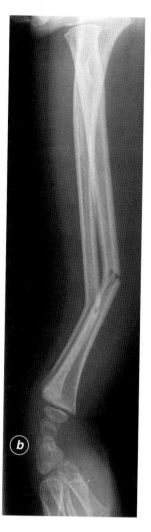

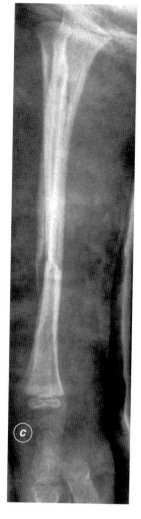

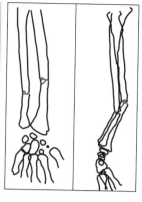

Figure 8.8 Antebrachial fracture, usually caused by a child falling. The frontal view shows the fracture lines, of both the radius and the ulna, but with what appears to be acceptable alignment *(a)*. The lateral view reveals malalignment *(b)*. After reduction, the lateral plane shows good alignment *(c)*. (Note: A frontal view must also be taken routinely after reduction).

ELBOW AND ARM

Monteggia Fracture !

The cause of Monteggia fractures is disputed, but they are probably the result of direct trauma or a fall. The injury consists of an ulnar fracture in the proximal third, with simultaneous dislocation of the proximal radius (figure 8.9). The injury is uncommon (7% of ulnar fractures and 0.7% of elbow injuries), but it may cause significant sequelae. The injury may also easily be overlooked, if–for example–only the wrist is imaged (and not the forearm and elbow) or if the position of the radial head is misinterpreted on X rays. The practitioner must also be aware of the possibility of an Essex-Lopresti fracture (defined as a fracture of the radial head, with simultaneous dislocation of the distal radioulnar joint) and of

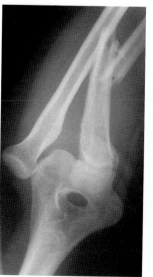

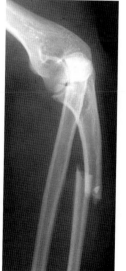

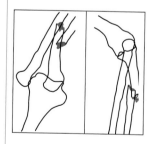

Figure 8.9 Monteggia fracture. Fracture in the proximal ulna with simultaneous dislocation of the radial head. These injuries may result from a fall or direct trauma.

a Galeazzi fracture (which is a fracture of the radial shaft, with simultaneous dislocation of the distal radioulnar joint). A Galeazzi fracture is caused by a fall on an outstretched arm. Because the patient's wrist symptoms dominate, it is easy to forget that the elbow joint needs to be examined clinically and, if necessary, radiographically.

- Symptoms and signs: Symptoms and signs include severe pain localized to the forearm, swelling, discoloration, malalignment, and significant functional impairment. The practitioner should be aware of injuries to the deep branch of the radial nerve and should test extension strength of the wrist.
- Diagnosis: The diagnosis is made by radiographic examination of the forearm on long film including the elbow joint in two planes. The practitioner should be aware that if a line is drawn through the shaft of the radius, it should always intersect the middle of the capitulum humeri in all planes. If this is not the case, the radial head is fully or partially dislocated.
- Treatment by physician: The patient with this type of injury must be referred to an orthopedic surgeon. The fracture must be reduced and its position monitored. If the radial head is insufficiently reduced, open reduction (and possibly fixation) becomes necessary.
- Treatment by physical therapist: Physical therapy provided should be similar to that discussed for the treatment of elbow dislocations.

Distal Biceps Tendon Rupture

Ruptures of the distal biceps tendon (figure 8.10) are very rare (only 3% to 10% of the biceps tendon ruptures), but without proper diagnosis and adequate treatment symptoms may become significant. The injury primarily affects men, and in 80% of cases it is localized to the dominant arm. The injury appears suddenly when the elbow is forcefully extended from a 90° flexed position while the elbow flexors work eccentrically. Pre-existing tendinopathy predisposes the tendon to rupture. Body builders are most susceptible to this injury. Anabolic steroid abuse significantly increases the risk of tendon ruptures.

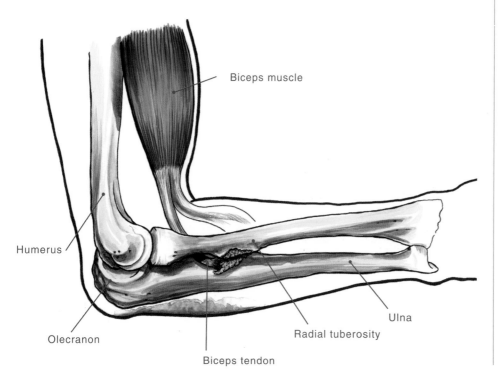

Biceps muscle

Humerus

Olecranon

Biceps tendon

Radial tuberosity

Ulna

Figure 8.10 Distal biceps tendon rupture, a rare injury, occurs in the radial tuberosity. It is palpated laterally while the forearm is pronated.

- Symptoms and signs: An athlete often reports sudden, sharp pain in the elbow, followed by discomfort in the forearm or the lower portion of the upper arm. The intense pain subsides within a few hours but is replaced by an aching pain that continues for weeks. Chronic pain may develop if the tendon is not sutured. The athlete will have reduced elbow flexor strength, but this tends to improve with time. A more limiting problem is relative weakness of supination, which contributes to reduced grip strength. Ecchymosis may track distally in the forearm. Upon activation of the biceps, a defect can be palpated in the distal biceps tendon, and flexion and supination strength is reduced.

- Diagnosis: The diagnosis is based on the symptoms and the clinical examination, but a standard X ray of the elbow is indicated. It is sometimes possible to see radiographic changes above the osseous prominence of the bicipital tendon insertion or signs of chronic cubital bursitis.

- Treatment by physician: Immediate surgical repair (within 7 to 10 days) is recommended for people with high activity levels who require full function of the arm. Conservative treatment will provide satisfactory function for about 50% of patients. Partial ruptures may heal without surgery.

Triceps Tendon Rupture

A rupture of the triceps tendon (figure 8.11) is also uncommon, but without proper diagnosis and adequate treatment, symptoms may become significant. The injury affects women almost as often as men (2 to 3). The injury mechanism is usually a fall on an outstretched arm (sudden eccentric loading of the elbow) or direct trauma. Previous tendinopathy predisposes the tendon to rupture. Body builders are most vulnerable to this injury. Anabolic steroid abuse significantly increases the risk of triceps tendon rupture.

- Symptoms and signs: The athlete complains of pain. If elbow extensor function is absent, a total rupture has occurred. Partial tendon tears will also result in weakness, however. Ecchymosis and swelling are common, and careful palpation may reveal a defect behind the olecranon.

- Diagnosis: The diagnosis is based on the patient's symptoms and clinical examination. A standard X ray of the elbow is also indicated. In 80% of cases, an avulsion from the olecranon is evident on the lateral X rays. The practitioner must distinguish clinically between partial tears and full-thickness tears (ruptures). The Thompson test used for Achilles tendon ruptures can also be used for triceps tendon ruptures. While supporting the arm and bending the elbow to 90°, the triceps muscle is squeezed quickly, and a reflex contraction will ensue that should result in visible elbow extension if the tendon is intact. Both MRI and ultrasound may be used to confirm the diagnosis.

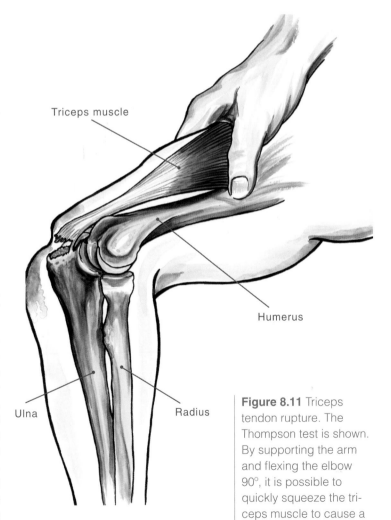

Triceps muscle

Humerus

Ulna

Radius

Figure 8.11 Triceps tendon rupture. The Thompson test is shown. By supporting the arm and flexing the elbow 90°, it is possible to quickly squeeze the triceps muscle to cause a reflex contraction. A lack of extension indicates a total rupture.

• Treatment by physician: Complete ruptures should be sutured immediately. Partial ruptures may be treated conservatively with active exercises that are within the limits of pain.

Acute Olecranon Bursitis

The olecranon bursa is vulnerable to injury from a blow or a fall, resulting in a hemorrhagic bursitis. If the synovial irritation persists, the condition may become chronic. Septic arthritis may occur without antecedent trauma. The bursa may rupture, causing swelling and pain in the upper arm or forearm.

• Symptoms and signs: Symptoms include tenderness, swelling, and fluctuation over the olecranon bursa. The skin is usually discolored. Septic bursitis causes rubor, local warmth, and fever. The practitioner must be aware that these symptoms can develop very quickly.
• Diagnosis: The diagnosis is usually based on the clinical history and the presence of fluctuation. Fever and an elevated CRP are signs of infection. If the diagnosis is unclear, aspiration is recommended. The aspirate will be clear or mixed with blood if the patient has sterile bursitis, whereas puss may be aspirated if the patient has septic bursitis.
• Treatment by physician: Other than protection against new trauma, no treatment is needed. If the patient is quite symptomatic, blood may be aspirated during the acute stage. This may be repeated as needed. If the patient has septic bursitis, the bursa must be incised and drained. Antibiotics are seldom needed. Nevertheless, a sample for Gram's stain and culture should always be taken.

Acute Vascular and Nerve Injury !

Acute vascular and nerve injuries are severe injuries that occur primarily in combination with serious upper arm, elbow, and forearm injuries. Minor trauma may also cause these types of injuries. Therefore, it is a good habit to always screen for vascular and nerve injuries whenever the elbow is examined, particularly before and after repositioning fractures or dislocations.

Acute vascular injury may involve torn vessels with a dramatic progression of subsequent symptoms, or it may involve thrombosis, which clinically may assume a more chronic course (e.g., thrombotic occlusion of the subclavian artery, in which symptoms are provoked by the use of the affected arm above the horizontal plane).

• Symptoms and signs: The earliest symptom of arterial damage is pain upon passive stretch of the affected area. The peripheral pulse will usually be weak or absent, the skin pale, and the skin temperature lowered. The musculature is weak and skin sensation is reduced in a "glovelike" distribution area.
• Diagnosis: Diagnosis is usually based on the clinical history of unusually severe pain and a weak pulse on exam. A radiographic contrast examination may confirm the diagnosis.
• Treatment by physician: Patients with a suspected vascular or nerve injury should be referred to a specialist for immediate evaluation.

Posttraumatic Stiffness !

Reduced elbow range of motion is common after an injury to the joint and may be disabling. A range of motion from 30° extension to 130° flexion and a combined pronation and supination of 90° is sufficient to perform activities of daily living. Special sports like gymnastics may require full extension, whereas athletes in sports such as ice hockey may continue their career with a reduced range of motion. The elbow is particularly vulnerable to posttraumatic stiffness, because of the unique tendency of the joint capsule to shrink, the short distance between the capsule and the muscle, and the great risk of comminuted fractures. The degree of stiffness is usually related to the extent of the trauma and how well the congruence of the articular surface can be restored.

- Symptoms and signs: The main sign is stiffness in the elbow. Pain indicates intra-articular injury, such as osteoarthritis.
- Diagnosis: The diagnosis is made clinically. Standard X rays of the elbow joint in two planes are necessary to demonstrate any osseous joint injury. A goniometer is used to measure the joint range of motion.
- Treatment by physician: The physician should instruct the patient in a stretching program 6 weeks after the acute trauma occurs. If results are unsatisfactory, surgery may be indicated. If surgery is required, it is usually necessary to release the adhesions by cutting the capsule anteriorly or posteriorly.
- Treatment by physical therapist: The physical therapist should instruct the patient in a home exercise program and should check to make sure that the exercises are done correctly, without provoking pain. Qualified therapists may attempt mobilization of the joint.

ELBOW AND ARM

Elbow Overuse Injuries

Stein Tyrdal

Occurrence

Although acute elbow injuries constitute a small portion (3% to 6%) of the total number of injuries in sport, there are several sports in which a significant number (40% to 75%) of athletes sustain overuse injuries to the elbow area during their sporting career. These injuries have a tendency to become chronic. In practice, the distinction between acute injuries and overuse injuries is negligible, and it is often of only academic interest whether the patient experiences the injury acutely or whether the injury is the result of short- or long-term overuse.

Differential Diagnosis

Table 8.3 provides an overview of the differential diagnosis for elbow overuse injuries. The practitioner should be aware that the athlete's symptoms might originate from several different parts of the elbow simultaneously. Patients with symptoms from multiple tendon insertions are more difficult to treat. In young, active patients, symptoms from several joints may be a sign of systemic disease, such as rheumatoid arthritis. Symptoms of hemophilia and tumors are often seen for the first time in connection with (minor) trauma. Children may sustain apophyseal fractures. Loose bodies with or without cartilage injuries may occur in isolation or in combination with ligament injuries or fractures.

Lateral (tennis elbow) and medial (golfer's elbow) tendinopathies are the most common overuse syndromes to affect the elbow, but ligaments (goalie's elbow), cartilage or bone (Little Leaguer's Elbow), and nerve tissue (entrapment syndromes) may also become symptomatic due to overload. Many activities may cause muscle soreness.

Most common	Less common	Must not be overlooked !
Lateral epicondylalgia (tennis elbow) (p. 209)	Triceps tendinosis (p. 214)	Ulnar stress fracture
Medial epicondylalgia (golfer's elbow) (p. 211)	Snapping triceps (p. 215)	
Team handball goalie's elbow (p. 212)	Ulnar nerve entrapment (p. 215)	
Cartilage injury (p. 213)	Radial nerve entrapment (p. 215)	
	Median nerve entrapment (p. 216)	
	Chronic compartment syndrome (p. 216)	
	Chronic olecranon bursitis (p. 217)	

Table 8.3 Overview of the differential diagnosis of elbow overuse injuries.

Tears of the muscle belly are rare. Tendon insertion sites are the most vulnerable locations for overuse pathology to develop, possibly because the muscle mass is relatively large compared to that of the tendon. Elbow pain may occur without obvious antecedant trauma (loose bodies, osteochondritis dissecans).

Diagnostic Thinking

The goal of the examination is to make the most precise diagnosis possible, so that it can be used as a basis for effective treatment. The examination should be conducted the same way every time, according to a standardized procedure, to avoid overlooking key symptoms and signs. The degree of functional impairment and the athlete's level of ambition help to guide the extent of the diagnostic workup. A decision should be made regarding the need for arthroscopy. An arthroscopic examination can be used to follow up on symptoms and findings that indicate intra-articular injuries. If no signs of elbow injury are found, the shoulder, neck, and wrist should be examined. If there are atypical signs, the practitioner must remember that tumors sometimes occur in the elbow. Because there are several nerves in this narrow anatomical region, a tumor can often result in nerve irritation.

Clinical History

The clinical history must be as short, clear, and concise as possible, but several factors need to be evaluated. Localization of the symptoms usually provides a good basis for evaluating which structure(s) are affected. The activity patterns and types of activity that provoke symptoms should be carefully charted. In addition, other factors that provoke or relieve symptoms should be noted. It is usually easier to find the cause(s) of the symptoms when the onset of pain is acute. The athlete should also be routinely asked whether he has problems with other joints.

The typical injury pattern differs for each sport (table 8.4). Therefore, it is important to record which sport the athlete is involved in to document the loading pattern preceding the current injury. Knowledge of the various sports and the associated loads makes it easier to determine which structures are involved. For example, most people think of the elbow joint as strictly a hinge joint, but when the elbow goes from full flexion to full extension, two other important movements take place simultaneously: the elbow's degree of valgar angulation increases and the forearm supinates. These observations help to explain why throwers often have medial pain and why a dislocation can result from a fall on an outstretched arm. Understanding that stretching the elbow is a combination of extension, valgus, and supination makes it easier to understand why the entire elbow may become painful from hyperextension overloading common to handball goalies, volleyball players, and gymnasts.

Sport	Most common injury
Golf	Medial epicondylalgia
Team handball (goalies)	Partial ligament injury due to hyperextension
Racket sports	Lateral epicondylalgia
Javelin	Medial ligament ruptures
Gymnastics	Anterior capsular injury due to hyperextension
Water skiing	Valgus injuries, chondromalacia
Weightlifting	Medial ligament rupture, ulnar neuritis
Volleyball	Partial ligament injury due to hyperextension

Table 8.4 The connection between various sports and typical injuries.

The activity that provokes the symptoms is often the one that causes them—for example, medial or lateral pain in the elbow, which is provoked by playing golf, may be medial or lateral epicondylalgia (figure 8.12). Each overuse injury tends to have a distinct pattern, and it is easier to make the diagnosis if the patient's history is precise.

Clinical Examination

Most structures in the elbow are superficial and easy to palpate. Good knowledge of anatomy is crucial to a meaningful clinical examination. It is recommended that the examination be performed in the same manner every time, so that necessary examinations are not overlooked or omitted. The anatomical structures that cause the symptoms are easiest to localize if the elbow is divided into four sections: the anterior section, the lateral section, the medial section, and the posterior section. The general examination technique for the elbow region is described under acute elbow injuries. Locking or crepitation during motion tests indicates the presence of loose bodies.

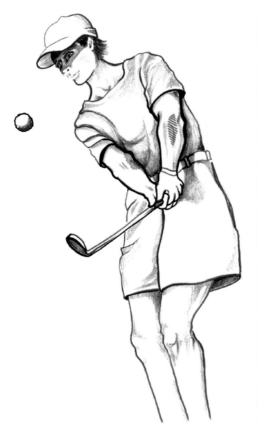

Figure 8.12 Injury mechanism in golf—medial and lateral epicondylalgia. Lateral epicondylalgia could occur in the golfer's left arm, which leads the motion, whereas medial epicondylalgia could occur in the right arm, which follows.

Specific tests. Varus and valgus stability are examined starting at 20° to 30° of elbow flexion (figure 8.13, a and b). If the elbow can be hyperextended, lateral elbow instability may also be tested on an extended elbow. The examiner should stress the elbow by locking the patient's forearm between the examiner's upper arm and thorax. Then the examiner should place the tip of their thumb into the joint space medially or laterally, and apply valgus and varus stress, respectively. The test is positive if there is a palpable, and possibly visible, opening of the joint with or without discomfort or pain. Varus instability is rare, but valgus instability may occur as a result of all types of valgus trauma (e.g., throwing or hyperextension trauma).

Valgus extension overload test. This test is used to demonstrate posteromedial osteophytes along the medial margin of the olecranon. This is seen as sequela after years of intensive throwing, and until now has only been described in American baseball pitchers. The elbow is placed in full extension, and the examiner then applies a valgus stress to the posteromedial edge of the olecranon. The test is positive if it causes discomfort and palpable posteromedial crepitation.

Radiohumeral chondromalacia. Degenerative changes in the radiohumeral joint may be demonstrated by starting at full extension. Palpate the radial head and apply steady pressure in supination and pronation. The test is positive if there is palpable crepitation, locking, and pain.

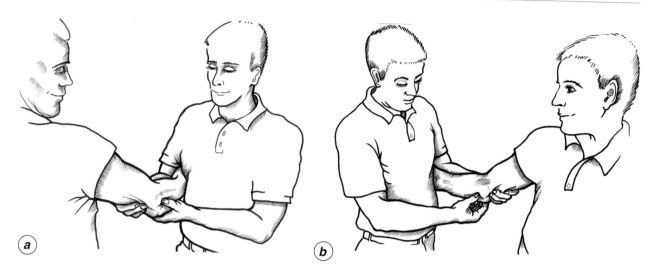

a   *b*

Supplemental Examinations

Radiographic examinations. A standard elbow series is taken with frontal and lateral views. Oblique X rays increase the sensitivity of detecting minor fractures, calcifications, or loose bodies.

Other diagnostic imaging methods:

- Fluoroscopy may be useful in evaluating instability, minor fractures, and interpositioned fragments.
- Arthrography (MRI or CT) may be useful if a total ligament rupture without dislocation is suspected. This exam should be ordered by an orthopedic surgeon. Leakage of contrast from the joint is considered an indication of a rupture. In practice, cross sectional imaging is seldom used. Indications for its use include acute ruptures without dislocation or preoperative evaluation of chronic ligament injuries. The method that currently provides the most relevant supplemental information is magnetic resonance arthrography. CT with contrast is an alternative if magnetic resonance imaging is not available.
- Stress radiography can be used to quantify (valgus) instability.
- Ultrasound is useful for demonstrating loose bodies and intra-articular fluid. Detecting pathological changes in tendons and ligaments requires an experienced radiologist.
- Scintigraphy provides a nonspecific image. The utility of scintigraphy in evaluating elbow injuries is unclear.

Figure 8.13 Technique for examining varus/valgus instability: With the elbow in 20° to 30° flexion, the examiner checks for varus *(a)* and valgus *(b)* instability by grasping the patient's right upper arm with his left hand. The examiner places the tip of his right thumb on the joint line laterally *(a)* or medially *(b)* and applies valgus and varus stress, respectively. The patient's forearm is locked between the examiner's own forearm and thorax. The test is positive if a palpable (possibly visible) joint opening is found.

Common Injuries

Lateral Epicondylalgia—Tennis Elbow

Repetitive and long-term loading may result in hyaline degeneration of the origin of the extensor tendons (figure 8.14). The histological changes are characteristic of tendinosis, and inflammatory cells are not found. The term epicondylalgia does not imply a specific cause for the symptoms. A 50% prevalence is reported among tennis players older than 30 years, with a peak between the ages of 35 and 50. The prevalence increases with age and career duration. Women and men are equally affected. Other athletes, including golfers, throwers, swimmers, fencers, and baseball players,

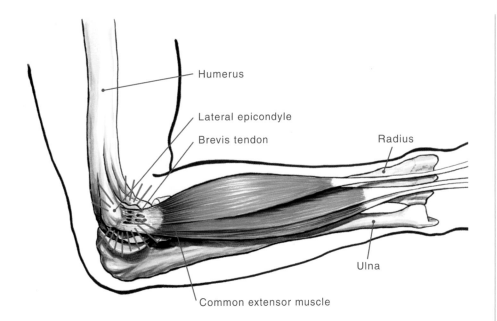

Humerus

Lateral epicondyle

Brevis tendon

Radius

Ulna

Common extensor muscle

Figure 8.14 Lateral epicondylalgia, usually caused by repetitive and long-term loading. The extensor tendon insertions undergo hyaline degeneration that may become visible macroscopically.

also have an increased incidence of lateral elbow pain. Lateral pain is 5 to 10 times more common than medial pain.

- Symptoms and signs: The predominant symptom is lateral elbow pain upon activation of the extensor muscles of the forearm.
- Diagnosis: The diagnosis is made clinically and is based on a typical history, tenderness at the origin of the extensor muscles, provocation of pain by extending the wrist or, alternatively, the second and third digits, against resistance.
- Treatment by physician: The physician should advise the patient to change his activity pattern and should provide information about proper technique and adapted equipment. NSAIDs may help in acute cases. Cortisone and local anesthetic may be injected under the extensor brevis, directly in front of, and distal to, the lateral epicondyle (figure 8.15). The injection is made into the triangular fatty tissue there and must not be made into the tendon itself. The fluid

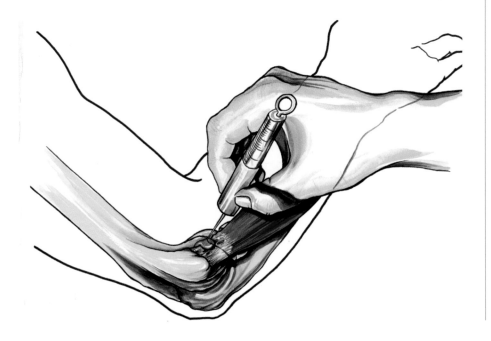

Figure 8.15 Injection technique for lateral epicondylalgia: cortisone mixed with local anesthetic is injected below the extensor longus tendon and above the extensor brevis tendon. The fluid is injected without resistance.

is injected without resistance. In order to stimulate healing, a needle can be used to make small holes in the periosteum on the anterior distal aspect of the lateral epicondyle under local anesthesia. Surgery may be indicated in resistant cases.

- Treatment by physical therapist: A program of eccentric strength training and stretching shows promising results. The patient should be instructed in a program of active exercises (that are within the limits of pain), stretching, and strength training. Playing technique should be reviewed, and a fitted orthosis (possibly tape) should be applied. The benefits of electrotherapy, ultrasound, and laser therapy are poorly documented. Extension splinting may be attempted for pain relief.

- Prognosis: The prognosis is generally good (50% to 70% healing), but it is best in cases with an acute onset due to a specific triggering event and prompt treatment. The condition can easily become chronic in cases where the cause is less clear, when symptoms are more diffuse, and when treatment was delayed. There is considerable risk of developing chronic symptoms with all types of enthesopathies (i.e., tendon insertion pain). In about 80% of cases, surgery successfully reduces symptoms, but only 50% to 60% of the patients become completely asymptomatic.

Medial Epicondylalgia—Golfer's Elbow

Medial epicondylalgia is a disorder characterized by pain localized to the origin of the wrist's flexor musculature on the medial epicondyle of the humerus (figure 8.16). The occurrence of the condition is reported to be 1/10 of the occurrence of lateral epicondylalgia. Histologically, it appears identical to tennis elbow–that is, hyaline degeneration of the tendon. Both golfers and tennis players may get both conditions. Medial epicondylalgia is also often seen in climbers. Practitioners should watch for simultaneous involvement of the ulnar nerve.

Figure 8.16 Medial epicondylalgia, usually caused by repetitive and long-term loading. The flexors and/or pronator tendon undergo hyaline degeneration that may be visible macroscopically.

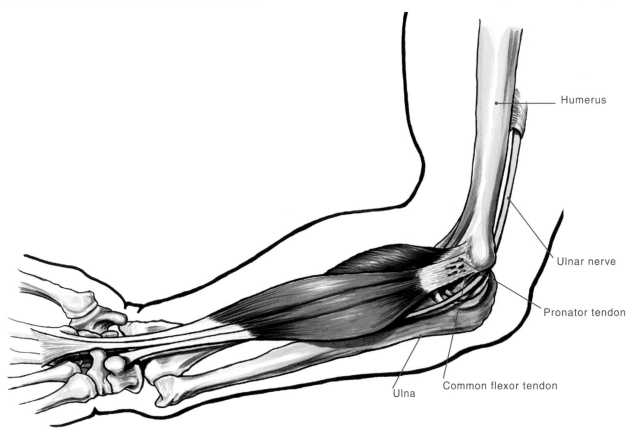

Humerus

Ulnar nerve

Pronator tendon

Common flexor tendon

Ulna

- Symptoms and signs: The principal symptom is medial elbow pain with activation of the flexor muscles in the forearm.
- Diagnosis: The diagnosis is made clinically based on a typical history, tenderness to palpation over the medial epicondyle, and provocation of pain when the wrist is flexed against resistance.
- Treatment by physician: The physician should advise the patient to change their activity pattern and should provide information about proper technique and appropriate equipment. In acute cases, NSAIDs may help. Cortisone and a local anesthetic may be injected above the insertion of the flexor and pronator muscles, anteriorly and distal to the medial epicondyle, taking care to avoid injecting the tendons themselves. The fluid should be injected without resistance. To stimulate healing, a needle can be used under local anesthesia to make small holes in the periosteum on the anterior distal portion of the medial epicondyle.
- Treatment by physical therapist: The patient should be instructed in a program of active exercises (that are within the limits of pain), stretching, and strength training. Playing technique should be reviewed, and a fitted orthosis (or tape) should be applied. The benefits of electrotherapy, ultrasound, and laser therapy are poorly documented.
- Prognosis: The prognosis is favorable for pain of acute onset with a specific identifiable cause that is treated promptly. The condition can easily become chronic in cases where the cause is less obvious, when symptoms are more diffuse, and when treatment was delayed. The risk of developing chronic symptoms is high with all types of enthesopathies (tendon insertion pain). In about 80% of the cases surgery alleviates the symptoms, but only 50% to 60% of the patients experience complete resolution of symptoms.

Handball Goalie's Elbow

Handball goalie's elbow is a syndrome that affects three of four goalies at some point during their playing careers. Shot blocking, resulting in elbow hyperextension, valgus stress, and supination of the forearm, can lead to partial ligament injuries in the elbow joint (figure 8.17). Field players in team handball and volleyball players may experience similar symptoms after blocking a ball with a hyperextended arm. The most common symptoms are pain and discomfort, weakness, numbness that radiates to the little finger, intermittent swelling with reduced range of motion, and locking.

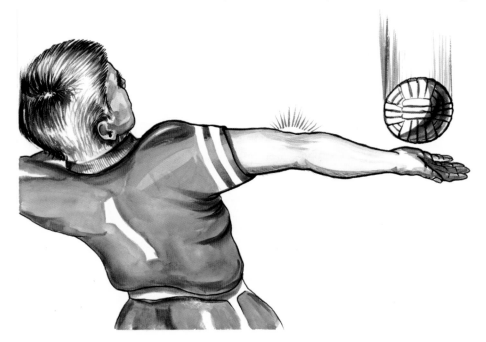

Figure 8.17 Handball goalie's elbow. The symptom is pain in one or more parts of the elbow. This syndrome results from blocking shots that cause hyperextension, valgus stress, and supination of the forearm. The drawing shows the goalie from behind and slightly above.

- Symptoms and signs: The major symptom is pain, usually located medially (50%). A small percentage of patients will have evidence of instability.
- Diagnosis: The diagnosis is made clinically, based on a good history and an adequate examination. X rays rarely demonstrate pathology. An MRI with contrast is the best means of documenting the underlying pathology.
- Treatment by physician: NSAIDs may help in acute cases. Surgery by a specialist may be considered in the case of long-lasting and significant symptoms.
- Treatment by physical therapist: The patient should be instructed in elbow, wrist, and forearm strength training. A fitted orthosis or the use of tape will help in 50% of cases.
- Prognosis: The prognosis is good. Permanent tissue damage occurs rarely. Only a small percentage of patients continue to suffer from symptoms after retiring from their sports career, although many end their career prematurely as a result of their symptoms. The risk of developing chronic sport-related symptoms is greater if the athlete is not treated adequately the first time.

Cartilaginous Injury

Cartilaginous injuries and degenerative conditions may be the result of long-term overuse, previous fracture, or prior dislocation (figure 8.18, a-c). Osteophytes along the posterior medial margin of the olecranon may develop after years of intensive throwing and primarily occur in American baseball pitchers. Degenerative changes in the radiohumeral joint are seen in throwers in other sports (e.g., javelin throwers) and after hyperextension trauma (e.g., handball goalies). Loose bodies can occur as the result of previous elbow trauma and from osteochondritis dissecans. In children, cartilage defects in the capitulum humeri may form spontaneously without trauma (Panner disease).

- Symptoms and signs: Symptoms include pain and locking.
- Diagnosis: An appropriate clinical history, documenting intermittent locking of the joint, and a thorough physical examination incorporating such tests as the valgus extension overload test and tests for radiohumeral chondromalacia and loose bodies, may indicate a cartilaginous injury. Radiography will seldom reveal localized cartilage injury but must always be performed if there is a suspicion of loose bodies. MRI arthrography is the best examination to rule out cartilage injury.
- Treatment by physician: NSAIDs may help when the condition is acute. Intra-articular cortisone injections may be used in an attempt to treat synovitis, but the outcome is controversial. Loose bodies can be surgically removed (by arthroscopy or arthrotomy). If additional loose bodies are formed (or overlooked), the procedure must be repeated.

Figure 8.18 Cartilage injury in a boxer's elbow. A loose body is located in the posterior and lateral portion of the humerus *(a)*. It is attached by scar tissue *(b)* and is arthroscopically removed using grasping forceps *(c)*.

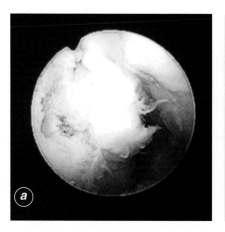
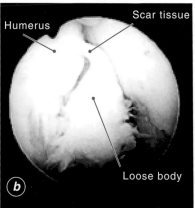
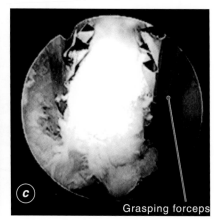

- Treatment by physical therapist: The patient should be instructed in active exercises that do not provoke pain.
- Prognosis: The prognosis is good if there are loose bodies that can be removed by arthroscopy and there is no cartilage injury. If the patient has osteoarthritis, the risk of developing chronic symptoms is great. The symptoms will depend on the amount and type of load on the joint.

Other Injuries

Triceps Tendinosis

Tendinosis of the triceps tendon at the site of insertion on the olecranon is relatively rare (figure 8.19).

- Symptoms and signs: Pain accompanies active elbow extension and palpation of the triceps tendon insertion behind the olecranon.
- Diagnosis: The diagnosis is suggested by a typical case history and by demonstrating pain during resisted elbow extension.
- Treatment by physician: The physician should advise the patient to alter their activity pattern and should provide information about proper technique and adapted equipment. NSAIDs may help in acute cases. Cortisone and a local anesthetic may be administered anterior to the tendon down toward the tip of the olecranon. The needle tip is inserted from the lateral side of the tendon. The injection must not be made into the tendon itself. The fluid must be injected without resistance.
- Treatment by physical therapist: The patient should be instructed in active exercises (that are within the limits of pain), stretching, and strength training. Technique should be reviewed. The benefits of electrotherapy, ultrasound, and laser therapy are poorly documented.

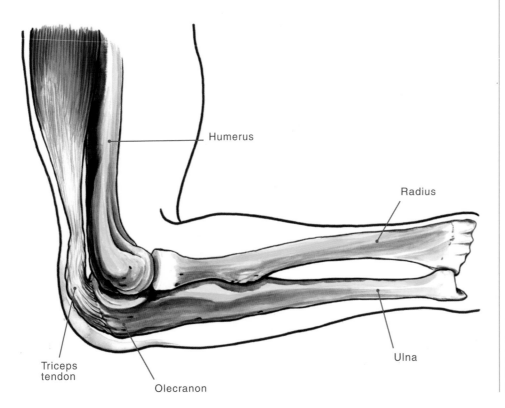

Humerus

Radius

Ulna

Triceps tendon

Olecranon

Figure 8.19 Triceps tendinopathy. The tendon becomes swollen and tender at the insertion to the olecranon.

Snapping Triceps

The feeling that something is slipping posteriorly and medially is usually caused by ulnar nerve subluxation or because part of the triceps tendon is slipping over the medial epicondyle. The phenomenon may also be due to an anomalous triceps tendon. The etiology is often unclear. The phenomenon usually occurs spontaneously during the second decade of life. Throwers and tennis players appear to be the most vulnerable.

- Symptoms and signs: The feeling that something is slipping may or may not be accompanied by pain.
- Diagnosis: The diagnosis is usually made on the basis of the clinical history and by demonstrating the slippage on physical exam.
- Treatment by physician: Surgery is the treatment of choice for intolerable symptoms.

Ulnar Nerve Entrapment

After carpal tunnel syndrome, ulnar neuropathy at the elbow is the most common peripheral nerve entrapment syndrome. Causes include (1) compression of the nerve due to external pressure or to scar tissue from a previous injury, (2) friction in the muscular tunnel distal to the medial epicondyle, (3) subluxation of the ulnar nerve, or (4) medial instability. The condition is seen most often in tennis players and in 60% of the patients who have had surgery for medial epicondylalgia.

- Symptoms and signs: Symptoms include paresthesias and numbness in digits IV and V of the hand. The Tinel sign is usually positive at the elbow. Nerve stimulation studies may be nondiagnostic at first, because the symptoms are intermittent. Symptoms usually intensify upon elbow flexion. Atrophy of the interossei muscles and weakened thumb-index finger pinch are late signs.
- Diagnosis: The diagnosis is made on the basis of a classical history and clinical evaluation. Numbness is easiest to test for on the two outermost joints of the little finger. Nerve stimulation studies can be used to confirm the diagnosis.
- Treatment by physician: Conservative treatment is indicated for patients with intermittent symptoms that occur with repeated elbow flexion and extension. In these cases, the patient's activity pattern should be modified to avoid provoking symptoms, and a straight night splint should be used for 2 to 3 months. Surgery is performed if conservative measures do not provide satisfactory symptom relief or if there is a progression of symptoms with motor involvement. The primary care physician can provide conservative treatment initially, but if these measures fail, the patient should be referred to a neurologist.

Radial Nerve Entrapment

Entrapment of the deep motor branch of the radial nerve may cause symptoms that resemble lateral epicondylitis. The condition, which has been described by several different names (atypical epicondylitis, posterior interosseous syndrome, and supinator syndrome), is caused by nerve compression due to a tumor or ganglion, synovitis, or spontaneous compression in the arcade of Frohse. Some authors have reported that radial nerve entrapment occurs in up to 5% of patients with tennis elbow.

- Symptoms and signs: There are two parts to the typical clinical scenario: (1) lateral, aching pain, often worse at night, which radiates down into the forearm and up into the upper arm and (2) weakness of the extensor muscles.
- Diagnosis: The diagnosis is usually made on the basis of an appropriate history, but clinically this condition is difficult to distinguish from tennis elbow. Three findings suggest entrapment of the radial nerve: (1) maximum tenderness deep in

the extensor musculature 2 cm distal and 2 cm medial to the lateral epicondyle, (2) increased pain upon resisted supination, and (3) pain provoked by extending the long finger against resistance while the elbow and wrist are held in extension. Electrodiagnostic therapy is rarely positive, but a neurologist should evaluate the patient before surgery is considered.

- Treatment: Alternative training may be attempted with a gradual resumption of sport activity. If this does not provide relief from symptoms, surgery is usually indicated. The difficulty lies in securing a definite diagnosis.

Median Nerve Entrapment

The median nerve can be compressed proximally at several sites (including the ligament of Struther's, within the pronator teres, or at the level of the anterior interosseous nerve) or distally (within the carpal tunnel). These two conditions are clinically distinct. Median neuropathy at the wrist (carpal tunnel syndrome) is discussed on pages 240 and 241.

- Symptoms and signs: Symptoms or proximal median nerve entrapment are often vague and include discomfort, weakness, and proximal forearm pain that is provoked by forearm pronation and weightlifting. Reduced skin sensation is a late sign.
- Diagnosis: Tinel's sign may be positive if percussion over the proximal course of the anterior interosseous nerve results in typical forearm systems. Palpation may reveal a tender lump in the proximal forearm as well. Pain can occasionally be provoked by resisted flexion of the long finger (with the elbow held at 90°).
- Treatment by physician: The physician may recommend a period of alternative training. Surgery can also be considered if conservative measures do not provide relief from symptoms.
- Prognosis: The outcome of surgery is usually good. The athlete usually returns to full activity in 6 weeks.

Chronic compartment syndrome

Chronic compartment syndrome in the forearm is a condition that can be seen in sports demanding prolonged static muscle contraction, (e.g., motorcycle riders competing in roadracing or motorcross). The condition can be difficult to distinguish from entrapment of the radial or median nerve.

- Symptoms and signs: The athlete describes gradually progressive cramp-like pain upon prolonged static arm use in addition to weakness and paresthesias in the forearm and all the fingers. Symptoms are usually relieved a few minutes after cessation of activity.
- Diagnosis: The pathogenesis is not known. Intramuscular pressure is usually normal (although in some individuals it may be elevated). The diagnosis is one of exclusion and is based primarily on the history (typically an elite motorcycle athlete complaining of numbness in the forearm and fingers with prolonged riding) as there are usually no findings of import on exam.
- Treatment: Surgery can be attempted if warranted by the degree of symptoms. Both fasciotomy through four small incisions and release of the radial and median nerves have been used with encouraging results.
- Prognosis: The prognosis is good after surgery. Athletes can usually return to sport two to four weeks after fasciotomy. Nerve release usually requires another two weeks of recovery.

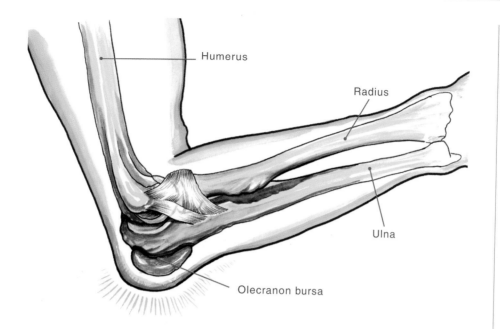

Figure 8.20 Olecranon bursitis, usually caused by a friction injury of the bursa, which swells up and becomes painful.

Chronic Olecranon Bursitis—Student Elbow

Acute bursitis may develop a chronic course, particularly if irritation continues (figure 8.20). It is often possible to palpate moveable fragments in the bursa, which usually represent synovial tissue or scar tissue.

- Symptoms and signs: Symptoms of chronic bursitis include tenderness and swelling above the olecranon with fluctuation, but without discoloration.
- Diagnosis: The diagnosis is usually made on the basis of an appropriate history and by demonstrating fluctuation of the bursa.
- Treatment by physician: Usually there is no need for treatment other than protection against new trauma. If symptoms and swelling are severe, serous fluid can be aspirated and cortisone injected. A compression bandage should then be applied to minimize swelling. Bursal injections often need to be repeated two to three times. If the problem continues, surgical removal of the olecranon bursa may be indicated.

Ulnar Stress Fracture !

Stress fractures in the elbow region are rare. The practitioner should distinguish between stress fractures that are caused by repetitive stress (e.g., in javelin throwers and baseball pitchers) and separation of the growth zones around ossification centers due to trauma (e.g., from one particular throw). Stress fractures may occur in all parts of the olecranon but are usually localized to the middle portion where there is often a natural lack of cartilage. Stress fractures become displaced only very rarely.

- Symptoms and signs: Symptoms include tenderness above the olecranon. Swelling and bruising are usually absent.
- Diagnosis: The diagnosis is made by scintigraphy or MRI. The fracture is usually not visible on plain X rays until late in the course.
- Treatment by physician: As is the case with other olecranon fractures, most stress fractures require surgery. Conservative treatment has been reported to be successful, but healing time is prolonged. If the tip of the olecranon has been avulsed or fragmented, it can be excised if it causes symptoms.

Rehabilitation of Elbow Injuries

Oddvar Knutsen and Stein Tyrdal

Goals and Principles

Table 8.5 outlines the goals for rehabilitation of acute elbow injuries.

During the initial phase of acute elbow injury rehabilitation, the goal is to gain control over pain and inflammation. This is accomplished by reducing activity or, if needed, by prescribing complete rest. If pain increases during an activity, the activity must be immediately discontinued and ice applied locally over the painful area for 15 to 20 minutes.

Pain is used to guide functional progression. A significant improvement in range of motion cannot be expected if strength training causes pain. The practitioner should be careful not to passively manipulate the joint overly aggressively because it may provoke inflammation or tissue tears with bleeding. The elbow's osseous contact surface, with its numerous small articular surfaces and increased susceptibility for developing intra-articular adherences, combined with the tendency of the anterior joint capsule to form adhesions and scar, makes the elbow particularly vulnerable to contracture. Extension is usually somewhat reduced. The risk of developing chronic instability is limited. However, the practitioner should be aware of the danger of recurrent dislocation during the period immediately after reduction and after removal of the brace or cast. This should be suspected if range of motion is severely restricted and is accompanied by pain. If dislocation can be ruled out, and range of motion is still significantly limited after 6 weeks, the therapist may begin specific mobilization of the joint and stretching within the limits of pain (flexion/extension and pronation/supination).

As range of motion gradually improves, the patient should begin light strengthening exercises (without external load) that are within the limits of pain. The number of repetitions should gradually be increased (up to 30 repetitions) before starting work against resistance. If there is no improvement in range of motion, the patient should work (in consultation

	Goals	Measures
Acute phase	Reduce pain and inflammation	PRICE
Rehabilitation phase	Normalize range of motion and strength in the elbow and wrist	Strength and stretching exercises
		Mobilize blood tissue and joints
Training phase	Complete healing of injured ligaments without the loss of mechanical stability or range of motion	Sensory motor exercises
	Return to sports-specific activity with gradually increasing load	Functional exercises
	Reduce the risk of reinjury	Eccentric strength exercises
		Sport-specific exercises

Table 8.5 Acute elbow injury rehabilitation goals and measures.

with the physician) with a qualified therapist who specializes in manual therapy. Tension band, weighted ball, or single hand manual resistance may be applied gradually. Elbow exercises with variations of forearm pronation and supination may be added gradually. The best endurance training is accomplished by using an arm ergometer, but prolonged activity in water or exercises with light external loads and numerous repetitions represent good alternatives. Bouncing balls, throwing and catching against a wall, and/or balancing on a soft balance mat provide important means of improving neuromuscular control.

During the final phase of rehabilitation, emphasis is placed on functional exercises to improve the athlete's ability to return to competitive activity. Exercises that require eccentric and plyometric muscle work are prioritized during this phase. Pace, speed, and degree of difficulty are increased until the competitive level is reached. The risk of chronic problems (e.g., loss of range of motion and pain) needs to be weighed against the benefit of being able to compete when considering returning to sport. The guiding principle should be for the athlete to resume her sport when she can safely tolerate loading during activity. In practice, this means a satisfactory clinical examination and pain-free simulated competitive training.

Preventing Reinjury

Prevention is important because elbow problems are very common in many throwing and racket sports. It is recommended that preventive measures be taken as long as the athlete has an active sport career. The following measures appear to be beneficial:

Warm-up. Athletes in all sports that put maximum stress on the elbow should warm up. Warm-up exercises should include throwing with progressively increasing speed and intensity, or (for team handball goalies) saving shots (of increasing intensity) from various positions on the court.

Strength training. Throwers should perform strength training for the elbow joint at least once a week for as long as they are active in sport.

Tape or orthosis. Athletes who have not been fully rehabilitated from previous injuries should protect themselves against new problems by wearing tape or a specially made orthosis until rehabilitation has been completed. Documentation for this is sparse, but there is little doubt that preventing recurrent episodes of pain helps to prevent acute injuries from developing into chronic injuries.

Exercise Program

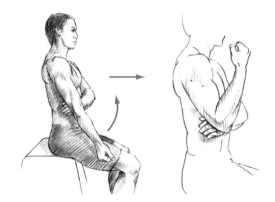

Exercise 8.1 Elbow flexion

- Starting position: Fully extend your elbow, then bend at maximum.
- Practice resistance with tension band or dumbbells.

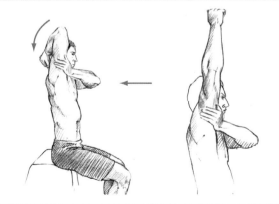

Exercise 8.2 Elbow extension

- Starting position: With your arm over your head and maximum flexion in the elbow, extend your forearm as far as possible.
- Practice resistance with tension band or dumbbells.

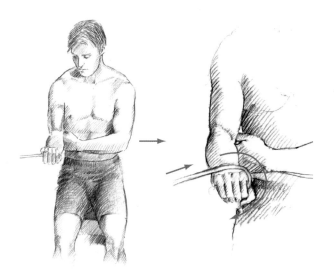

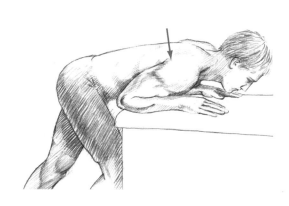

Exercise 8.3 Supination and pronation in the forearm

- Rotate your forearm in supination and pronation; hold your elbow at 90° flexion.
- Practice resistance with a tension band or traction apparatus.

Exercise 8.4 Stretching to increase elbow joint flexion

- Lower yourself toward a table or "fall" into a wall.

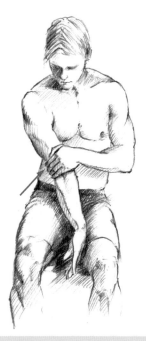

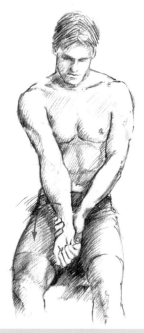

Exercise 8.5 Elbow flexor muscle stretching

- With your hand against your thigh, stretch as shown to increase elbow joint extension.
- Use your other hand to increase the extension.

Exercise 8.6 Stretching to increase supination in the elbow or forearm

- With your forearm next to your upper body, position yourself as shown in the figure.
- Supinate and extend your elbow with the help of your other hand.

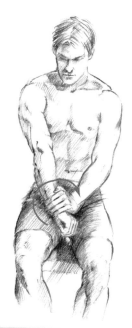

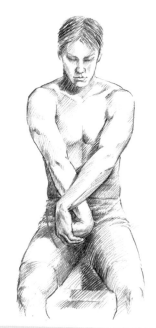

Exercise 8.7 Stretching to increase pronation in the elbow or forearm

- With your upper arm next to your upper body, position yourself as shown in the figure.
- Pronate and extend your elbow with the help of your other hand.

Exercise 8.8 Stretching for extensors in the forearm or wrist

- Start by flexing fingers II to V, palmar flex your wrist (the right one here).
- Increase stretching using your other hand.

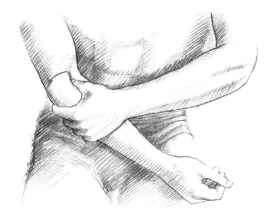

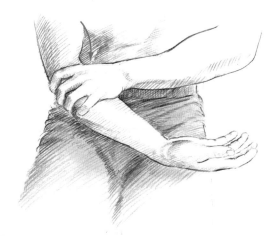

Exercise 8.9 Mobilization of extension in the elbow joint (radial humerus)

- Hold the upper part of your forearm, elbow at about 30° flexion.
- Press downward using the thumb of your other arm, directly above the proximal part of the radial head; try to hold for 5 seconds. Repeat several times.

Exercise 8.10 Mobilization of extension in the elbow joint

- Thenar pushes the ulna downward as shown in the figure; hold for 5 seconds, and repeat several times.

Wrist, Hand, and Fingers   9

Hand and Wrist Injuries

Jan-Ragnar Haugstvedt

Occurrence

Hand injuries represent 20% to 25% of all injuries that are treated at emergency clinics. The injury panorama ranges from "innocent" sprains to complicated fracture-dislocations. An injury causing stiffness of the wrist that eventually results in a fusion as a consequence of a missed diagnosis or inappropriate treatment produces greater medical disability than does loss of the anterior cruciate ligament in the knee. Therefore, the physician must strive to provide an accurate diagnosis and treatment of hand and wrist injuries.

Differential Diagnosis

Table 9.1 provides an overview of relevant hand and wrist injury diagnoses. The most common injury is a sprained wrist. The athlete falls and puts her hands out for protection, resulting in twisting, stretching, or hyperextension. This mechanism of injury may cause a contusion or strain injury of the musculature or a sprain of the capsular apparatus.

Major forces may cause ligament or skeletal injury. A partial ligament tear causes pain, swelling, and discoloration of the skin but no signs of instability or fracture. Fractures are more common in the elderly than in the young because the quality of the bone is better in younger people. Depending on the force at the time of the injury, a fracture of the distal forearm or a ligament injury within the carpus with or without a fracture of the carpal bones may result. The practitioner must remember that a scaphoid fracture may be easily overlooked on initial exam and thus should maintain a high index

Most common	Less common	Must not be overlooked !
Wrist sprain (p. 230)	Distal radius fracture (p. 231)	Scaphoid fracture (p. 234)
	Carpal bone fracture (p. 235)	Carpal dislocation (p. 241)
	Ligament injuries in the wrist (p. 236)	
	Injury of the distal radioulnar joint (p. 237)	
	Triangular fibrocartilage complex tear (p. 239)	
	Tendon injuries (p. 239)	
	Nerve entrapment (p. 240)	

Table 9.1 Overview of the differential diagnosis of injuries and disorders in the hand and wrist.

of suspicion for the diagnosis on subsequent follow up. If missed and left untreated, scaphoid fractures may precipitate changes in the wrist and carpus that could necessitate surgery.

People in all age groups may sustain a distal radioulnar joint (DRUJ) and/or triangular fibrocartilage complex (TFCC) injury concomitantly with a wrist fracture. These injuries are often overlooked because an arthroscopic examination, considered the gold standard for diagnosing intra-articular injuries of the radiocarpal joint, is rarely performed acutely. Studies have shown that more than 70% of patients with a distal radius fracture simultaneously sustain a TFCC injury. If a patient has wrist pain after healing a fracture of the distal radius, an undiagnosed injury of the TFCC may be the cause.

Acute tendon injuries at the wrist level without a simultaneous open wound are very rare. Occasionally, the extensor pollicis longus (EPL) (the long extensor tendon of the thumb) will spontaneously rupture.

Diagnostic Thinking

Upon initial inspection of the hand and the wrist, the physician should first look for deformity. If present, deformity or malalignment may indicate a fracture or dislocation. A classic "dinner fork" or "bayonet" deformity on the distal forearm is typical of a distal radius fracture. The physician should look for swelling or bruising, indicating bleeding from a fracture or a severe ligament sprain. If there is deformity or swelling, the patient should be referred for a radiographic examination. The same is true if signs of instability are found during the clinical examination.

Generally, however, deformity, major swelling, or definite signs of instability are uncommon—quite unlike tenderness from direct palpation. Tenderness to palpation is suggestive of a sprain (an injury of the soft tissue and the ligamentous capsular apparatus). A sprain should be considered a diagnosis of exclusion that is used when the patient indicates mild discomfort and pain but when no evidence of instability or skeletal damage is found during an objective examination that includes radiography.

If a patient returns several days or a week after an injury complaining of persistent pain and discomfort, the patient should be referred to a specialist for radiographic and clinical examination.

After falling on his hand with great force, the patient may have major swelling over the wrist, pain on attempted active range of motion, and tenderness on palpation with or without simultaneous passive range of motion. These symptoms and findings are suggestive of a ligament injury in the wrist or a carpal bone fracture. It is impossible to distinguish between a fracture and a ligament injury by means of a clinical examination alone, and in fact the patient often may have a combination of the two diagnoses. The patient must be referred for a radiographic examination in which additional views (other than standard posterior-anterior (PA) and lateral views) may be requested. The area of maximum tenderness should be described to guide the radiologist in focusing on the area that needs to be examined. If the patient is suspected of having, or is found to have, a carpal bone fracture or a ligament injury in the wrist, he should be referred to a specialist for further diagnostic evaluation and treatment.

In the case of an open wound, particularly one caused by a sharp object, the possibility of a tendon and/or nerve injury should always be considered. Each tendon should be examined separately. An injury to the median nerve will result in impaired sensation of the thumb, index finger, middle finger, and the radial half of the ring finger. The athlete will typically notice this numbness shortly after being injured, prompting him to seek medical advice. However, an ulnar nerve injury at the wrist might be overlooked. Ulnar neuropathy may result in significant weakness and eventual atrophy of the intrinsic muscles of the hand. Therefore, thorough examination of sensory perception and muscle function should be performed whenever the history or mechanism of injury is suggestive of possible nerve injury. The reduction of nerve function should not be "observed" but rather documented by careful *clinical examination*. If reduced function in one or more tendons is found upon clinical examination, or the patient indicates reduced sensation in all or part of his hand, he *must* immediately be referred to a hand surgeon for further treatment.

Clinical History

The mechanism of injury—such as a fall on an extended (figure 9.1) or flexed hand while the hand is either pronated or supinated; a direct blow; or twisting of the wrist, with a strong extension or flexion moment at the wrist—may provide a clue as to the type of injury sustained. Other diagnostic clues include deformity, significant swelling, or an audible "crunch" at the moment of injury. Has the injury resulted in ecchymosis or tendon or nerve dysfunction?

A fall on an outstretched hand may cause a fracture through the distal radius. The type of injury caused by a fall depends on (1) the position of the hand at the time of the fall, (2) the direction and intensity of the forces occuring during the fall, and (3) the age of the person falling (related to bone quality). Several types of fractures have been described and classified according to a variety of systems, but in practice most classification systems are of little value clinically. In addition to a fracture, depending on the mechanism of injury, the athlete may also sustain ligament injury that could result in instability of the wrist and/or the DRUJ.

A scaphoid fracture is the most common type of carpal fracture. As is the case for a fracture of the distal radius, the mechanism of injury is typically a fall on an extended hand. Scaphoid fractures are more common in young, active men. Children and the elderly may sustain them as well, however. A scaphoid fracture may be associated with other injuries of the wrist, such as a dorsal avulsion fracture or a transverse fracture of the triquetrum. The hook of the hamate (projecting into the palm of the hand) may be fractured during golf or as a result of a strong blow from a racket or club held in the athlete's hand. A direct blow to the ulnar side of the hand may also cause a fracture of the pisiform bone. Isolated fracture of the other carpal bones occurs infrequently.

Several ligaments stabilize the various carpal bones to each other and to the

Figure 9.1 Typical mechanism for wrist injury: falling on an extended hand can cause a distal radius fracture, a fracture in the carpus, or a ligament injury in the wrist.

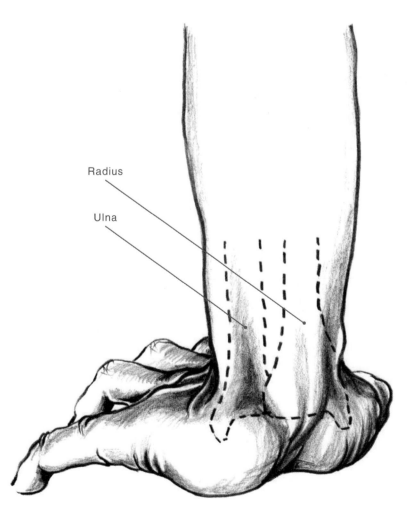

Radius

Ulna

radius and the ulna. Depending on the mechanism, direction, and force of the injury, various ligaments may be torn. Falling on a hyperextended, ulnar-deviated, and slightly pronated hand may cause a significant ligament injury in the wrist. The ligament injury may occur alone or in combination with a fracture or dislocation of one or more carpal bones. For example, the scapholunate ligament may rupture, there may be a fracture of the scaphoid, the lunotriquetral ligament may be torn, the triquetrum may be broken, or the lunate may dislocate. Alternatively, a combination of these injuries can occur. Other ligaments may also be injured, but they are rarely diagnosed and treated as isolated injuries.

The TFCC is one of the most important structures in the wrist. It consists of a meniscus-like articular disk, in addition to the palmar and dorsal radioulnar ligaments. The TFCC may be injured, particularly if the mechanism of injury involves a combination of rotation and hyperextension of the wrist. TFCC injuries are also frequently seen in combination with fractures of the distal radius.

Clinical Examination

Inspection. Bruising of the skin and swelling may indicate bleeding, which accompanies ligament injuries, dislocations, and fractures. Similar types of injuries should also be suspected if malalignment or malrotation are observed. A fractured distal radius is often accompanied by obvious deformity (typically a "dinner fork" or "bayonet" deformity). A single finger observed persistently in a flexed position may indicate an injury to the finger's extensor apparatus, while a finger observed in an extended position, with a lack of tension on the flexor side of the finger, may indicate injured flexor tendons. If there is an open wound, the possibility of nerve injury should be considered.

Palpation. Find the point of maximal tenderness and palpate it to determine whether the swelling is soft (e.g., hematoma) or hard (e.g., bone) and if the pain radiates in a consistent fashion. By examining an injured finger, it is possible to feel the motion of fractured phalange(s) or the instability that may result from a fracture or a ligament injury.

Nerve function. Nerve injury in the hand or at the wrist level reduces sensation in all or part of the hand. In addition, there may be a loss of motor (muscle or tendon) function. By touching the skin with a cotton ball, a paper clip, or some similar object, it is possible to evaluate the patient's sensation. This is typically tested for on the palmar (flexor) side of the hand. The *median nerve* innervates the entire thumb, the index finger, the middle finger, and the radial side of the ring finger. The distal motor portion of the median nerve may be injured as a result of wrist trauma, resulting in weakness of thumb opposition (i.e., the thumb cannot be flexed and rotated into the hand so that the tip of the thumb comes into contact with (and in the same plane as) the tip of the little finger) (figure 9.2, a-d).

If there is an injury to the *ulnar nerve* at the wrist, the patient may lose sensation in the little finger and in the ulnar side of the ring finger. In addition, the intrinsic muscles of the hand may be dysfunctional. The ability of the patient to adduct and to abduct her fingers as well as to extend her proximal interphalangeal (PIP) joint (a function of the hand intrinsic muscles) (figure 9.2) will be reduced. In addition, there is reduced strength in the adductor pollicis longus muscle, leading to loss of the ability to hold a piece of paper between the thumb and index finger when the thumb is extended and pressed against the index finger's metacarpophalangeal (MCP) joint. This latter finding is termed Froment's *signe de journaux*.

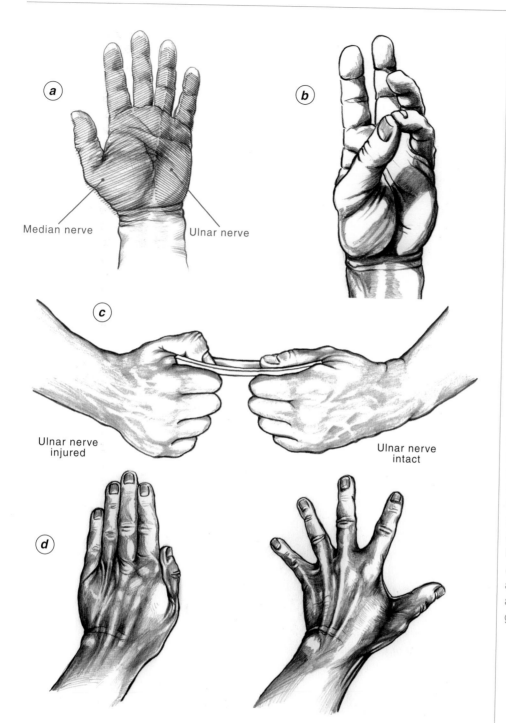

Figure 9.2 Median and ulnar nerves—innervation areas and functional tests. The median nerve innervates the thumb, the index finger, the middle finger, and the radial side of the ring finger (red) on the palm of the hand, whereas the ulnar nerve innervates the ulnar side of the ring finger and the little finger (blue) *(a)*. If the median nerve is intact, the thumb can be rotated and flexed towards the pulp of the little finger (function of the opponens pollicis muscle) *(b)*. If the ulnar nerve is intact, it can activate the adductor pollicis longus muscle, so that it is possible to hold a piece of paper between an extended thumb and the index finger. If the ulnar nerve is injured, the paper can be held using the flexor muscles of the thumb (which are innervated by the median nerve) *(c)*. An intact ulnar nerve allows normal abduction and adduction of the fingers *(d)*.

Range of motion. Wrist extension is normally about 70°, flexion is about 80°, and pronation and supination are both close to 90°. Normally, the wrist can be deviated radially to approximately 20°; ulnar deviation is approximately 30°.

Tendon function. Tendon ruptures at the wrist level rarely occur in the absence of a simultaneous open wound. However, after a radius fracture, the EPL tendon may tear at Lister's tubercle (a bony prominence on the dorsal side of radius just proximal to the wrist). The examining physician may test for EPL function by asking the patient to place the palm of his hand flat on a surface and then lift his thumb from the surface. This movement is not possible if the EPL tendon has been seriously injured (see figure 9.9).

Supplemental Examinations

Radiographic examination. A radiographic examination is necessary if the patient has pain, swelling, and tenderness in the wrist after being injured. A wrist fracture is usually visible on "standard" X rays (posterior-anterior [PA] and lateral views should always be taken as a minimum). On the lateral view, the articular surface of the distal radius normally shows 10° to 12° of palmar tilt. In the PA view, the articular surface of the ulna and the radius should be nearly congruent. The radioulnar inclination (examined on a PA view reflecting the angle between a line running through the distal radial and ulnar corner of the radius and another line perpendicular to the longitudinal axis of the radius) should be about 22°.

Fractures and fracture-dislocations involving the carpus may be difficult to diagnose both clinically and radiographically. Hence, any indicated additional examinations will be very useful.

- If injuries of the wrist are suspected, at least four different radiographic views of the carpus should be performed:
  1. A PA view. This is obtained when the styloid process of the ulna and the styloid process of the radius are as far apart as possible.
  2. A true lateral view. When the palmar edge of the pisiform is between the palmar edge of the capitate and the scaphoid, the view is within about 10° of a true lateral view.
  3. A PA view with the hand in a fist and at maximum ulnar deviation. This allows the scaphoid to extend, producing a good image of the bone and making a possible dissociation between the scaphoid and the lunate easier to see.
  4. An oblique view with the hand in 45° of pronation.
- If there are tenderness and swelling in the wrist, particularly in the anatomic snuffbox, and the initial radiographs are read as negative, the patient should return for repeat examination within 5 to 10 days. At that time, a second set of radiographs consisting of several different views (preferably the previously mentioned four views) should be taken.
- Magnetic resonance imaging (MRI) and computed tomography (CT) with various cross sections may also demonstrate a scaphoid fracture, or other fractures within the wrist. These may also be demonstrated by means of ultrasonography or a bone scan. For optimal results, the additional examinations require a radiologist with both interest and experience in the method used and the equipment necessary for completing the requested examination. It might be of great help to discuss available methods with the radiologist in advance of requesting the images.
- Experience and several studies have demonstrated that wrist arthroscopy is the "gold standard" if soft-tissue injuries (e.g., intercarpal ligament injuries or TFCC ruptures) are suspected.
- Fluoroscopic visualization of the wrist may be helpful in demonstrating ligament injuries if no dislocated bones are demonstrated by routine radiographs. Videofluoroscopy should make it possible to visualize instability between the carpal bones.
- Arthrography (radiographic examination after injection of contrast) may demonstrate ligament injuries.
- Bone scan may demonstrate significant bony pathology.

Common Injuries

Wrist Sprain

Wrist pain may be caused by a fall on an extended hand or by a direct blow to or twisting of the wrist in combination with an extension or flexion moment. Most people who fall and injure themselves do not seek medical assistance because their symptoms are moderate and generally temporary. Typically, the fall results in a contusion of the soft tissue or an injury to the joint capsule. The accompanying swelling and pain usually subside after a few days.

A sprain of the wrist is a diagnosis of exclusion, most often employed when the X rays do not demonstrate any direct signs of a fracture or indirect signs of a ligament injury (e.g., dislocation of intact bones). Pain caused by a capsular injury is subjective and varies from patient to patient.

- Symptoms and signs: Patients experience pain, tenderness, swelling, and limited range of motion.
- Diagnosis: If there are signs of discoloration (bruising), swelling, malalignment, or instability, the patient should be referred for a radiographic examination. If no objective signs of a fracture or a ligament injury are found during the clinical examination, but the patient complains of a great deal of pain, he should also be given a radiographic examination. If pain and swelling do not improve within a week, the patient should be referred for radiographs, possibly with additional radiographic examinations as indicated. A clinical examination may demonstrate swelling and reduced range of motion, but a sprain is often considered to be a diagnosis of exclusion after additional examinations have "ruled out" other injuries.
- Treatment by physician: The recommended treatment is PRICE, nonsteroidal anti-inflammatory drugs (NSAIDs), and possibly immobilization in a cast for a few days. Gradual retraining and (possibly) taping or use of a brace is also recommended when resuming sporting activities.
- Treatment by therapist: A physical therapist may tape the patient or adjust a brace to prepare him to return to sport activities.
- Prognosis: The prognosis for a simple sprain is good, and if other injuries have been excluded, the athlete should be expected to resume sport activities within 1 to 2 weeks.

Other Injuries

Fracture of the Distal Radius

A fall on an extended hand may result in a fracture through the distal radius. The type of injury caused by a fall depends on (1) the position of the hand at the time of the fall, (2) the direction and magnitude of the force, and (3) the age of the person who falls (related to bone quality). The most common type of fracture (a Colles' fracture) runs through the distal metaphysis of the radius, causing a dorsal angular deformity known as a "dinner fork" deformity (figure 9.3, a and b). A palmar angulated fracture of the distal radius is known as a Smith's fracture (or a reverse Colles' fracture) (figure 9.4, a and b).

A Colles' fracture (or Colles-type fracture) often causes shortening of the radius, dorsal angulation of the distal articular surface (normally 10° to 12° of palmar tilt), reduction of the radioulnar inclination (measured on a PA view as the angle between a line running through the distal radial and ulnar corner of the radius and another line that is perpendicular to the longitudinal axis of the radius—normally 22°), or a combination of these malalignments. Normally, nearly 80% of the force from the wrist is transferred to the forearm through the radiocarpal joint, whereas slightly more than 20% is transferred through the ulnocarpal joint. Changes in normal anatomy of the wrist due to injury alter the transfer of force across the carpus, and the cartilage will undergo wear and tear in various locations. If there is shortening of the radius of 5 mm (or more), a

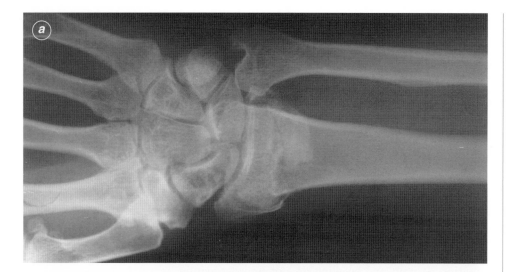

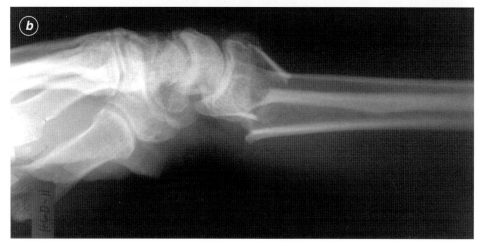

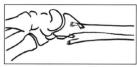

Figure 9.3 Colles fracture ("fractura radii typica"). Shortening of the radius *(a)* and dorsal displacement of the distal articular fragment *(b)*.

change occurs in the DRUJ and the TFCC. If dorsal angulation in the radiocarpal joint increases, there is a corresponding increase in force transferred to the ulnar. Major portions of the remaining force transferred between the radius and the wrist will be between the dorsal side of the scaphoid and the radius, causing cartilage degeneration in that location. To prevent this, the physician should correct malalignment caused by a fracture.

• Symptoms and signs: The patient has pain from her wrist, where a classic deformity (figures 9.3 and 9.4) is often found. The hand may be held in a slightly flexed and pronated position, while the distal ulna seems to protrude somewhat. Swelling and tenderness are essentially universal findings, and palpation will cause pain. Use of the hand is limited by pain and immobility, and symptoms of compression of the median nerve and/or the ulnar nerve may exist. There may be tenderness and possibly instability of the distal end of the ulna.

• Diagnosis: Although the diagnosis is often made on the basis of a clinical examination alone, patients who have wrist pain in association with a deformity of the carpus should be referred for a radiographic examination to confirm the suspected diagnosis of fracture. A radiographic examination should likewise be performed if there is any doubt about the presence of a fracture. One PA and one lateral view often suffice, but the physician may need to request various additional views and possibly a CT scan if the first views are difficult to read or otherwise inconclusive.

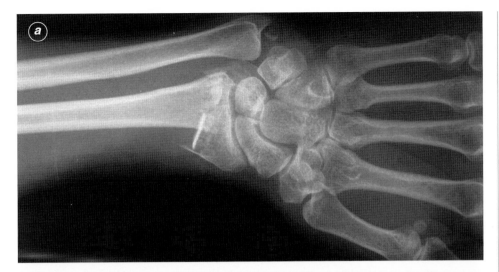

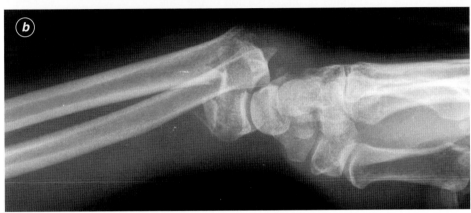

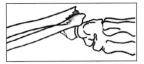

Figure 9.4 Smith fracture ("fractura radii atypica"). Shortening of the radius *(a)* and palmar displacement of the distal articular fragment *(b)*.

WRIST, HAND, AND FINGERS

• Treatment: The goal of the treatment is to restore normal alignment if possible. If there is any angulation, the fracture must be reduced. It is difficult to provide definite guidelines for the degree of acceptable angulation. This depends on the age of the patient and to some degree the attitude of the attending physician. For patients younger than 30 years of age, only anatomic position (i.e., a palmar tilt of 10° to 12° on a lateral view) should be accepted. The radius should not be shortened. If an X ray taken during a check-up one week postinjury demonstrates that the fracture has been redisplaced, the patient should be referred for surgical evaluation. The same rule applies if there is radial shortening of 3 to 5 mm. In an older patient, 10° to 15° of dorsal tilt and shortening of 3 to 5 mm are generally acceptable. Even greater displacement is tolerated in patients older than 75 years. If the physician is inexperienced in treating fractures of the distal radius, the patient should be referred to an orthopedic or hand surgeon. If repositioning succeeds, a well-molded cast is applied to prevent the fracture from dislocating again. Follow-up X rays are taken after the repositioning and application of the cast as well as 1 and 2 weeks after the initial treatment. If the wrist dislocates again while casted, the physician may attempt further reduction; but this often fails, and surgery should be considered. Many fractures return to the initial position (shortening and angular displacement) during the period when the patient is wearing a cast. As a consequence, some authors consider surgery the treatment of choice if shortening and dorsal angulation of the radius occur. Whenever a physician is in doubt, he should consult a hand surgeon. If an intra-articular fracture with incongruity of the articular surface and/or a major displacement that cannot be reduced has occurred, surgery should be considered mandatory. Surgical options include closed, open, or arthroscopic-assisted reduction in combination with some type of osteosynthesis such as percutaneous pinning, an external fixator, or screws and a plate. The choice of surgical treatment depends on the age of the patient and the type of fracture. Depending on age, fracture type, and the type of treatment used, the wrist must be immobilized from 4 to 6 weeks. External fixation devices should be removed earlier. A feared complication of distal limb injuries is reflex sympathetic dystrophy (RSD), which causes intense pain and swelling and reduced function of the hand and fingers. Patients who develop this complication should immediately be referred to a hand therapist with experience in treating RSD.

• Prognosis: Fractures of the distal radius where normal alignment and bone length are reestablished usually result in a pain-free and well-functioning wrist. However, many patients experience pain and discomfort in the wrist for up to a year after the injury, and all patients should therefore be informed regarding potential complications influencing outcome. If normal anatomy is not reestablished, reduced range of motion in the radiocarpal joint and in the DRUJ (rotation) may occur. A corrective osteotomy and/or a resection of a smaller or larger portion of the ulna may be performed if indicated. After many years of malalignment, osteoarthritis may develop, making arthrodesis a possible treatment alternative. However, the best prognosis results from optimal initial care and from restoring normal wrist anatomy after injury.

Scaphoid Fracture !

A scaphoid fracture is the most common type of fracture in the carpal bones (figure 9.5). As in the case of a fracture of the distal radius, the mechanism of injury is typically a fall on an extended, radially deviated hand. Most athletes who sustain a scaphoid fracture by this mechanism are young, active men, but children and the elderly may also sustain this type of fracture. The blood supply to the scaphoid comes from branches of the radial artery that enter the bone distally and palmarly, which has clinical significance for the healing of scaphoid fractures. Fractures in the distal half of the bone usually heal without problems, but healing may be difficult in the proximal pole due to interruption of the blood supply. A fracture of the scaphoid may be associated with other injuries in the wrist.

• Symptoms and signs: The patient complains of pain and weakness in her hand and may refer to a remote trauma. The injury may have been originally diagnosed as a sprain, but the symptoms have not resolved. Tenderness and pain in the anatomic snuffbox are common.

• Diagnosis: Tenderness in the anatomic snuffbox immediately after the injury should heighten suspicion of a scaphoid fracture. Although distal radius fracture can be excluded radiographically, a scaphoid fracture may not. If a scaphoid fracture is suspected on clinical examination (i.e., tenderness in the anatomic snuffbox), a cast should be applied, even if

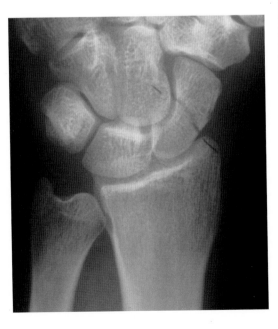

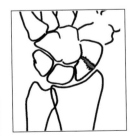

Figure 9.5 Scaphoid fracture, the most common fracture in a carpal bone.

the radiographic examination is normal. The patient should be seen for a follow-up within 5 to 10 days. If a fracture is still suspected, the patient should be reimaged, and additional examinations (such as CT scan, MRI, bone scan, or ultrasound) should be considered to demonstrate the suspected pathology in the scaphoid.

- Treatment: If the fracture is minimally displaced (≤1 mm) and there is no axial angulation, the fracture can be treated with immobilization. A short arm cast is used for this injury, immobilizing the thumb to the IP joint and leaving the other fingers free from the MCP joint distally. Because the circulation in the scaphoid is poor, healing time may be prolonged. The cast should therefore be worn for a minimum of 12 weeks. Several studies have shown that some scaphoid fractures take longer than 12 weeks to heal. Serial radiographs are imperative to confirm healing or to determine whether further casting is required. Less than 12 weeks of casting may result in delayed union or development of a pseudoarthrosis. Nondisplaced, stable scaphoid fractures that are surgically treated by screw fixation and casting heal faster than those that are treated by casting alone. Therefore, active athletes with this type of fracture should have surgery performed to allow them to return to the sport activity as quickly as possible. Displaced (>1 mm) and angulated scaphoid fractures should be referred for surgical evaluation. If a pseudoarthrosis develops, surgery may be attempted even several years after the primary fracture. When surgery is performed, any malalignment should be corrected, and bone should be transplanted and fixed using pins or screws. The patient must wear a cast for a minimum of 12 weeks after surgery.
- Prognosis: The prognosis is good if initial patient care is adequate. The physician must confirm that the fracture has healed, clinically and radiographically, before the athlete is allowed to return to sport activity. Surgically treated pseudoarthrosis also has a relatively good prognosis. If secondary changes develop in the wrist, such as osteoarthritis, the patient must be referred to a specialist for surgical evaluation.

Carpal Bone Fracture

If a patient has wrist pain after trauma, the possibility of a carpal bone fracture should be considered. The most common fractures have already been discussed. During the clinical examination, the most tender area can be identified, along with any areas of contusion and swelling. This information may be important in helping the radiologist determine what views to take in order to demonstrate any fractures. An isolated fracture of a carpal bone (other than the scaphoid) is rare. Avulsion fractures from dorsal radiotriquetral or lunotriquetral ligament injuries, or an occasional transverse fracture within the body of the triquetrum may be seen. If this occurs, the patient will have maximum soreness on the dorsal and ulnar side of the wrist. A golfer or other athlete who uses a racket or club may injure the hook of the hamate (which projects into the palm of the hand). This causes distinct soreness on the ulnar side of the palm. Direct blows to the ulnar side of the hand may cause a pisiform fracture. If a carpal bone fracture is demonstrated, the patient should be referred to a specialist for further diagnostics and treatment.

- Symptoms and signs: Symptoms include pain, soreness, and swelling, possibly combined with functional limitation.
- Diagnosis: A clinical examination may cause the suspicion of a fracture, but the diagnosis is made by radiographic examination. If a fracture in the wrist is suspected, several views are needed. In addition, CT, MRI, or other imaging studies may be indicated. If the hook of the hamate is injured, a carpal tunnel view should be requested to demonstrate a freely projecting hamulus (hook). Similarly, special views can be requested to evaluate the pisiform bone.
- Treatment: An isolated, nondisplaced fracture through the triquetrum, hamate, or pisiform may be treated with a cast or splint for 4 to 6 weeks. Patients with

fractures through other bones in the wrist should be referred for appropriate evaluation and treatment. These fractures are often part of a larger injury, and the treatment alternatives include open repositioning of displaced bones, repair of ligaments, osteosynthesis using pins or screws, and casting for 8 to 12 weeks. If there are late symptoms from a hamate or pisiform fracture, the hook of the hamate or the pisiform may be surgically removed without causing any discomfort.

- Prognosis: The prognosis depends entirely on the type of fracture, when the injury is diagnosed and treated, and on the type of treatment provided. The patient may fully recover but may also end up with persistent pain (osteoarthritis) from displaced carpal bones that may eventually make some type of arthrodesis necessary. The patient, the physical therapist, and the physician will need to discuss every case individually to determine when the athlete may resume sport activity.

Ligament Injury in the Wrist

A number of ligaments stabilize the various carpal bones in relation to each other and to the radius, ulna, and the metacarpal bones. Some of the interosseous ligaments are strongest on the palmar side, whereas others have greater dorsal strength. If there is a strong blow to the hand, usually caused by a fall on a hyperextended, ulnar-deviated, and somewhat rotated hand, then a fracture, a ligament injury, or a combination of the two may occur. Ligament injuries, with or without dislocation of the carpal bones, may be difficult to diagnose. The most common injuries are to the scapholunate or lunotriquetral ligaments (figure 9.6, a and b).

- Symptoms and signs: Pain, swelling, tenderness, and restricted range of motion are symptoms of ligament injuries in the wrist.

Figure 9.6 Scapholunar and lunotriquetral ligament injuries. When both ligaments are injured, the lunate bone becomes unstable and may become dislocated. Most commonly, only one of the ligaments ruptures. The wrist and carpus are seen from the dorsal side, with intact ligaments *(a)*. If an athlete falls on an extended hand, the ligaments in the carpus may rupture (as seen from the palmar side) *(b)*.

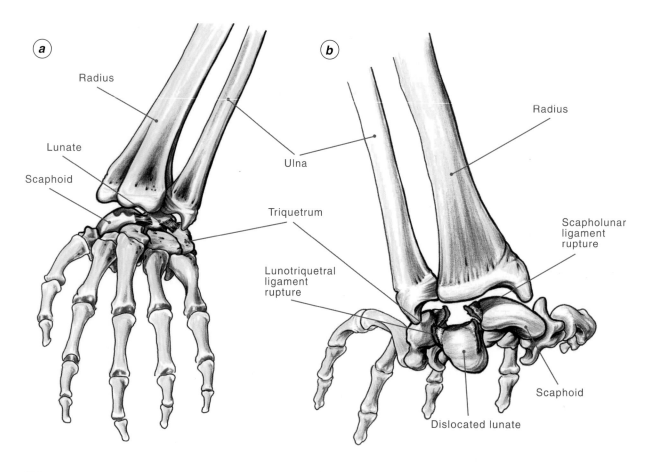

- Diagnosis: The diagnosis is based on the location of any resultant instability and tenderness in the wrist. During the acute phase it is difficult to perform a clinical assessment of the various carpal ligaments ("everything hurts"), but such testing is often possible later on. Therefore, if the mechanism of injury suggests significant force was involved and on exam there is a great deal of swelling and pain, a ligament injury should be suspected, and the patient should be referred to a hand surgeon for further evaluation. There are numerous examples of experienced radiologists overlooking obvious deformities in the wrist. Therefore, patients who seek medical attention after several weeks of pain, discomfort, clicking, and a feeling of "give way" in the wrist should be referred to a hand specialist. Radiographic imaging may demonstrate increased distance between the involved carpal bones as a sign of ligament disruption. Views of the wrist obtained with the hand in a position of maximum radial and ulnar deviation may demonstrate increased distance between the scaphoid and the lunate, whereas views of a supinated hand may demonstrate increased distance between the carpal bones on the ulnar side of the carpus. However, partial ligament ruptures often occur, potentially resulting in dynamic instability. The patient may complain of pain, clicking, and a feeling of something "going out of joint" when he rotates his hand. In this situation, radiography (PA and lateral views) may be unremarkable, and even MRI and CT are of limited help. Arthrography or fluoroscopic visualization of the wrist while the patient's hand is being rotated may demonstrate any instability. However, arthroscopy is the only method of simultaneously visualizing the various ligaments and assessing carpal stability. Arthroscopy is the best way to diagnose the extent of a ligamentous injury.
- Treatment: The patient should be referred to a hand surgeon. Generally, surgical treatment includes repositioning and fixation of the bones and repair of the ligaments. In case of an old injury with established instability and damage to adjacent cartilaginous surfaces, reconstruction of the ligaments or other procedures (capsulodesis, tenodesis, or arthrodesis) may be indicated. The wrist should be immobilized in a cast for 6 to 12 weeks.
- Prognosis: With early treatment, normal anatomy can be reestablished with a good outcome. The usual sequelae for the athlete include limited range of motion (and sometimes pain) in the wrist. Sport activity should be restricted for at least 3 months.

Distal Radioulnar Joint Injury

Forearm rotation takes place at the proximal and distal radioulnar joints (DRUJ). There is a concave articular surface (the sigmoid notch) on the distal radius, where the head of the ulna (which is convex toward the radius) articulates. Motion at the DRUJ is a combination of rotation and translation. Stability of the DRUJ depends in part on the skeleton and in part on the soft tissues (i.e., the triangular fibrocartilage complex (TFCC), the ulnocarpal ligaments, the extensor carpi ulnaris tendon, the pronator quadratus musculature, and the interosseous membrane). Trauma to the wrist may cause a DRUJ injury. This could be a soft-tissue injury or a soft-tissue injury combined with a fracture (figure 9.7, a and b). The fracture may be an intra-articular radius fracture that engages the sigmoid notch or a fracture through the styloid process of the ulna.

- Symptoms and signs: Symptoms and signs are pain in the wrist, particularly on the ulnar side, and reduced forearm rotation combined with instability or increased motion of the head of the ulna.
- Diagnosis: Patients suspected to have a DRUJ injury should be referred for an X ray or a CT scan of the wrist (which provides the best overview of the joint). A

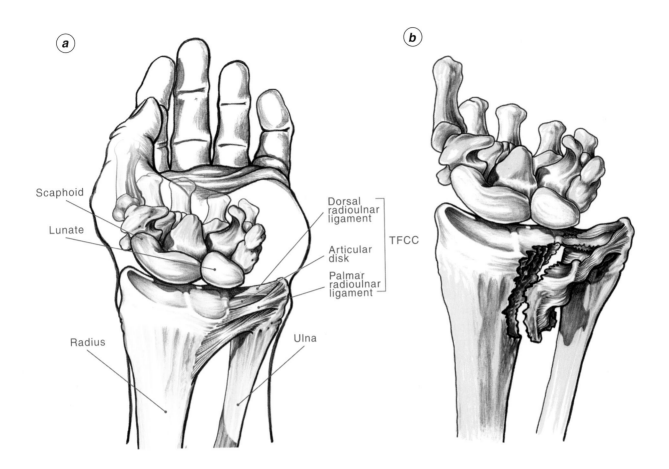

Scaphoid

Lunate

Radius

Dorsal radioulnar ligament

Articular disk

Palmar radioulnar ligament

TFCC

Ulna

Figure 9.7 Distal radioulnar joint injury. The wrist, seen from the palmar side, with an intact triangular fibrocartilage complex (TFCC) *(a)*. Intra-articular radial fracture that engages the articular surface of the distal radioulnar joint, and the TFCC *(b)*.

CT scan directly demonstrates the congruence in the DRUJ and any dislocation of the radius relative to the ulna. The uninjured side should be imaged for comparison. An isolated soft-tissue ligamentous injury that causes instability of the DRUJ may be diagnosed by clinical examination. Stability should be examined in a neutral rotational position and at maximal supination and pronation. These tests also need to be compared to the uninjured side. If instability or dislocation is suspected or demonstrated, the patient should be seen by a hand surgeon.

- Treatment: The physician should refer the patient to a hand surgeon for treatment. Surgery is performed on a fracture to ensure congruence in the DRUJ, whereas a ligament injury may be repaired by open or closed repositioning of the joint, followed by possible suturing of the ligament and immobilization for 6 weeks with a high cast (above elbow level to prevent rotation of the forearm). For an old injury, an attempt may be made to reconstruct the skeletal structure in the distal radioulnar joint. Other options include a limited resection of the distal end of the ulna or reconstruction of the ligaments using a free tendon graft.
- Prognosis: Results are good when acute injuries are treated, and the athlete may resume sport activity after about 12 weeks. If the patient has an old injury, function (forearm rotation) and pain will determine the need for surgical intervention. If surgery is performed, the situation may improve but the prognosis is indefinite.

Triangular Fibrocartilage Complex (TFCC) Rupture

Several structures contribute to stability in the DRUJ and in the ulnocarpal joint. A key structure is the TFCC. It consists of a meniscus-like structure, the articular disk, and the palmar and dorsal radioulnar ligaments. Hyperextension and rotation of the wrist contribute often to injury of the TFCC (figure 9.8). TFCC injuries also occur in combination with radius fractures. In addition, degenerative changes occur in the central part of the TFCC as the patient ages. Traumatic ruptures tend to occur peripherally.

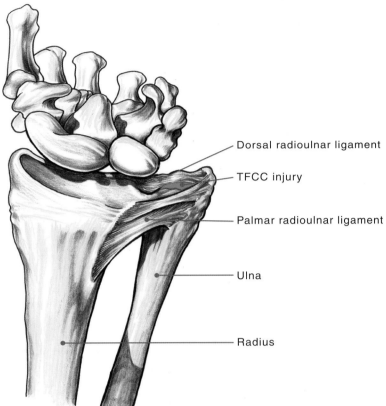

- Dorsal radioulnar ligament
- TFCC injury
- Palmar radioulnar ligament
- Ulna
- Radius

Figure 9.8 Triangular fibrocartilage complex rupture.

- Symptoms and signs: Symptoms and signs include ulnar-sided wrist pain, particularly upon forearm rotation and with ulnar deviation of the wrist. In a slightly flexed position, the injured wrist is often tender to palpation along the sheath of the flexor carpi ulnaris tendon. The patient may experience clicking, but real locking is less common.
- Diagnosis: An injury of the TFCC may be suspected, based on the mechanism of injury and the clinical examination. Patients with vague ulnar-sided wrist pain, possibly accompanied by clicking or a clicking sensation, should be further evaluated. An MRI examination is highly dependent on the radiologist's interpretation of the different views, and different findings from MRI and surgery are often reported. A negative MRI does not exclude a TFCC injury, and wrist arthroscopy should be considered the gold standard for diagnosing pathology.
- Treatment: Degenerative changes with central defects in the TFCC may be arthroscopically resected so that a loose flap does not interpose in the joint and cause pain. Avulsion from the radius is seldom repaired (because of the poor blood supply in this part of the cartilage, reducing the chance of healing). Conversely a peripheral ulnar avulsion may be sutured using an arthroscopic-assisted suture technique. Resection of a central injury does not require immobilization, whereas a repair requires 6 to 8 weeks of immobilization in a cast.
- Prognosis: Studies have shown that patients with central (usually degenerative) ruptures that are resected and peripheral ruptures that are repaired are generally pain free and satisfied. Patients with central injuries may resume sport activities immediately. Athletes who have undergone a repair of the TFCC should not return to sport for 12 weeks after surgery.

Tendon Injury

Tendon injuries at the wrist level rarely occur without a simultaneous open wound. One exception, which is not uncommon, is rupture of the extensor pollicis longus tendon in connection with a radius fracture (figure 9.9, a and b). Fracture is believed to increase pressure within the EPL tendon sheath where it curves around Lister's tubercle (a bony prominence on the doral side of radius proximal to the wrist), thereby creating an area of reduced circulation, which makes the tendon prone to rupture.

WRIST, HAND, AND FINGERS

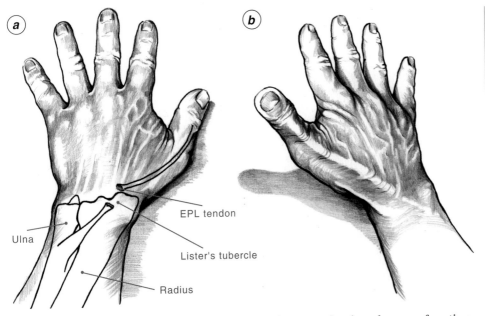

EPL tendon

Ulna

Lister's tubercle

Radius

Figure 9.9 Extensor pollicis longus (EPL) rupture. To test for EPL tendon function, the patient places the palms of both hands on a table-top and lifts his thumbs off the surface. If the EPL tendon is ruptured, he will not be able to do this *(a)*. If the tendon is intact, the contours of the tendon can be observed and palpated *(b)*.

- Symptoms and signs: Tenderness, swelling, weakness, and reduced range of motion.
- Diagnosis: The best way to test for extensor pollicis longus (EPL) function is to have the patient place the palm of her hand on a surface and ask her to lift her thumb off that surface. She cannot do this if the EPL tendon is ruptured.
- Treatment: If there is a suspected or a diagnosed tendon injury, the patient should be referred for surgery. It may be difficult to suture together the frayed ends of a ruptured EPL tendon directly. If so, one surgical alternative is transposition of one of the index finger's extensor tendons (the extensor indicis proprius tendon) to the thumb's extensor tendon. Flexor tendons are put in a dynamic casting for 4 weeks, while extensor tendons are immobilized for 5 weeks after surgery.
- Prognosis: Prognosis is good after surgical treatment. A flexor tendon does not have normal strength for active grip until 12 weeks after the injury. If an injury of the extensor tendons has occurred, sport activity may be resumed after 8 weeks.

Nerve Entrapment

The median and ulnar nerves may both be subjected to pressure at the wrist level (figure 9.10). The most common nerve entrapment is the result of compression of the ulnar nerve, such as might be caused when a cyclist holds onto the handlebars. Ulnar neuropathy may cause reduction of sensation in the little finger and the ulnar half of the ring finger, and it may also reduce the function of the hand intrinsic muscles (figure 9.2). The patient may as a result experience difficulties with fine motor activity. Pressure on the median nerve typically causes numbness and tingling ("the fingers are

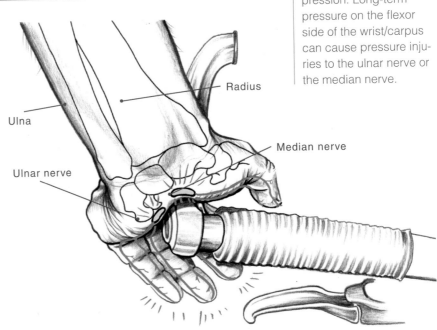

Radius

Ulna

Median nerve

Ulnar nerve

Figure 9.10 Nerve compression. Long-term pressure on the flexor side of the wrist/carpus can cause pressure injuries to the ulnar nerve or the median nerve.

asleep") of the thumb, index finger, long finger, and the radial half of the ring finger (figure 9.2).

- **Symptoms and signs:** The patient may experience tingling and numbness radiating into various fingers and reduced hand function. The patient may report that his hand is "butter-fingered" (i.e., he tends to drop objects).
- **Diagnosis:** Mild tapping (with a finger) over the affected nerve can cause radiating pain, discomfort, or paresthesias corresponding to the course of the affected nerve (referred to as a positive Tinel sign). Compression of the median nerve at the wrist will not significantly reduce muscle function. Compression of the ulnar nerve may reduce the patient's ability to abduct and adduct her fingers and may cause atrophy in the hypothenar area and in the area between the first and second fingers (i.e., the hand appears "flat").
- **Treatment:** The most important aspect of treatment is to avoid putting pressure on the affective nerve. The symptoms may gradually disappear on their own. Alternatively, a surgical procedure releasing the ligament compressing the nerve may be performed.
- **Prognosis:** The prognosis is good if the nerve compression has not persisted for a long time.

Carpal Dislocation !

The practitioner should recognize the possibility of carpal dislocation with or without a simultaneous fracture through the carpus (figure 9.11). A perilunar (fracture) dislocation could be a midcarpal, a transscaphoid perilunate, a palmar, an axial, or a radiocarpal dislocation. The mechanism of injury and symptomatology is the same

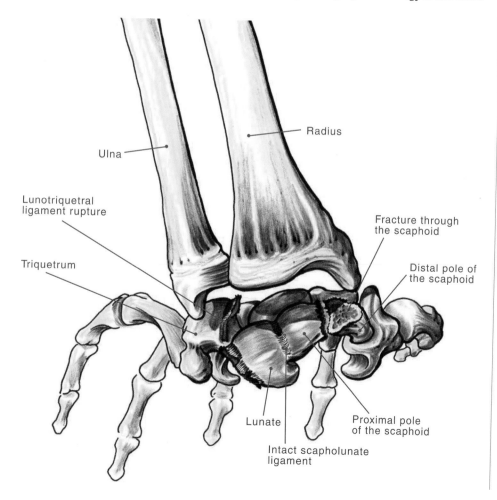

Radius

Ulna

Lunotriquetral ligament rupture

Triquetrum

Fracture through the scaphoid

Distal pole of the scaphoid

Lunate

Proximal pole of the scaphoid

Intact scapholunate ligament

Figure 9.11 Carpal dislocation. Forceful trauma to the carpus can cause various types of fractures, dislocations, or combinations thereof. In the transscaphoid perilunar dislocation shown, a fracture through the scaphoid and a rupture in the lunotriquetral ligament have occurred. However, the scapholunate ligament is intact, so that the proximal part of the scaphoid is dislocated at the same time as the lunate.

as for an isolated carpal fracture or ligament injury. A carpal dislocation is rare, and it is often overlooked at first. Therefore, if a carpal dislocation is suspected, the patient should be referred to a hand surgeon for further diagnostics and treatment.

The prognosis is best with early diagnosis and treatment; late treatment often makes surgical intervention necessary, which in turn will likely limit wrist motion. If there are large deformities that have existed for a long time and caused osteoarthritis in several joints, the patient may end up with some type of a limited carpal arthrodesis or even a total wrist fusion.

Finger Injuries

Jan-Ragnar Haugstvedt

Incidence

Finger injuries frequently occur as a result of various types of sport activities, particularly ball sports such as volleyball, basketball, and team handball. Sprain injuries occur most commonly and usually require only symptomatic treatment. More significant injuries, such as dislocations, ligament injuries, or fractures require referral to an orthopedic or hand surgeon for definitive management.

Differential Diagnosis

Table 9.2 lists various finger injuries. The most common are sprains, but fractures, dislocations, and ligament injuries are not uncommon sports injuries. Tendon injuries are less common. Although diagnosing and treating finger injuries is often straightforward, some cases require additional diagnostic testing or special treatment.

Diagnostic Thinking

The physician should examine the injured finger for open wounds (suggesting possible tendon or nerve injury), swelling and bruising (indication of bleeding, as in the case of ligament injuries, dislocations, and fractures), malalignment (for fractures and/or dislocations), and specific muscular weakness (for tendon injury). If the athlete reports reduced sensation in the injured finger, the patient should be referred to

Most common	Less common	Must not be overlooked !
Sprain (p. 247)	Finger fracture (p. 248)	Interposed soft tissue after dislocations (p. 255)
	Metacarpal fracture (p. 248)	Rotary malalignment with finger fractures (p. 249)
	Bennett's fracture (p. 248)	
	Reversed Bennett's fracture (p. 248)	
	Collateral ligament ruptures in the PIP and MCP joints (p. 250)	
	Collateral ligament ruptures in the MCP joint of the thumb (p. 251)	
	Mallet finger (drop finger) (p. 253)	
	Tendon rupture (p. 252)	
	Pulley rupture (p. 254)	
	Finger joint dislocation (p. 255)	
	Nerve injury (p. 255)	

Table 9.2 Overview of the differential diagnosis of finger injuries.

a hand surgeon. Injury of a dorsal digital nerve (especially of the radial nerve) may not need to be repaired because this injury usually causes only minor discomfort for the patient. However, injuries of the digital nerve on the palmar surface of a finger *should* be referred for prompt surgical evaluation and treatment (within 1 to 2 weeks). There is no need for further observation. A compression (closed) injury, however, may be observed for 2 weeks before referring the patient for surgical evaluation. The patient should also be referred to a hand surgeon if a lack of flexion or extension of one or more fingers is found.

If a patient exhibits swelling and bruising, function of the affected digit should be tested. The easiest way to do this is to ask the patient to make a fist and then extend her fingers. The physician examines for tenderness and stability. If active or passive finger motion is painful, and if instability is present (or suspected), the patient should be referred for radiographic evaluation. Similarly, if the patient has obvious malalignment, fracture, or dislocation, she should be referred for a radiographic examination. Although a dislocated joint may be immediately reduced, afterwards the patient should be referred for a radiographic examination to verify the reduction and to rule out a fracture combination. Depending on the results of the radiographic examination, a finger fracture may be treated by immobilization alone or the patient may be referred for surgery.

Clinical History

In most cases, information about the mechanism of injury reveals a great deal about the type of injury incurred. Direct trauma to one or more fingers or force applied in the axial direction may cause an avulsion of a tendon insertion or a dislocation of a finger joint. The patient probably has suffered a dislocation and/or a fracture if side-to-side trauma has resulted in malalignment (e.g., a finger pointing in the wrong direction). If a dislocation was reduced, information on how the reduction was performed should be included in the patient's case history. For example, in a hyperextension trauma of the PIP joint with a resultant tear of the volar tendon plate, the finger will be dorsally dislocated and a flexion maneuver will be required to reduce the finger. Did the athlete (or others) hear a crack or other sound indicating tearing of soft-tissue or fracture of bone? Did the swelling or ecchymosis occur immediately, indicating a ligament injury or a fracture?

Clinical Examination

Inspection. Bruising and swelling may indicate bleeding, such as that caused by ligament injuries, dislocations, and fractures. Fracture may also be suspected if there is deformity with malalignment or rotary deviation. A single finger observed in a persistently flexed position suggests an injury to the finger's extensor apparatus, whereas a finger observed to be in a persistently extended position (the dorsum of the hand against the surface) with a lack of tension on the flexor side of the finger suggests an injury to the flexor tendons. If there is an open wound, the possibility of nerve and tendon injuries should always be considered.

Palpation. The physician should examine the point of greatest tenderness and determine whether the swelling is "soft" (as in the case of a hematoma) or "hard" (as in the case of a displaced bone). Exerting pressure on the injured finger makes it possible to verify instability from fractures or from ligament injuries.

Nerve function. A laceration or a crush injury may result in a loss of sensation in the finger. The motor nerve branches originate more proximally in the hand and forearm and therefore peripheral nerve injury is unlikely to be the cause of motor dysfunction following a finger injury. Sensation is easily assessed by touching one side of the finger with a cotton ball or the end of a paper clip or pen and comparing the response to the contralateral side or an uninjured digit on the same hand. The median nerve innervates the thumb, index finger, middle finger, and the radial side of the ring finger, whereas the ulnar nerve innervates the ulnar side of the ring finger and the entire little finger (figure 9.2).

Range of motion. The normal range of motion in the four fingers is full extension (i.e., to 0° in the metacarpophalangeal (MCP), the proximal interphalangeal [PIP] and the distal interphalangeal [DIP] joints). It should be possible to flex all three joints to 90° on the individual fingers. A somewhat simplified assessment of available finger flexion is to ask the patient to make a fist to see whether the fingertip of each digit can reach the distal palmar crease. The IP joint of the thumb is extended to 0° and flexed to 90°, whereas the MCP joint is extended to 0° and flexed to 50°-60°. In some people, hyperextension of the finger joints could be considered normal. In others, however, hyperextension of the affected joint may be a sign of injury (e.g., avulsion of the volar tendon plate in the PIP joints). The physician should compare motion to that of the other fingers and ask if motion has changed after the injury.

Tendon function. Tendon injuries can often be diagnosed by inspection. For example, if the patient can flex the IP joint of his thumb, the long flexor tendon of his thumb is intact. The flexor tendons of the fingers need to be tested individually (figure 9.12, a and b). The attachment of the flexor digitorum superficialis is palmar and proximal on

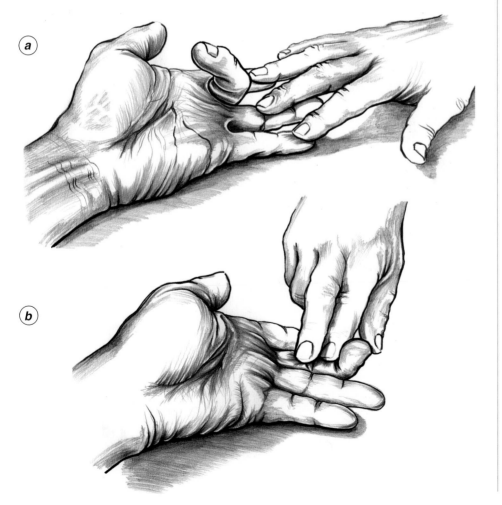

(a)

(b)

Figure 9.12 Function test of the deep and superficial flexor tendons. During testing of one of the superficial flexor tendons, the adjacent fingers are locked in full extension while the patient flexes the proximal interphalangeal (PIP) joint (a). When testing the deep flexor tendons, the proximal part of the finger is immobilized in the extended position while the patient flexes the distal interphalangeal (DIP) joint (b).

WRIST, HAND, AND FINGERS

the middle phalanx, and its function is tested by holding the other three fingers locked in an extended position while asking the patient to flex the PIP joint of the examined finger. The attachment of the flexor digitorum profundus is palmar and proximal on the distal phalanx, and the function is tested by fixing the middle phalanx (keeping the PIP joint in an extended position) of the finger to be examined and asking the patient to flex the DIP joint. If an extensor tendon injury is suspected, ask the athlete to fully extend the injured finger. When the long extensor tendon of the thumb (EPL) is involved, the best way to determine if the EPL is intact is to ask the patient to place the palm of her hand on a surface and to then lift her thumb off that surface. This is not possible if the EPL tendon has ruptured.

Testing of stability. When examining the stability of the collateral ligaments, one should remember that the ligaments of the fingers have different origins and insertions in the MCP joints than in the PIP joints. In the MCP joints, the lateral ligaments are tight when the fingers are flexed to 90°, whereas they are relaxed when the fingers are extended. For this reason, the lateral ligaments of the MCP joints should be tested with the MCP joints in a flexed position. The opposite is true of the PIP joints, where the lateral ligaments are tight when the fingers are extended (0°) and more relaxed when the PIP joints are flexed. Therefore, the lateral ligaments of the PIP joints should be tested with the PIP joints in the extended position. The collateral ligaments of the MCP joint in the thumb should be tested both in a fully extended position and in a slightly flexed (20° to 30°) position (figure 9.13).

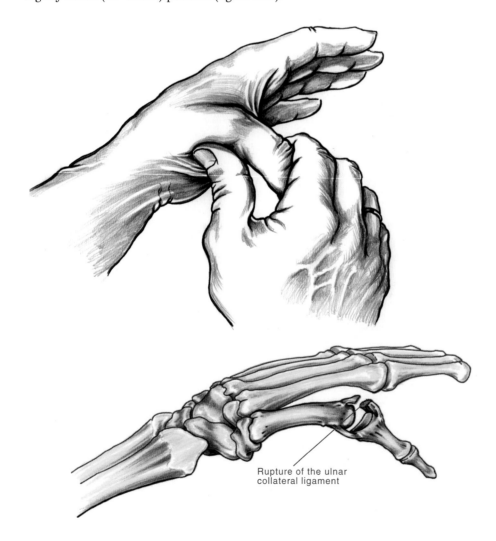

Rupture of the ulnar
collateral ligament

Figure 9.13 Stress test of the thumb's MCP joint. When the ulnar collateral ligament is ruptured, lateral instability increases in comparison with the non-injured hand.

The clinical assessment of stability is made more difficult by the individual variation that exists. Therefore, it is important to compare the injured digit with adjacent fingers or (best of all) with the corresponding digit on the opposite, uninjured hand. The most reliable testing is usually performed immediately after the injury occurs. The patient does not feel the same degree of pain as she would later on, when it may be necessary to use local anesthesia for adequate testing.

Supplemental Examinations

Radiographic examination. Even if the patient has been given a thorough clinical examination, it is not always possible to exclude subtle skeletal injury without additional testing. It is generally very important to the patient's future hand function that the physician recognize a skeletal injury (e.g., avulsion of a tendon or ligament at the point of insertion) as early as possible so that proper treatment can be provided. If there is doubt, the patient should be referred for an additional examination. No one benefits from a wait-and-see attitude. For example, in children, a fracture may begin to heal after 2 weeks, and delaying the definitive diagnostic examination may result in the need to reopen a fracture line so that it can be properly reduced. Generally, routine radiographic examinations, using several views (always a minimum of two), will confirm a suspected fracture. If there is doubt, additional oblique views should be requested. Stress radiographs (i.e., X rays taken while static force is applied to the injured finger) may make it possible to expose instability. Corresponding views of the other (uninjured) hand should always be taken for comparison.

Other examinations, such as MRI, CT scans, and bone scan, are not commonly used in the evaluation of finger injuries. MRI may provide information about interposed soft tissue in a joint after a dislocation, but in general advanced cross sectional imaging should be requested only by a hand surgeon. Ultrasonography is potentially useful in diagnosing a fracture but is best used to confirm a suspected tendon rupture or a pulley rupture.

Common Injuries

Sprains

The most common finger injuries are caused by a blow to a finger caused by a fall, a ball or puck hitting the finger; a finger getting stuck in equipment; or a finger attempting to grab the jersey of a teammate or opponent. A sprained finger is swollen and is painful and sore on palpation. Range of motion may be limited as the result of a partial lesion of the joint capsule or of a ligament.

- Symptoms and signs: Pain, swelling, tenderness, and limited range of motion (particularly flexion), are common findings, but joint instability is rare.
- Diagnosis: If there is malalignment and palpation causes pain, a fracture should be suspected and the patient should be referred for a radiographic examination. If the radiographic examination is normal and the finger is stable in flexion and extension, the patient may have a sprain. A sprain is a diagnosis of exclusion: radiographs should be normal, the finger should be stable, with intact sensation and preserved tendon function. Mild swelling and some soreness are common. The diagnosis is based largely on the clinical examination, but a radiographic examination is necessary to exclude fracture.
- Treatment by physician: The recommended treatment by a physician is PRICE treatment, NSAIDs, and possibly immobilization in a cast, brace or tape for a few days. It is often useful to "buddy tape" the injured finger to an adjacent finger when resuming activity.

• Prognosis: The prognosis is good. However, it may be a long time before the range of motion (particularly flexion) of a sprained PIP joint has returned to normal. The PIP joint may look swollen for a long time (up to a year) without anyone finding anything wrong or being able to give any specific treatment. Sport activity that is within the limits of pain can normally be resumed as soon as pain allows, usually within a few days, provided that the finger is buddy taped to an adjacent finger for support.

Other Injuries

Finger Fracture

Direct or indirect force to a finger may cause ligament injury, fractures, or a combination of the two. In this section, two special fractures involving the base of the first and fifth metacarpals—Bennett's fracture (figure 9.14 a) and the reversed Bennett's fracture (figure 9.14 b)—are discussed. In these fractures, a small fragment of the base of the first or fifth metacarpal is avulsed. This fragment represents an important site of ligament insertion. The bone fragment remains in place while the remainder of the phalanx is out of position and must be reduced. The athlete may also sustain other transverse, oblique, spiral, intra-articular, or comminuted finger fractures.

• Symptoms and signs: Symptoms include pain, tenderness, swelling, and malalignment.
• Diagnosis: Radiographs are essential to verify the suspected fracture. For individual fractures (such as a reversed Bennett's fracture) a CT scan may be helpful

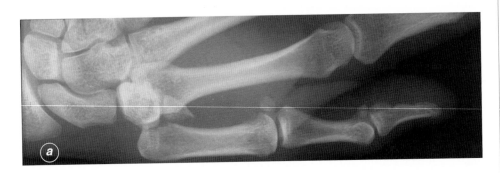

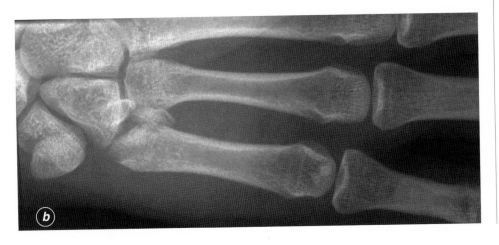

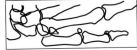

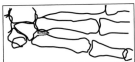

Figure 9.14 Bennett fracture *(a)*: Avulsion fracture of the base of the first metacarpal. Reversed Bennett fracture *(b)*: Avulsion fracture of the base of the fifth metacarpal. The small triangular bone fragments are "in place" while the body of the metacarpal bones is dislocated and must be reduced.

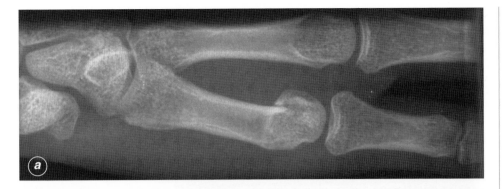

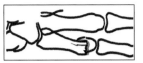

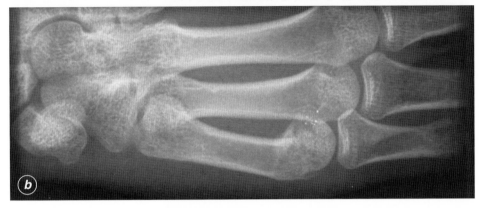

Figure 9.15 Transverse fracture of the fifth metacarpal. Frontal *(a)* and oblique lateral *(b)* views demonstrate a distal subcapital fracture. However, it is not possible to obtain a direct lateral view of these fractures. Therefore, it must be noted that malalignment could be significantly greater than what is revealed by the lateral views.

in demonstrating the fracture dislocation. To examine the finger for possible malrotation, the physician should ask the patient to make a fist. The nails of the four fingers are normally in the same plane, the fingertips merging towards the scaphoid.

- Treatment of transverse fractures (figure 9.15): These are usually stable fractures that can be treated by immobilizing the finger (e.g., buddy taping it to an adjacent finger). However, transverse fractures (e.g., of the middle phalanx) can be greatly displaced due to the action of tendons (the flexor digitorum superficialis muscle). If the fracture is displaced, it it must be reduced and the finger immobilized in a cast for 3 to 4 weeks. If reduction fails, surgery is necessary.

- Treatment of oblique and spiral fractures (figure 9.16, a and b): These are often shortened and involve malrotation. The position cannot be maintained after reduction, and as a consequence, these fractures should be treated surgically—for example, by percutaneous pinning. Prompt reduction and stable fixation facilitate healing and permit the athlete to resume training more quickly. Fractures that are not treated surgically should be checked by a second radiographic examination after 1 week.

- Treatment of intra-articular fractures (figure 9.17, a and b): Comminuted fractures compromising joint congruity should be referred to a hand surgeon for definitive treatment.

- Treatment of Bennett's fracture and reversed Bennett's fracture: These fractures require surgery.

- Prognosis: Usually short-term immobilization and early rehabilitation are required to achieve good functional results. If the fracture is properly reduced and stabilized, rehabilitation may begin after 3 to 4 weeks of immobilization, resulting in a favorable prognosis. If initial treatment is inadequate, there may be a prolonged rehabilitation period keeping the athlete from participating in sports activities. Surgery may eventually be required to correct any deformity that has resulted. Tendon injuries with concomitant fractures are challenging because of adhesions

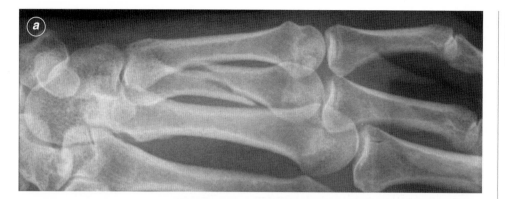

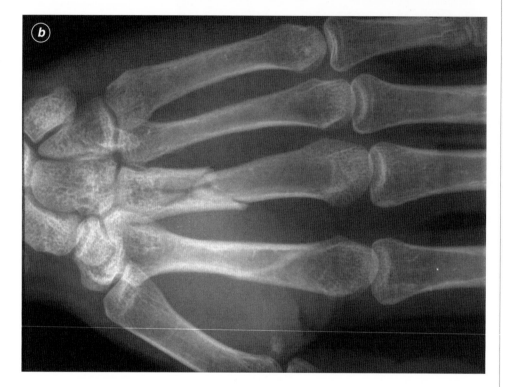

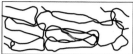

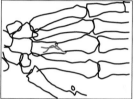

Figure 9.16 Oblique and shaft fractures. These fractures often cause shortening and/or malrotation of the finger and, therefore, require surgery.

between the skeleton and the tendon and may require long-term rehabilitation under the supervision of a hand therapist. The patient usually can return to sport activity after 4 to 6 weeks, depending on the type of fracture, the response to treatment, and the sport involved.

Rupture of the Collateral Ligament of the PIP and MCP Joints

The collateral ligaments in the finger's PIP and MCP joints may be injured by direct side-to-side trauma or when the finger gets caught on an object.

• Symptoms and signs: Patients experience pain, tenderness, and swelling, as well as reduced active joint flexion.
• Diagnosis: The diagnosis is based on soreness and pain upon palpation and on tests of the stability of the involved joint. A complete ligament rupture may cause instability. A radiographic examination is indicated to rule out avulsed bone fragments; these occur rarely in the PIP joint but are somewhat more common in the MCP joint.

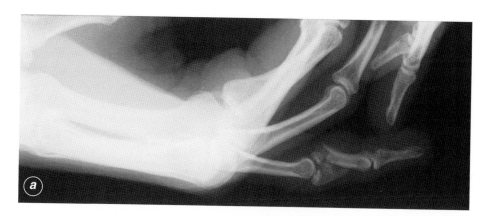

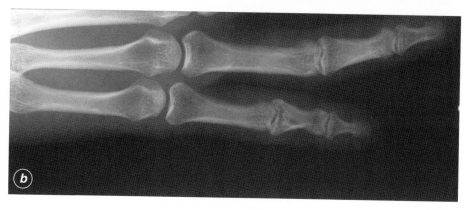

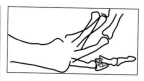

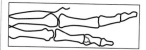

Figure 9.17 Intra-articular fracture. These fractures require exact repositioning to provide good function and to prevent the development of arthrosis. Surgery is usually necessary.

- Treatment: The injured finger is immobilized to an adjacent finger for 1 to 3 weeks, and then free exercise is allowed. If significant swelling and pain occur, immobilization in a cast may be indicated for a few days: placing the MCP in 90° flexion and fully extending of the PIP and DIP joints. A fracture may be an indication for open reduction and fixation of the bony fragment followed by immobilization for 3 to 4 weeks.
- Prognosis: The prognosis is generally good, but, as in the case of a sprain, it may take a long time for range of motion to return to normal. The PIP joint may be swollen for up to one year. Buddy taping the affected finger to an adjacent finger for a few more weeks is a good prophylactic measure, particularly in ball sports such as team handball or volleyball, where there is considerable risk of reinjury.

Rupture of the Collateral Ligament in the MCP Joint of the Thumb—Skier's Thumb

The most common mechanism of injury is falling while skiing, causing trauma to the thumb with increasing stress leading to a possible rupture of the ulnar collateral ligament (figure 9.18).

- Symptoms and signs: Symptoms and signs include pain upon thumb motion, as well as swelling (bleeding) and soreness to palpation on the side of the thumb corresponding to the injured collateral ligament. Soreness is often also present on the palmar side of the thumb's MCP joint (simultaneous injury of the palmar tendon plate).
- Diagnosis: It is best to examine the injury immediately after the accident occurs, when the proper diagnosis can be made on the basis of the clinical examination alone. By moving the thumb in a radial direction away from the rest of a stabilized hand, stability of the ulnar collateral ligament is tested (figure 9.13). The

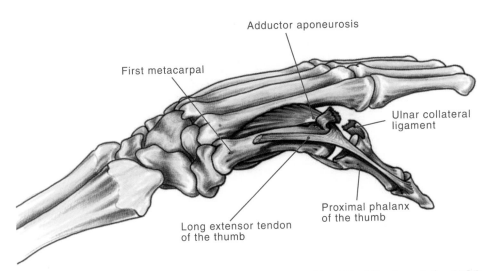

First metacarpal

Adductor aponeurosis

Ulnar collateral ligament

Long extensor tendon of the thumb

Proximal phalanx of the thumb

Figure 9.18 Rupture of the ulnar collateral ligament in the thumb's MCP joint (skier's thumb). The ulnar collateral ligament usually ruptures at the insertion to the proximal phalanx, sometimes with a bone fragment that is avulsed. A midsubstance rupture may also occur so that the proximal part of the ligament becomes displaced by the adductor aponeurosis (as shown). These ruptures will not heal without surgery.

thumb should be examined both fully extended and in 20° of flexion at the MCP joint. Slightly increased laxity followed by a *distinct stop* is often interpreted as a partial (incomplete) ligament tear. If there is increased laxity without a distinct stop, the patient should be referred for stress radiographic evaluation and examination by a hand surgeon. Similar X ray views of the other, uninjured thumb should be taken for comparison. The patient should also be examined in a similar fashion if an injury of the radial collateral ligament is suspected clinically.

- Treatment: A partial tear (distinct stop while testing) may be treated by immobilization in a cast for 4 to 6 weeks. If there is an avulsion fracture with displacement of the ligament insertion, surgery is required. If there is no fracture, but definite instability is detected, surgery is required as well. This is particularly true of the ulnar collateral ligament, where the mechanism of injury may involve the ruptured ligament becoming "caught" by the aponeurosis of the adductor pollicis longus, preventing the ligament ends from healing without surgery. After surgery, the patient needs to be casted for 5 to 6 weeks. Injuries to the radial collateral ligament are less common and have traditionally been treated conservatively (with a cast for 5 to 6 weeks). "Combination" injuries to the radial collateral ligament and the volar tendon plate are not uncommon. The current tendency is to perform surgery on these injuries (as in the case of the ulnar collateral ligament injury).
- Prognosis: The prognosis is good with proper treatment. When casting is completed, the patient may benefit from a protective brace when resuming sport activity after about 8 weeks.

Tendon Rupture

If there is a wound, a rupture of the extensor or flexor tendons should be suspected, depending on the location of the injury. A tendon rupture without an open wound is rare, but a flexor tendon may rupture if sufficient force is applied against resistance (e.g., finger flexion against resistance). Flexor tendon injury may also occur due to extreme loading, as in the case of mountain climbing. The EPL tendon may rupture as the result of a radius fracture (figure 9.9).

- Symptoms and signs: Symptoms include pain, tenderness, mild swelling, and reduced tone in the injured muscle-tendon unit. A persistently extended or flexed IP joint that cannot actively be moved in the opposite direction is often a sign of a tendon rupture.
- Diagnosis: The clinical examination serves as the basis for making the diagnosis. Ultrasonography may help, and radiography may demonstrate an avulsed bone fragment.

- Treatment: Surgery is the recommended treatment.
- Prognosis: The prognosis is good if surgery is performed. The athlete may return to sport activity 8 weeks after an extensor tendon injury, but full loading is not allowed until 12 weeks after a flexor tendon injury.

Mallet Finger—Drop Finger

If a ball (e.g., handball, basketball, or volleyball) hits the very tip of a finger, or if the finger is suddenly subjected to an external load that forces the extended IP joint into flexion, the extensor tendon inserting onto the dorsal side of the distal phalanx (figure 9.19, a-b) may be injured.

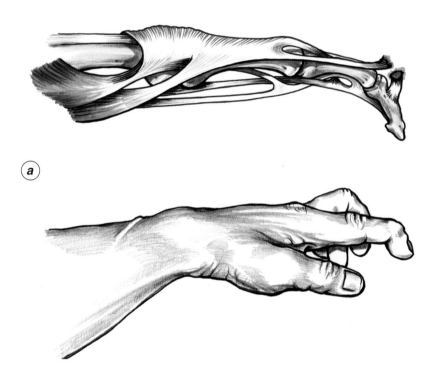

(a)

- Symptoms and signs: Symptoms include tenderness, mild swelling, possible ecchymosis as a sign of bleeding, and pain. The DIP joint of the affected finger remains in a flexed position and may only be extended passively, not actively.
- Diagnosis: The diagnosis is made clinically, but a radiographic examination should be obtained to exclude fracture.
- Treatment: If there is an avulsion fracture of the extensor tendon insertion involving one-fourth to one-sixth of the articular surface, surgery should be performed on the finger within a few days. Otherwise,

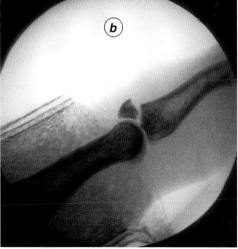

(b)

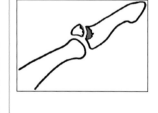

Figure 9.19 Mallet finger. Mallet finger can be treated conservatively in case of a torn tendon insertion, if the skeleton is intact (a). Always take an X ray to exclude skeletal injury. If there is a fracture injury, the patient must be evaluated for surgery (b).

a drop finger can be treated with a splint that immobilizes the DIP joint in an extended (or slightly hyperextended) position, while allowing free motion in the

PIP and MCP joints. The brace should be worn day and night for 6 to 8 weeks, and then it should be worn as a night splint for a few more weeks. If there is no fracture, surgery does not improve outcome.

- Prognosis: The prognosis is good. Improvement is gradual; it may, however, take 6 to 12 months before the DIP joint can be fully extended actively. Even a several-month-old drop finger injury may be treated as described with a good result. Sport activity may be resumed after about 10 weeks, but it is recommended that the finger be protected with tape or a splint.

Pulley Rupture—Tendon Sheath Injury

Pulleys are thickened areas within the flexor tendon sheath, located in specific spots along the course of the tendon. They serve the purpose of keeping the tendon in place next to the bony skeleton, thereby preventing "bowstringing" of the affected tendon (figure 9.20). The finger's flexor tendons may rupture as a result of extreme loading (such as mountain climbers impose on their fingers).

- Symptoms and signs: Pain, tenderness, and swelling on the palmar side of the finger are typical findings.
- Diagnosis: The diagnosis is based on localized pain upon palpation over the pulley, and pain with active flexion motion of the affected finger. If several pulleys are torn, the flexor tendon may be palpated as a bowstring in the subcutaneous tissue. A trained radiologist should be able to visualize the ruptured pulleys on ultrasonography.
- Treatment: If a bowstring is palpated, the patient should be referred for surgical repair or reconstruction. There is no effective treatment other than surgery. The patient should be informed about the cause of the condition.
- Prognosis: The prognosis is good. After pulley reconstruction, adhesions might develop that could reduce the flexion of the affected finger. The patient should wait 8 to 10 weeks after surgical intervention before resuming sport activity.

Figure 9.20 Pulley rupture. Extreme pulling of the flexor tendons of the finger, such as when mountain climbing, may cause the sheath of the flexor tendons to rupture.

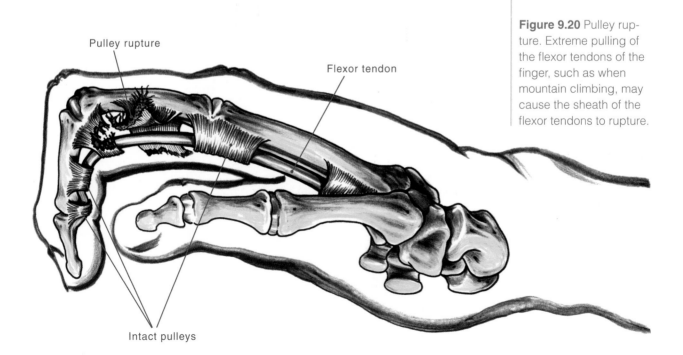

Pulley rupture

Flexor tendon

Intact pulleys

Finger Joint Dislocation

Dislocation of a finger joint (figure 9.21) is a relatively common injury resulting from participation in various ball sports. Dislocation of the little finger or thumb is most common, but any joint of any finger can be dislocated.

- Symptoms and signs: Symptoms include swelling, tenderness, deformity, and limited range of motion.
- Diagnosis: The diagnosis is based on the presence of malalignment and instability, or a history thereof. Radiographic examination is necessary to rule out associated fractures.
- Treatment: Reduction of a dislocated finger by axially distracting the finger immediately after the injury has occurred is usually a simple procedure. A *radiographic examination should be performed to confirm the reduction* and to rule out fracture. The finger should be immobilized by casting or buddy-taped to an adjacent finger for 3 to 4 weeks, after which exercises may begin. The injured finger should subsequently be taped to an adjacent finger for a few more weeks upon resumption of sport activity. The PIP joints in particular, but also the MCP joints, may be dorsally dislocated as a result of traumatic hyperextension. *Interposition of the* patient's *volar tendon plate or flexor tendons* may also occur, making closed reduction impossible and necessitating surgery. Surgery should also be considered for a fracture dislocation.
- Prognosis: The prognosis is generally favorable, but active range of motion is often reduced (particularly in PIP joints) for several months after the injury. Swelling in the joint may persist for up to a year. Sporting activity may be resumed 5 to 6 weeks after the injury occurs, but the finger should be protected by buddy taping.

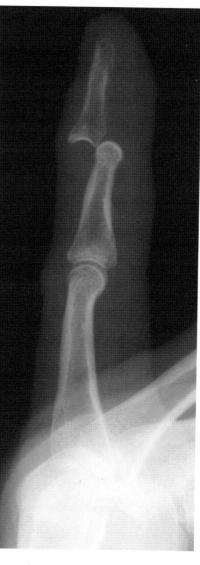

Figure 9.21 Dislocation. Forceful trauma to a finger may cause dislocation of a finger joint, as shown in the DIP joint of this little finger.

Nerve Injury

Digital nerve injuries tend to occur in association with open wounds. Digital nerve compression may impair sensation, even though nerve continuity is retained. Injuries to terminal branches of the radial nerve, located dorsally in the fingers are usually not repaired, as they cause only minor inconvenience to the patient. However, an injured digital nerve on the palmar side of the finger *should* be referred for surgical treatment as soon as the injury is diagnosed (preferably no later than 1 to 2 weeks after injury). There is no reason for a longer period of "observation." The patient may indicate whether sensation differs between the radial and ulnar sides of each finger, when examined as previously described. The physician also should compare the injured hand to the uninjured hand. If the patient indicates reduced sensation in all or part of his hand, he *should* be referred for surgery.

WRIST, HAND, AND FINGERS

Rehabilitation of Hand and Finger Injuries

Oddvar Knutsen and Jan-Ragnar Haugstvedt

Goals and Principles

Table 9.3 lists the goals of acute hand and finger injury rehabilitation.

A combination of several measures is needed to rehabilitate major hand and finger injuries. It is preferable for an experienced hand therapist to administer or direct this therapy. A well-functioning hand must have motion, stability, strength, and sensation and must be pain free. When stabilizing surgery is necessary, systematic conservative rehabilitation must follow, with the goal of achieving good long-term results.

During the acute phase, it is important to control pain and inflammation by cooling with ice, elevating the hand or providing compression to control swelling, and resting the hand from activities that cause pain. During the rehabilitation phase, braces, splints, or taping to an adjacent finger are often used to facilitate resumption of active assisted mobilization of joints with the greatest possible joint motion. If a joint is stable, early mobilization is recommended. If there is considerable swelling, compression may be used. The patient can accomplish this by wearing fitted compression gloves, individually adjusted finger stockings (or Coban), or Tubigrip on his hand or wrist. Elastic bandages about 2.5 cm wide are well suited to fingers.

	Goals	Measures
Acute phase	Reduce pain and inflammation	PRICE
Rehabilitation phase	Normalize movement and strength in the hand and finger joint	Strength and stretching exercises
	Normalize endurance and coordination	
Training phase	Complete healing of injured ligaments without the loss of mechanical stability or movement	Functional exercises
		Sport-specific exercises
	Practice training in sport activity while gradually increasing load	
	Reduce the risk of reinjury	

Table 9.3 Goals and measures for rehabilitation of acute hand and finger injuries.

Contrast bath treatment provided prior to joint mobilization helps to minimize any discomfort associated with passive mobilization. Two bowls of water, one with ice and the other with hot water, should be used. The hand or fingers should be immersed for 45 seconds in the hot water and then for 15 seconds in the cold water, and the angle should be repeated 10 to 15 times. Electrical stimulation may also help mobilize intra-articular fluid. If pain increases during activity, the activity must be stopped immediately and ice applied locally to the painful area for 15 to 20 minutes.

To avoid overloading the tendons, isometric or concentric exercises are recommended for strength training during the initial training phase. Toward the end of the training phase, eccentric exercises are incorporated, so that the athlete is ready to meet the requirements of the sport. Progressive loading of the tendons is achieved in this manner. In addition to a general warm-up, specifically warming the injured muscles and tendons is necessary during the training phase before beginning functional exercises. After training, ice may be applied locally, to help prevent the recurrence of symptoms.

For the hand, the function of the thumb is the most important thing to normalize because it provides a "backup" for the fingers. A "rubber sponge" can be used to facilitate gripping function during the start-up phase of rehabilitation.

Exercise Program

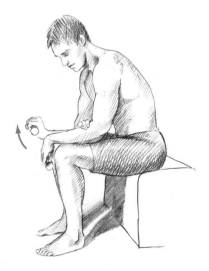

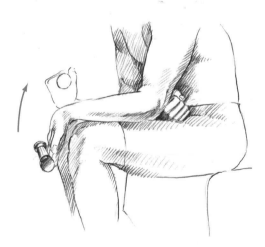

Exercise 9.1 Strengthening the extensor muscles of the wrist

- Lift your hand gently, as shown in the figure.
- Hold for 1 second.
- Lower your hand.

Exercise 9.2 Strengthening the flexor muscles of the wrist

- Lift your hand gently, as shown in the figure.
- Hold for 1 second.
- Lower your hand.

WRIST, HAND, AND FINGERS

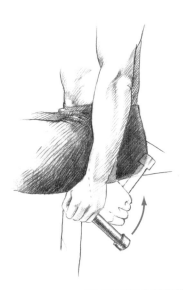

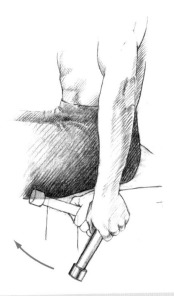

Exercise 9.3 Strengthening the ulnar muscles of the wrist

- Hold the end of a dumbbell or bottle; lift.
- Hold for 1 second.
- Lower gently.

Exercise 9.4 Strengthening the radial muscles of the wrist

- Hold the end of a dumbbell or bottle; lift.
- Hold for 1 second.
- Lower gently.

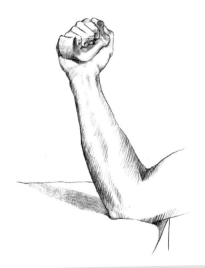

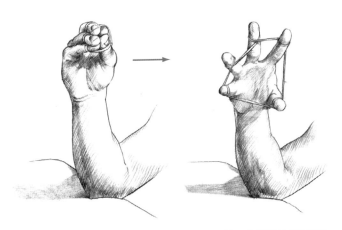

Exercise 9.5 Strengthening the flexor muscles of the fingers

- Grasp a foam rubber grip.
- Hold for 3 to 5 seconds.

Exercise 9.6 Strengthening extensor muscles of the fingers

- Wrap a tension band around each finger once, and spread your fingers.
- Hold for 3 to 5 seconds.

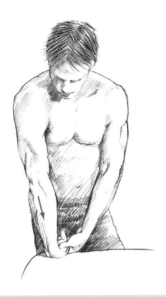

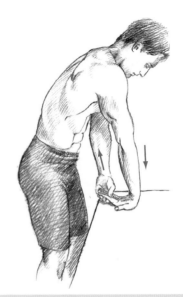

Exercise 9.7 Stretching the extensor muscles of the wrist

- Place your wrist on a table or chair, and use your other hand to flex your fingers in toward your hand to get maximum stretching effect.
- Hold for up to 1 minute.

Exercise 9.8 Stretching the flexor muscles of the wrist

- Place your wrist against a table or bench, and lift your fingers off the table using your other hand to achieve the best possible stretching effect.
- Hold for up to 1 minute.
- Remember to extend your elbow.

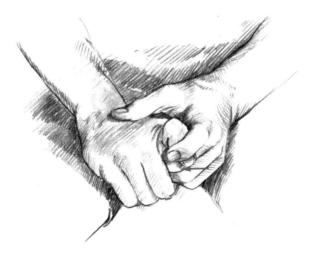

Exercise 9.9 Stretching the small muscles of the second to the fifth digits (dorsal interossei muscles)

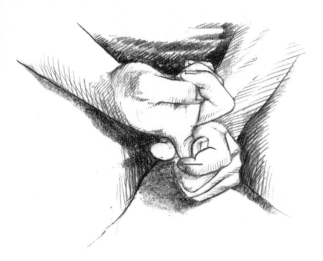

Exercise 9.10 Stretching the small muscles of the second to the fifth digits (lumbrical muscles)

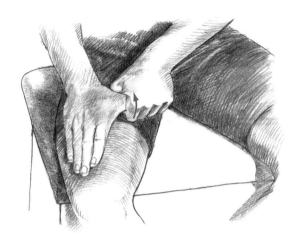

Exercise 9.11 Stretching the thumb's grasping muscles

Acute Injuries to the Pelvis, Groin, and Hip

Torbjørn Grøntvedt

Occurrence

Athletes frequently sustain acute injuries of the pelvis, groin, and hip girdle. Soccer and ice hockey players, cross-country skiers (especially freestyle), speed skaters, hurdlers, high jumpers, and horseback riders are particularly vulnerable. A 1980 Swedish study found that 5% of all injuries sustained by soccer players involved the pelvic and inguinal regions.

Differential Diagnosis

The most frequent acute injuries involving the pelvic, inguinal, and hip regions of athletes are strains of the adductor longus, rectus femoris, rectus abdominis, and the iliopsoas muscles. Although fractures do occur among young athletes, they are most common in the elderly—usually physically inactive individuals with osteoporosis. Avulsion fractures almost always occur in young, pubertal athletes, when muscle strength develops rapidly and while the tendinous insertion is still relatively weak, particularly in the apophyseal areas. Acute traumatic bursitis occurs exclusively in the greater trochanteric bursa, because it is the only superficial bursa in the pelvic region.

Table 10.1 lists these and other conditions resulting in acute pain in this area. Good, working knowledge of the regional anatomy coupled with a thorough examination generally leads to the proper diagnosis and are therefore keys to successful treatment of these disorders.

Most common	Less common	Must not be overlooked !
Adductor longus strain (p. 266)	Other adductor strain (p. 271)	Hip joint dislocation (p. 272)
Rectus femoris strain (p. 268)	Gluteal muscle strain (p. 271)	Epiphyseolysis of the femoral head (p. 274)
Iliopsoas strain (p. 269)	Sartorius strain (p. 271)	Appendicitis (p. 270)
Rectus abdominis strain (p. 270)	Gracilis strain (p. 271)	Diverticulitis (p. 270)
Proximal femur fracture (p. 271)	Tensor fascia lata strain (p. 271)	Kidney stone (p. 270)
Pelvic fracture (p. 271)	Avulsion fractures (p. 273)	Torsion of the testis
Coxitis (serous/purulent)	Acute trochanteric bursitis (p. 275)	Torsion of the testicular appendices
Acute disk prolapse (p. 126)	Injury to the acetabular labrum (p . 272	

Table 10.1 Overview of the differential diagnosis of acute injuries in the pelvic, groin, and hip region.

Diagnostic Thinking

Relatively few diagnoses involve acute localized pain in the pelvic, inguinal, and hip regions. The clinical history often provides significant diagnostic clues, both for muscle strains and fractures. Strains occur most frequently in the adductor musculature, particularly the adductor longus.

The adductor muscles adduct (and to some degree flex and externally rotate) the hip, a function that is particularly important in soccer. Kicking the soccer ball with the inside of the foot, frequent and rapid changes of direction, and tackling with an abducted leg all result in major loading and a correspondingly high frequency of injuries. As a result, strains are occasionally so small that they cause few initial symptoms. Therefore, the athlete neglects the pain and continues the sport activity. Acute injuries therefore often evolve into chronic disorders that may be much more difficult to treat than the original muscle injury. Early diagnosis and appropriate and adequate treatment are thus crucial to good outcomes.

If the patient has a fracture, he usually is in so much pain that the diagnosis is obvious. However, avulsion fractures with slight dislocation are not usually very symptomatic. In such cases, the practitioner must be aware of this possible diagnosis and test the muscle group involved by loading the painful area during the clinical examination.

A hip joint dislocation is a rare injury, triggered by major trauma and characterized by severe pain and typical positioning of the affected lower extremity. Epiphyseolysis, on the other hand, is usually not overly painful. Pain caused by slipped capital femoral epiphysis is nearly always referred to the medial side of the knee. If a child has pain in this area, it is necessary to assess hip joint range of motion in order to determine if such motion induces more pain.

Clinical History

Numerous potential diagnoses can be excluded by means of a thorough clinical history, in which the injury mechanism is carefully recorded. An acute groin strain is usually caused by a sudden, forceful hip abduction movement in opposition to adductor activation. The athlete often feels something tearing in the medial aspect of her thigh, and subsequent attempts at adduction will trigger pain in the affected area.

A similar mechanism applies to avulsion fractures. It is always the weakest link in the chain that breaks, and in adolescents who are undergoing a growth spurt the tendon insertion at the apophysis is often weaker than the muscle belly or the tendon itself. Pain localization indicates which growth plate may have been injured.

Direct trauma to the greater trochanteric region (e.g., from a fall), may cause acute trochanteric bursitis or a fracture of the proximal femur or of the pubic rami. However, a much greater load is required to cause a pelvic fracture. Such high-energy trauma may result, for example, from a fall while downhill skiing or from a motocross accident.

Clinical Examination

Inspection. If the patient has an acute muscle injury, examination may reveal localized swelling or possibly muscle defects, which can be accentuated by muscle activation. Local ecchymosis tracking distally may also be present if there is an intermuscular injury with ruptured muscle fascia and resultant bleeding into the subcutaneous tissue. This type of discoloration usually appears about 3 days after the injury occurs. If the patient sustains a major injury of the gluteal musculature, the Trendelenburg test may be positive. The back, especially the lumbar spine, should also be examined.

In the case of displaced fractures of the proximal femur, the affected lower extremity will be externally rotated and shortened to some extent, whereas a fracture in the pelvic girdle usually does not cause any visible outward signs of injury (other than possible contusion marks).

Traumatic hip joint dislocations always occur posteriorly, causing the hip to be held in a flexed, adducted, and internally rotated position. In thin individuals, incongruence above the hip joint should be clearly visible. Epiphyseolysis that has progressed to some extent will also result in visible incongruence.

Palpation. Careful palpation of an injured muscle shortly after the injury has occurred may reveal a tender defect in the muscle belly corresponding to the site of the strain. Eventually, this defect will fill with blood and edema fluid that are gradually replaced by scar tissue. Such scar tissue may be somewhat sensitive and firm on palpatory exam of the muscle belly.

If the patient has a fracture, palpation may reveal evidence of hematoma in the area of the fracture. Unstable pelvic fractures may be demonstrated by gently pressing on both anterior superior iliac crests at the same time. If the patient has an "open book" injury, pathological movement can be easily felt between the two halves of the pelvis.

Specific testing. If a muscle has been significantly injured, testing of the affected muscle against resistance would trigger pain corresponding to the area of the injury. With simultaneous palpation, the defect or area of scar tissue can be localized, and it will be possible to estimate the extent of the muscle injury. A subtotal or total rupture of the muscle will appear as an asymmetrical bulge with muscular activation. Pain at the site of muscle insertion in young patients who are not fully grown may indicate an avulsion fracture.

Other types of fractures in the area usually cause so much pain that specific testing is impossible. However, impacted fractures of the neck of the femur and simple fractures of the pubic rami may be relatively asymptomatic. Passive hip joint movement, particularly internal and external rotation, will cause pain if there is a fracture of the neck of the femur, and bimanual pressure over the greater trochanter will trigger groin pain when there is a fracture of the pubic bone.

Supplemental Examinations

Radiographic examination. If there is a history of major trauma to the pelvic region, particularly from a high-energy impact (e.g., from motor sports or downhill skiing), X rays should be taken to rule out fractures or dislocations. If an avulsion fracture is suspected in a young athlete, X rays can usually confirm the diagnosis. However, the radiographic examination request form should include a description of which apophysis may be involved, so that it can be properly imaged. If there is even the slightest indication of an epiphyseolysis of the head of the femur, the patient must be sent for immediate radiographic examination in addition to follow up and further evaluation and treatment by an orthopedic surgeon.

Computerized tomography (CT). CT scans of the pelvic, inguinal, and hip regions are often performed in case of major trauma, to define the injuries in greater detail. Otherwise, CT scans are rarely useful for routine evaluation of sports injuries in this area.

Magnetic resonance imaging (MRI). MRI is occasionally useful for injuries in this area, particularly for soft-tissue diagnostics. Muscle strain injuries and their size can be clearly demonstrated, both during the acute phase and during the scar-tissue phase. MRI is particularly useful for deep muscle groups, such as the iliopsoas.

Skeletal scintigraphy. Bone scan imaging is seldom useful in diagnosing acute injuries in the pelvic, inguinal, and hip regions. An exception occurs when an avulsion fracture is suspected but is difficult to clearly project on plain films. If the bone insertion is torn, scintigraphy will produce strong contrast enhancement that corresponds to the affected and acutely injured apophysis.

Ultrasound examination. In experienced hands, ultrasound is an excellent tool for diagnosing muscle strains. It provides a good imaging of the size of the injury and associated hematoma. Ultrasound also aids in the localization of deep injuries. Later, scar changes will be found in the muscle belly, and it is also possible to demonstrate early calcium deposition (myositis ossificans).

Common Injuries

Adductor Strains

Adductor strains are the most common soft-tissue injuries in the pelvic, inguinal, and hip regions, particularly of the pectineus, adductor brevis, longus, magnus, and gracilis muscles. Strains occur primarily in the proximal portion of the adductor longus, at the muscle-tendon junction, or at the insertion on the pubic bone (figure 10.1). The injury mechanism is usually a strong hip abduction movement, simultaneous with eccentric activation/overload of the adductors–for example, from tackling in soccer. Overloading the adductor muscles, such as from repeated strong abduction and adduction movements in skating or freestyle cross-country skiing, may also result in relatively minor strains in the affected area. Complete ruptures of one or more of the adductor muscles can also occur. Clinically, these ruptures nearly always occur distally (at the femoral insertion or in the distal muscle belly itself).

- Symptoms and signs: The injured athlete recalls a sudden intense pain in the groin or, in the case of significant strains, more distally on the medial aspect of the thigh. Attempts at continued activity cause the pain to recur. Eventually, the injured area swells and may become bruised superficially over the subsequent 2-3 days following injury if intermuscular bleeding has occurred. If a rupture of the distal muscle tendon junction has occurred–for example, of the adductor longus–the athlete may have surprisingly little pain. In most cases, the diagnosis is not made until the athlete begins to activate the muscle during the rehabilitation sequence. In the case of a serious adductor strain injury, a relatively large soft-tissue mass will be visible on the proximal medial part of the thigh when the hip is adducted against resistance.
- Diagnosis: The clinical history combined with a thorough physical examination should reveal the diagnosis. During the acute stage, a defect that corresponds to the rupture can often be palpated, but bleeding and edema will cause this defect to swell quickly. When the adductors are activated against resistance, the patient will complain of pain corresponding to the area of rupture, and the affected muscle will be weakened. If the slightest indication of a malignant soft-tissue disorder is present, the "tumor" must be examined by MRI.
- Treatment by physician: During the acute stage, the injury is treated according to the RICE principle. The patient may be given nonsteroidal anti-inflammatory drugs (NSAIDs) for a short period (2 to 3 days). This therapy will reduce the inflammatory response and, consequently, the extent of scar tissue formation in

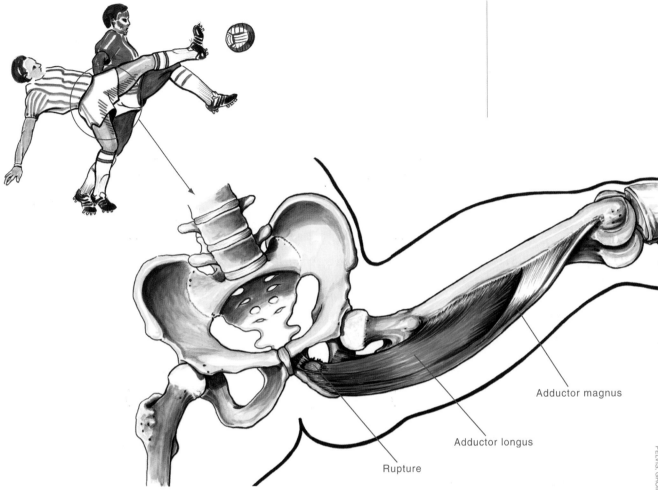

Figure 10.1 Adductor rupture. Soccer players often sustain acute partial ruptures of the adductor longus.

Adductor magnus

Adductor longus

Rupture

the area, and will have an analgesic effect. If diagnosed early, total distal ruptures may be treated by surgical reinsertion to the femur.

- Treatment by physical therapist: As soon as the pain begins to abate, the athlete must begin to actively exercise the injured musculature. The progression of the activity must not be too rapid. Hence, the athlete must be carefully followed and must train the entire time without, or with only minimal, pain. If rehabilitation progresses too quickly, injuries in this region have an expressed tendency to become chronic. Some therapists recommend careful isometric exercises for the adductors in the early stages of rehabilitation. However, in our experience after 3 or 4 days the athlete may begin careful, active strength training, accompanied by careful stretching. If flexibility of the muscle groups on both sides is full and pain free, strength training can be increased to full loading. The goal is for the patient to have normal muscle length and strength before returning to his sport. Neuromuscular training (balance training) of the hip and groin musculature may begin as soon as symptoms permit. In addition, the patient must undergo a period of controlled functional training in the relevant sport before returning to full training and competition. If long-term stiffness and moderate pain in the inguinal region are present, applying heat packs locally before training may have a therapeutic effect. Wearing Neoprene pants has the same effect, particularly at the start of functional training. To maintain the best possible general strength and physical condition, the athlete must be instructed in alternative types of training. Bicycling and swimming (not breaststroke) are normally tolerated well, and training by running straight ahead can be started as soon as pain allows. General strength training for the rest of the body is started as soon as the patient is able to perform the exercises without local pain. Total ruptures may be treated conservatively in the same manner as acute proximal injuries, with stretching and strength training. Functional loss of strength in the adductors will usually be insignificant after adequate rehabilitation.

- Prognosis: The amount of time needed for rehabilitation varies greatly, depending on whether intermuscular or intramuscular bleeding occurred at the time of injury. If blood is allowed out of the muscle belly, the inflammatory response and, consequently, scar tissue formation will be significantly reduced. The athlete may then count on 3 to 6 weeks of rehabilitation, depending on the extent of the injury. When the hematoma remains within the muscle belly, rehabilitation usually takes twice as long (up to 12 weeks). Patience and caution are key elements in successful retraining. If the athlete ignores their pain, the likelihood that the injury will develop into a chronic, painful, difficult-to-treat condition is high. The risk of developing myositis ossificans increases when the rehabilitation of more distal ruptures with associated intramuscular bleeding is too vigorous. This heterotopic ossification may cause chronic pain in the area, making surgical removal necessary.

Rectus Femoris Strain

The rectus femoris muscle originates at the anterior inferior iliac spine and inserts at the tibial tuberosity via the patellar tendon. The rectus femoris flexes the hip and extends the knee, and athletes strain this muscle more often than any other muscle (figure 10.2). Total ruptures usually occur somewhat distally, and commonly occur at the junction of the muscle distally with the quadriceps tendon. Partial ruptures usually occur at the proximal musculotendinous junction (figure 10.2). The injury normally occurs when the athlete has his hip extended and the knee flexed and then forcefully flexes his hip while extending the knee–for example, when kicking a soccer ball with the dorsal side of the foot and with the ankle in plantar flexion. The rectus femoris muscle may tear, especially if the athlete encounters sudden, unexpected resistance through the range of motion.

- Symptoms and signs: Proximal partial tears typically result in acute, intense pain radiating toward the groin. More distal strains generally cause less intense pain, particularly if the muscle tendon junction is torn.

Figure 10.2 Rectus femoris strains. Strains may result in partial or complete tears. Partial ruptures usually involve the proximal muscle-tendon junction whereas the less common total ruptures usually occur distally.

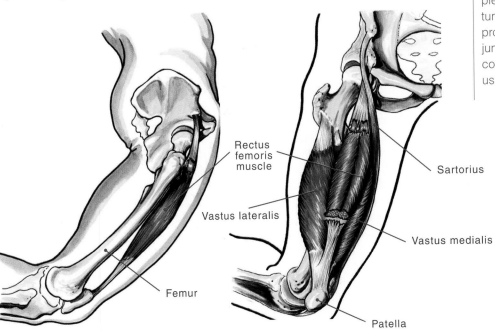

Rectus femoris muscle

Sartorius

Vastus lateralis

Vastus medialis

Femur

Patella

- **Diagnosis:** Depending on the extent of the injury, it may be possible to palpate a tender defect in the muscle belly during the acute phase. Active knee extension will be restricted and painful, and knee extension strength will be reduced. If the injury results in intermuscular bleeding, the skin above and distal to the site of the injury will become ecchymotic within 2 or 3 days. In the case of a total rupture, it should be possible to palpate the distal end of the muscle belly, which should be somewhat mobile. Minor ruptures, particularly those that occur at the muscle tendon junction, may be difficult to palpate. Ultrasonography may be useful in diagnosing such cases.
- **Treatment:** Treatment for partial ruptures of the rectus femoris is the same as for ruptures of the adductor longus. If a total rupture of the muscle-tendon junction has occurred, the athlete should be offered surgical repair. Postoperatively, the patient is provided with a long orthosis that locks the knee in extension for 3 to 4 weeks. Thereafter, careful and gradual flexibility and strength training may begin.
- **Prognosis:** The prognosis for partial ruptures is good, provided the patient receives adequate conservative therapy. The athlete is usually able to return to full sport activity after 4 to 6 weeks. If activity starts prematurely, particularly if the rupture occurs close to the muscle tendon junction, there is a greater risk of developing chronic tendinosis. After surgical repair of a total rupture, the athlete can normally return to his sport after about 8 to 12 weeks. Stretching and strength training of the quadriceps are essential components of the rehabilitation of overlooked total ruptures. There is surprisingly little function loss once retraining has been completed.

Iliopsoas Muscle Strain

The iliopsoas muscle consists of three muscles (the psoas major, the psoas minor, and the iliacus), and has a broad origin from the L1 to L5 transverse processes and the inside of the ala of the ilium. The muscles are retroperitoneal in location and insert jointly on the lesser trochanter of the femur. The iliopsoas is the strongest hip flexor. Strains of this muscle (figure 10.3) typically occur as a result of forced flexion of the hip against resistance, such as when kicking a soccer ball or during intensive sit-up training with the hips extended.

- **Symptoms and signs:** Ruptures of the muscle belly are uncommon. When they do occur, the athlete complains of pain located deep in the abdomen, radiating inferiorly toward the inguinal ligament. A large hematoma may develop causing pressure on the surrounding nerves (the lateral femoral cutaneous nerve of the thigh, ilioinguinal, genitofemoral, and femoral nerves) resulting in a sensory deficit and possibly weakness of the quadriceps. These symptoms are usually transient and resolve as the hematoma is resorbed. If the strain injury is localized to the muscle tendon junction, the pain is more centrally located in the groin. Total ruptures of the iliopsoas seldom occur.

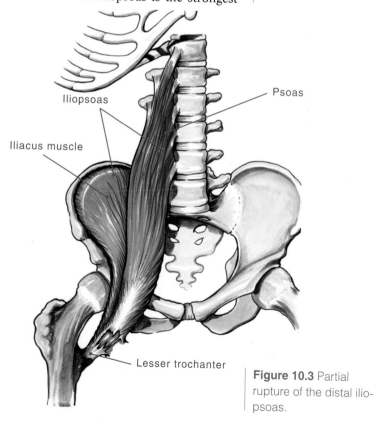

Figure 10.3 Partial rupture of the distal iliopsoas.

- Diagnosis: The patient indicates pain corresponding to the area of the muscle injury when she flexes her hip against resistance or when she raises her leg with the knee extended while sitting on a chair. Patients with proximal strains tend to be tender to palpation but do not demonstrate rebound tenderness of the lower abdomen (i.e., there is no peritoneal irritation). In the case of a partial rupture of the distal iliopsoas, bimanual palpation over the lesser trochanter may trigger significant pain. The most critical diagnoses that need to be excluded are appendicitis, diverticulitis, strangulated hernia, kidney stones, and a rupture of the rectus abdominis muscle.
- Treatment: Treatment is typically conservative, as in the case of a rupture of the adductor longus. If rehabilitation is too aggressive or if the athlete returns to sport activity too early, a partial distal rupture may develop into chronic tendinosis.
- Prognosis: The prognosis is good with proper rehabilitation.
- Prophylaxis: Regular stretching and strength training of the hip flexors is particularly important in specific sports in which athletes are vulnerable to hip flexor strains, including soccer, high jumping, hurdle jumping, and rowing.

Rectus Abdominis Muscle Strains

The rectus abdominis originates at the xiphoid process and from the cartilage of the 5th through the 7th ribs, and inserts into the pubic bone. Its main function is flexion of the spine, pulling the sternum toward the pubic bone. Partial tears of the muscle belly or at the distal musculotendinous junction are common, although complete ruptures are rare (figure 10.4). Sports in which athletes are particularly vulnerable to this injury are tennis, weightlifting, rowing, and soccer (e.g., when training for shooting or heading the ball).

- Symptoms and signs: The athlete feels sudden intense pain corresponding to the area of the muscle injury. Attempting to further load the muscle reproduces the pain.
- Diagnosis: During the acute stage, a tender defect in the muscle that corresponds to the area injured may be palpable. The defect will gradually fill up with blood and edema that fibroses into firmer scar tissue. The fascia over the rectus abdominis is thick, so it rarely ruptures. Therefore, most strain injuries result in intramuscular hematomas. Having the athlete simultaneously lift her head and leg from a prone position can test muscle function. The most important diagnoses to exclude are appendicitis and diverticulitis.
- Treatment: Treatment for an acute strain of the rectus abdominis is essentially the same as for an acute strain of the adductor longus (page 266). If symptoms are ignored and the athlete returns to sport activity too quickly, partial tears of the distal muscle-tendon junction may develop into a chronic tendinosis. Such chronic tendenopathies are typically difficult to treat and often slow to heal.
- Prognosis: The prognosis is good with prompt intervention, including proper rehabilitation. The athlete must not be allowed to return to sport activity before he is pain free during stretching, strength training, and weight bearing.

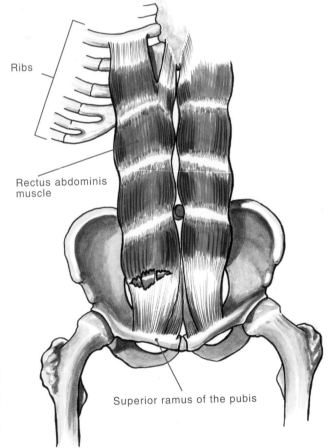

Ribs

Rectus abdominis muscle

Superior ramus of the pubis

Figure 10.4 Partial tear of the distal right rectus abdominis muscle.

- Prophylaxis: Prophylactic measures include regular strength training and stretching of the abdominal musculature. For recurring injuries, it is essential that technique (e.g., the tennis serve) be carefully evaluated and corrected if flaws are detected.

Other Injuries

Injuries to Other Muscles in the Inguinal and Hip Region

Other muscles, such as the gracilis, sartorius, tensor fasciae latae, and the gluteal muscles, may also be injured. The physician must perform a thorough examination, including palpation and specific tests, to determine which muscle or muscle group has been injured. The principles for treatment and prophylactic measures are the same as those for the treatment of an adductor longus rupture.

Fractures of the Proximal Femur

Fractures of the proximal femur (the femoral neck and the trochanteric region) occur frequently in the elderly but rarely in young people. Nevertheless, young athletes may occasionally sustain a fracture in this area. The mechanism of injury is often a fall resulting in direct trauma to the area around the trochanter—for example, on the skating rink, during downhill skiing, or from a bicycling crash in which the athlete's shoes are locked in the pedals.

- Symptoms and signs: Patients feel intense pain when attempting to move or load the hip.
- Diagnosis: If a displaced fracture has occurred, the lower extremity generally is shortened and externally rotated, and direct pressure over the trochanter region or any attempted hip movement results in severe pain. A radiographic examination confirms the diagnosis.
- Treatment: Treatment is always surgical, with reduction and osteosynthesis.
- Prognosis: The prognosis is variable, particularly for displaced fractures. About 20% of the patients develop osteonecrosis of the femoral head with segmental collapse of the articular head, and 10% to 20% of the fractures do not heal. In such cases, additional surgical intervention may be required, including arthrodesis (immobilization of the joint) or total hip arthroplasty. In recent years, total hip replacement has become more common among younger patients, because the long-term results are good.

Pelvic Fractures

Pelvic fractures or acetabular fractures are very rare in athletes but can occur after high-energy injuries, such as those caused by motor sports or downhill skiing accidents. Dislocated hip joints are often accompanied by acetabular fractures. Pelvic fractures may be divided into stable and unstable fractures. Stable fractures affect only part of the pelvic girdle, usually the inferior and superior pubic rami on one side. In unstable fractures, the entire pelvic girdle is broken. This either results from an anterior fracture and posterior dislocation of the sacroiliac joint, or when the pelvic girdle is fractured in two places. Most pelvic fractures are stable.

- Symptoms and signs: Pain in the pelvic area upon loading is the most common symptom.
- Diagnosis: Bimanual pressure on the iliac crest triggers pain in the pelvis. This type of pressure makes it possible to get an impression of whether the fracture is stable or unstable. X rays and CT scans are mandatory for confirming the diagnosis and demonstrating the extent and stability of the fracture.

• Treatment: The only treatment required for a stable fracture is a brief period of symptom-limited weight bearing as tolerated. The prognosis for stable fractures is very good. Because the pelvic area has a good blood supply, these fractures heal quickly. The athlete is usually training again within 4 to 6 weeks. Unstable fractures are potentially life threatening because of major bleeding (usually into the retroperitoneal space). These fractures require rapid surgical treatment, either by external screws into the pelvic crest and attached to a solid frame or by internal fixation with plates and screws. Pelvic fractures that affect the acetabulum require surgical repositioning and fixation if the articular surface is significantly incongruent or a large posterior edge fragment has been knocked off. The prognosis for these fractures is less definite, and major injuries of the acetabulum often result in premature development of osteoarthritis of the hip.

Hip Joint Dislocation !

Hip joint dislocations are generally caused by high-energy accidental trauma (e.g., motor sports and downhill skiing accidents). The mechanism of injury is usually indirect trauma (e.g., a hard blow to the knee area that dislocates the hip posteriorly). Part of the hip socket can be fractured and displaced to the rear as a consequence of posterior dislocation.

• Symptoms and signs: An athlete who has a posteriorly dislocated hip is typically in a great deal of pain, and the affected lower limb is adducted, flexed at the hip, and internally rotated.
• Diagnosis: Attempts to range or move the affected hip joint trigger significant pain, and elastic resistance may be felt. The dislocation may injure the sciatic nerve, and its function should always be examined before reduction. An X ray confirms the diagnosis.
• Treatment: A dislocated hip must be reduced as quickly as possible, but typically not at the scene of the injury. Reduction requires adequate anesthesia and muscular relaxation. After reduction, a CT scan of the joint must be obtained to rule out an acetabular fracture. If present, large fragments must be surgically fixed, so that congruence of the articular surface is reestablished and the risk of an unstable hip is minimized.
• Prognosis: The blood supply to the femoral head may be damaged as a result of dislocation, and segmental collapse of the femoral head may result. The risk of ischemia increases significantly if the dislocation remains unreduced for more than 6 hours. The prognosis is good if reduction occurs quickly and the blood supply is maintained. The injured hip should not bear weight for 4 to 6 weeks, and the patient should not anticipate returning to full activity until approximately 3 months after the injury.

Injury to the Acetabular Labrum

Forceful loading of the hip joint combined with translational force (e.g., trauma that results in subluxation) may injure the acetabular labrum (figure 10.5). The labrum is a rim of fibrocartilage (located along the edge of the acetabulum), which serves to extend the depth of the acetabulum by a few millimeters.

• Symptoms and signs: Symptoms include a sudden, pricking pain during hip movement, possibly accompanied by a click or a sensation of locking. Pain may linger for some time after these episodes.
• Diagnosis: Hip rotation may trigger the patient's pain, particularly by abduction combined with internal rotation. X rays are usually negative, whereas an MRI examination (preferably with contrast) may prove diagnostic.

- Treatment: The preferred treatment is typically arthroscopic debridement of the torn labrum.
- Prognosis: The prognosis is good if the hip joint has escaped additional injury. After surgery, the athlete usually returns to full activity after 4 to 6 weeks.

Avulsion Fractures

Avulsion fractures most commonly occur at apophyses. Apophyses are secondary ossification centers that contribute to peripheral growth of bone. The apophysis is separated from the rest of the bone by a growth plate and serves as the origin or site of insertion for muscles or tendons. Boys between the ages of 13 and 17 are at greatest risk for avulsion fractures. During periods of rapid growth, the growth plate is weak in comparison to the muscle inserting at the apophysis. Consequently, strong muscular activation may exert sufficient traction on the related apophysis to cause fracture through the growth plate (figure 10.6).

Avulsion fractures may occur in six different locations in each half of the pelvis (the affected muscle or muscle group is indicated in parenthesis): the iliac crest (abdominal musculature), anterior superior iliac spine (sartorius muscle), the anterior inferior iliac spine (rectus femoris muscle), the ischial tuberosity (hamstring musculature), the lesser trochanter (iliopsoas muscle), and the greater trochanter (gluteus medius and gluteus minimus muscles). Avulsion fractures off the iliac crest or the anterior inferior iliac spine will only be minimally displaced because the surrounding soft tissues hold the avulsed fragment in place, whereas avulsion injuries of the other apophyses may be more significantly displaced.

- Symptoms and signs: The patient experiences pain of acute onset that corresponds to the site of the avulsion. Minimally displaced fragments may cause relatively little pain. A major avulsion injury results in intense pain, comparable to that caused by other fractures. The athlete usually cannot tolerate loading or movement of the affected area.

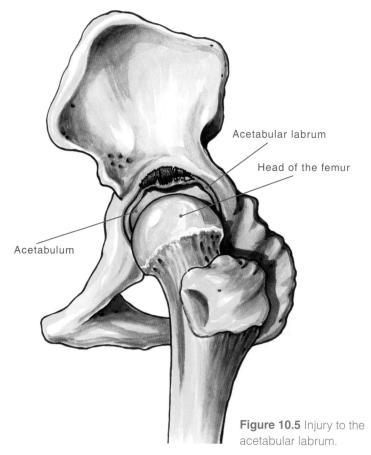

Figure 10.5 Injury to the acetabular labrum.

Acetabular labrum

Head of the femur

Acetabulum

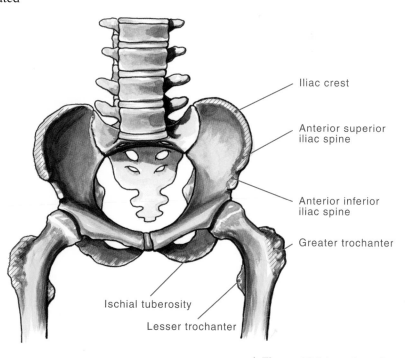

Iliac crest

Anterior superior iliac spine

Anterior inferior iliac spine

Greater trochanter

Ischial tuberosity

Lesser trochanter

Figure 10.6 Location of avulsion fractures in the pelvic and hip areas.

PELVIS, GROIN, AND HIP

• Diagnosis: The diagnosis of an avulsion fracture is based on an appropriate clinical history combined with findings on palpation of the painful area and the result of specific muscle testing. A radiographic examination usually confirms the diagnosis, but images should always be compared to the healthy side. Oblique images are often needed to freely project the avulsed apophysis. On occasion, a CT scan or skeletal scintigraphy is necessary.

• Treatment: Treatment is usually conservative with a period of non-weight bearing and prescription of analgesics. Major avulsion injuries (i.e., more than approximately 2 cm) of the apophyseal fragment may be an indication for surgical reduction and fixation. This is particularly true of the greater trochanter, to avoid gluteal failure.

• Prognosis: The prognosis is good in most cases. Normally, the apophysis heals within 4 to 6 weeks and the athlete can return to his sport again after a few more weeks of stretching and strength training of the affected muscles. Painful pseudoarthrosis occasionally develops between the avulsed fragment and the rest of the bone. In such cases, surgical fixation of the apophysis is necessary.

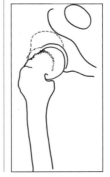

Epiphyseolysis of the Femoral Head—Slipped Capital Femoral Epiphysis !

Epiphyseolysis of the femoral head results in slippage in the growth plate located between the neck and the head of the femur (figure 10.7). It tends to occur during the adolescent growth spurt (between the ages of 12 and 15), often in connection with minor trauma, such as jumping from a height. The disorder may also occur ideopathically (i.e., without known antecedent cause).

• Symptoms and signs: Pain is localized to the groin or more often to the inside of the knee, particularly with weight bearing.

• Diagnosis: Findings from the clinical examination include limited hip rotation that is associated with pain. Radiographic examination in two planes will demonstrate the slippage. If there is the slightest indication of epiphyseolysis, the patient must be sent for X rays and a prompt evaluation by an orthopedic surgeon.

• Treatment: Recommended treatment includes surgical fixation of the femoral head. The less slippage of the epiphysis, the better the prognosis, and so prompt intervention is recommended. Some orthopedists routinely perform prophylactic fixation of the femoral head on the opposite side because of the significantly increased risk of developing contralateral epiphyseolysis. However, it is more common to provide the patient and her parents with detailed information so that they can seek medical assistance as soon as symptoms appear.

• Prognosis: The prognosis is favorable with minimal slippage and early fixation. If there is major dislocation, the head and neck of the femur often become deformed, increasing the risk of developing early osteoarthritis of the hip joint.

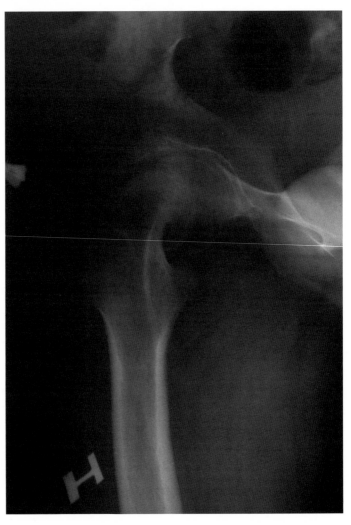

Figure 10.7 Epiphysiolysis of the femoral head.

Acute Trochanteric Bursitis

The trochanteric bursa is the only superficial bursa in the pelvic and hip region. Therefore, the bursa may be subjected to direct trauma, such as that caused when a handball player falls on her hip. This may cause crushing of part of the mucous membrane in the bursa, resulting in bleeding and inflammation.

- Symptoms and signs: The patient complains of pain and perhaps swelling over the greater trochanter. The pain may radiate inferiorly along the lateral side of the thigh, occasionally prompting clinicians to mischaracterize the pain as sciatica.
- Diagnosis: The diagnosis is based on tenderness and swelling over the greater trochanter. Adduction and rotation of the hip with the knee extended will trigger pain. Ultrasound and MRI examinations may demonstrate a thickened wall and an increased amount of fluid in the bursa.
- Treatment: The recommended treatment is restricted weight bearing, NSAIDs, and alternative training. If this regimen is not carried out thoroughly, the symptoms may become chronic (page 290).

Pain in the Pelvic, Groin, and Hip Region

Torbjørn Grøntvedt

Occurrence

Chronic painful conditions in the pelvic, inguinal, and hip region are among the most difficult injuries to deal with in sport traumatology, both with respect to diagnosis and treatment. These injuries occur frequently, especially in sports such as soccer and ice hockey. The symptoms caused by chronic groin injuries are often diffuse and uncharacteristic and may seemingly appear in several areas at the same time. For example, pain that primarily originates from a particular muscle group will often trigger secondary pain from other areas because of improper loading. Therefore, these injuries represent a significant diagnostic challenge. Good outcomes are dependent upon an accurate initial diagnosis.

Most common	Less common	Must not be overlooked ❗
Adductor tendinosis (p. 281)	Iliopsoas tendinosis (p. 283)	Iliopectineal bursitis (p. 290)
Rectus femoris tendinosis (p. 283)	Trochanter tendinosis (p. 284)	Gluteal bursitis (p. 291)
Rectus abdominis tendinosis (p. 283)	Typical snapping hip (p. 291)	Atypical snapping hip (p. 292)
Trochanteric bursitis (p. 290)	Pubic rami stress fracture (p. 286)	Myositis ossificans (p. 284)
Femoral neck stress fracture (p. 286)	Femur shaft stress fracture (p. 286)	Injury to the acetabular labrum (p. 272)
Osteitis pubis (p. 286)	Groin insufficiency (Gilmore's groin) (p. 288)	Prostatitis
Inguinal hernia	Nerve entrapment (p. 292)	Osteochondritis dissecans coxae
Femoral hernia	Referred pain from the back (p. 113)	Tumors
Obturator hernia	Sacroiliac joint pain	
Hip osteoarthritis	Sequelae from injuries	
	Pelvic insufficiency (symphysis pubis pain and/or sacroiliac joint pain)	
	Hypermobility	
	Ankylosing spondylitis	
	Sacroiliitis	
	Legg-Calvé-Perthes Disease	
	Gynecological disorders	

Table 10.2 Overview of the differential diagnosis of chronic injuries in the pelvic, groin, and hip region.

Differential Diagnosis

Table 10.2 provides an overview of the current differential diagnosis of conditions that may produce chronic pelvic, inguinal, and hip region pain. The most common of these diagnoses is tendinopathy of the adductor longus, the rectus femoris, the rectus abdominis, the iliopsoas, and the gluteus medius muscles. Formerly, pain ascribed to tendons was described as tendonitis. However, histologic examinations have not demonstrated obvious inflammatory changes in the affected tendons, other than possibly at the very outset of the degenerative process. Subsequent microscopic examination demonstrates degenerative granulomatous change in the tendinous tissue. Therefore, the term *tendinosis* is preferred instead of *tendonitis*, because it more accurately describes the observed pathological changes. The causes of the pain during and after loading are unclear. The most likely etiology is the release of noxious chemical substances from the degenerating tendinous tissue that irritate the nerve endings in the tissue around the tendons.

Athletes often have chronic changes in the trochanteric bursa, although the other bursae in the region are rarely affected.

Classic snapping hip syndrome often occurs in young, thin women, such as ballet dancers and gymnasts, whereas atypical snapping hip is a rare disorder that may affect all age groups and both sexes.

Stress fractures of the proximal femur and the pubic rami (particularly the inferior ramus) often occur in athletes who primarily train and compete on hard surfaces. Osteitis pubis is strictly an overuse condition in athletes (particularly soccer players) who have strong, short muscles in the groin area. The same is true of groin insufficiency (Gilmore's groin).

Diagnostic Thinking

A large number of overuse disorders may cause chronic pain in the pelvic, inguinal, and hip region. The practitioner must be familiar with the natural history of the various conditions from onset of symptoms to recuperation. If deviation from the anticipated course has occurred, further evaluation of the patient is indicated, so that one or more conditions within the differential diagnoses in the area may be definitely excluded. This is particularly true of tumors, which may also occur in young patients.

Clinical History

Several potential diagnoses can initially be excluded by means of a thorough history, in which special circumstances surrounding the initial onset of symptoms are documented. Chronic groin strains usually begin with an acute muscle rupture on the medial aspect of the thigh. Often this is initially such a minor problem that the patient may have trouble remembering it. Patients describe classic snapping hip as a painful click over the hip, and if the patient has chronic trochanteric bursitis, the clinical history often includes frequent trauma (falls) on the lateral hip girdle. If the tensor fascia lata muscle is too tight, it may precipitate bursitis, a snapping hip, or runner's knee. If the patient has a stress fracture of the pubic rami, the pain will also have a relatively acute onset, but in this case the triggering event is often running a long distance on a hard surface. Osteitis pubis and groin insufficiency result in gradually progressive, diffuse groin pain, initially during and eventually after weight bearing. Probably the most classic symptom of piriformis syndrome is pain at the ischial tuberosity when the patient sits with his hips slightly hyperflexed—for example, when driving a car for a long time. An acetabular labrum injury may cause painful clicking and locking in the hip, usually with the pain localized to the groin or to the inside of the thigh.

Referred pain is typical of several disorders in the pelvic and inguinal region—meaning that the patient experiences pain in an area other than where the pain originates. This is particularly true of sacroiliac joint and sacroiliac ligament-related pain.

Clinical Examination

Inspection. The pelvis and hips should be examined from both the front and from the back while the patient is standing and walking. A patient who walks with toe-in may have increased femoral neck anteversion. If a stress fracture has occurred in one of the pubic rami or in the neck of the femur, the patient will be able to pinpoint the location of the pain with weight bearing either to the groin or to the medial side of the thigh. By hopping on the affected lower extremity, the patient's pain is further provoked, making it easier to localize (positive "hop test"). The physician should also examine the patient's back, particularly the lumbar spine.

Palpation. The presence of anisomelia (leg-length discrepancy) can be approximated while the patient is standing with his knees extended and while bearing weight equally on both feet. The pelvis must not be rotated when this measurement is taken. If the patient has lumbosacral back pain, the physician should palpate the insertion of the erector spinae on the sacrum and the iliac crest. The spinous processes of L4 and L5 should be palpated to check for spondylolisthesis between L5 and the sacrum. If spondylolisthesis is found in that location, the spinous process of L4 will be displaced in a position that is anterior to L5. Sacroiliac joint arthritis or overuse of the posterior sacroiliac ligaments will be painful upon palpation over the joint or ligaments. Single limb weight bearing, or a compression test of the sacroiliac joints (pressing the crests of the iliac bones firmly towards each other), may also trigger sacroiliac joint pain if the SI joint is involved.

If a groin hernia is suspected, the external inguinal opening is palpated while the patient coughs. If the patient has manifest hernia, it will be possible to palpate the hernial sac. A patient with groin insufficiency will indicate more pain on the affected side than on the opposite, nonaffected side. It may be possible to palpate a femoral hernia immediately distal to the inguinal ligament beside the vessel/nerve stem.

With the patient in the supine position, the physician should palpate the various muscles and muscle insertions while loading the suspected muscle group. Pain may be a sign of chronic inflammation at the myotendinous insertion, while a defect or tender infiltrate in the muscle belly indicates a muscle tear, possibly with scar tissue formation.

Palpation over the greater trochanter will trigger pain if the patient has trochanteric bursitis or classic snapping hip.

Pressure over the lateral cutaneous nerve of the thigh where it passes under the inguinal ligament immediately medial to the anterior superior iliac spine may increase the symptoms of meralgia paresthetica.

Specific Testing

The shape of the hip joint (ball-and-socket joint) enables it to move in every direction. The joint capsule is relatively loose to allow great mobility but is solidified and strengthened by three ligaments—the iliofemoral, the pubofemoral, and the ischiofemoral ligaments. These three ligaments prevent (in order) extension, abduction, and internal rotation from becoming too excessive. Hip joint stability is primarily a factor of the depth of the acetabulum and the strength of the muscles that control articular movement.

The concept of femur anteversion refers to the angle formed by the femoral neck and the condylar plane of the femur (figure 10.8). Normally, this angle measures about 15°. Increased anteversion results in increased internal rotation of the femur, and consequently the patella will be located too far medially. Walking and running with toe-in is the most characteristic clinical finding, in addition to reduced external rotation of the hip. Femoral anteversion is an important cause of chronic overuse disorders in the lower extremities.

Passive hip range of motion (including flexion, abduction, adduction with slight flexion, internal rotation, and external rotation at about 90° flexion) is tested with the patient in a supine position. Comparison to the opposite side is essential.

The practitioner should test the sacroiliac joint by applying strong pressure posteriorly (toward the anterior superior iliac spine), bilaterally, or by forceful passive abduction of a flexed hip. If the joints or the surrounding ligaments are affected, these tests may trigger sacroiliac pain. However, sacroiliac joint pain tends to be somewhat nonspecific, and it is therefore difficult to consistently and reproducibly examine the sacroiliac joint region.

Specific muscle groups, such as the hip flexors (iliopsoas and rectus femoris), the hip abductors (gluteal muscles), the hip adductors, the internal and external rotators of the hip, and the abdominal muscles, should be tested against resistance. Pain at the muscle insertion suggests tendinosis and possibly an avulsion fracture in adolescent patients.

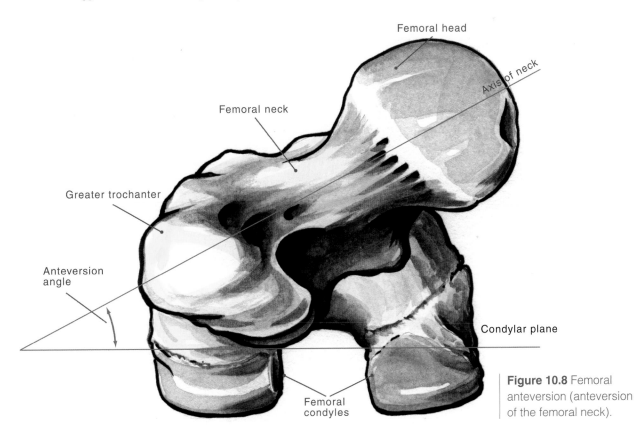

Figure 10.8 Femoral anteversion (anteversion of the femoral neck).

While in the prone position, the patient is tested for passive hip mobility, including extension, internal rotation, and external rotation with the hip extended. Increased femoral anteversion causes increased internal hip rotation (often up to 90°), whereas external hip rotation is correspondingly reduced or discontinued. Normally, internal and external hip rotations are about equal and depend on joint laxity. Pain at the ischial tuberosity produced by extending and internally rotating the hips while in a prone position suggests the diagnosis of Piriformis syndrome. Piriformis syndrome is also characterized by asymmetric flexibility of the hips, with restricted internal rotation on the affected side.

The quadriceps and hamstring may be tested against resistance while the patient is in the prone position. Muscle defects or scar tissue in the hamstrings can often be palpated by contracting the hamstrings against resistance. Strength of the short rotator muscles of the hip should be tested with the hip extended and the knee joint flexed to 90°.

The Ludloff test (figure 10.9a) is a specific test for the iliopsoas muscle. The test isolates the iliopsoas by flexing the patient's hip to about 90° and internally rotating the femur against resistance or by lifting her leg with her knee extended while sitting on a chair. Production of deep groin pain during this test implies that the muscle's tendinous insertion onto the lesser trochanter is affected (a positive Ludloff sign).

The Thomas test (figure 10.9b) assesses the flexibility of the iliopsoas. The test is performed with the patient supine, with his buttocks close to the edge of the examination table. Both lower extremities are maximally flexed at the hip and knee, and then one lower limb is extended while the other is held in flexion. Incomplete inability to fully extend the hips is suggestive of a contracted or inflexible iliopsoas. Pressing on the patient's thigh and passively forcing the hip further into extension will trigger pain if the iliopsoas is affected.

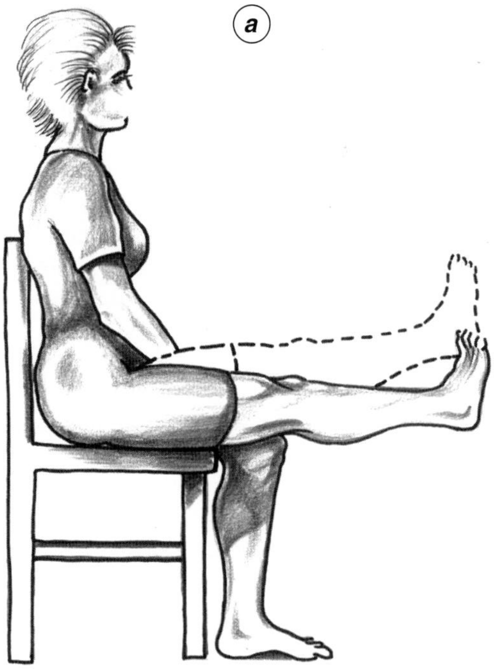

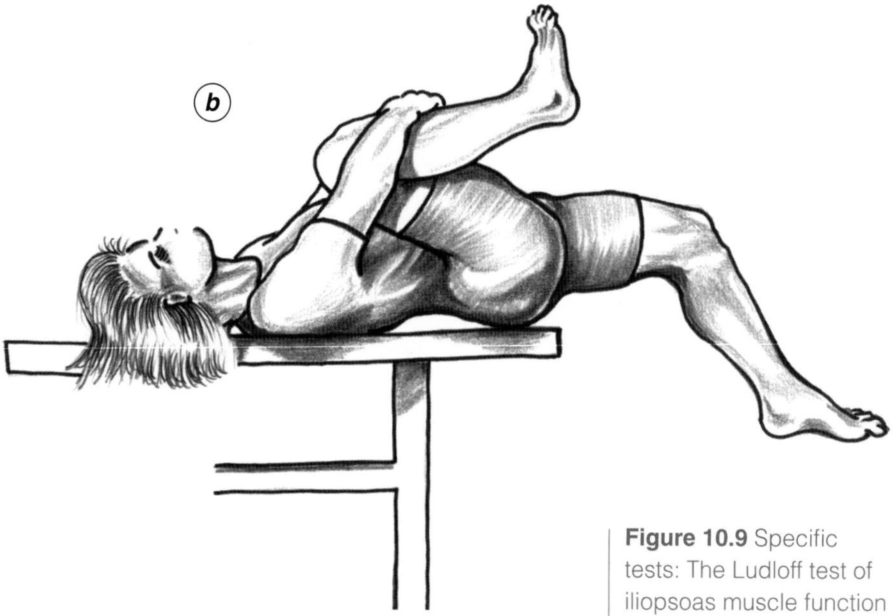

Figure 10.9 Specific tests: The Ludloff test of iliopsoas muscle function (a) and the Thomas test of iliopsoas flexibility (b).

Supplemental Examinations

Radiographic examination. Stress fractures can be diagnosed by means of a radiographic examination but often not until some time after the fracture occurred, when callus begins to form around the narrow fracture cleft. If the patient has osteitis pubis, the pubic bone will appear moth-eaten on X ray. If they persist long enough, chronic tendinosis or bursitis may cause calcium deposition at the muscle insertion or in the affected bursa. These calcium deposits often look like gray shadows on an X ray of the injured area. Myositis ossificans may have a similar appearance. Indefinite painful conditions in the pelvic, inguinal, and hip regions should be evaluated radiographically to rule out bone tumors or other elements of the differential diagnosis (e.g., hip joint osteoarthritis, osteochondritis dissecans coxae, and ankylosing spondylitis).

CT. If lumbar spondylolysis is suspected without radiographically demonstrable spondylolisthesis, a CT scan can clearly demonstrate the fracture cleft. If the etiology of pelvic regional pain is uncertain or indefinite, CT scanning of the entire area may be indicated, particularly if a tumor is suspected.

MRI. Tendinosis and bursitis may be demonstrated on MRI. If a patient has osteitis pubis or a stress fracture, MRI will demonstrate edema and changes in the bone structure of the affected area. MRI is the examination of choice for evaluating tumors.

Skeletal scintigraphy. Skeletal scintigraphy (bone scan) is almost immediately positive in the case of stress fractures, and it is the best diagnostic tool for demonstrating stress injury of bone. Scintigraphy reveals diagnostic findings in patients with osteitis pubis or acute spondylolysis. Scintigraphy is also a sensitive technique for evaluating bone tumors, whether malignant or benign (such as osteoid osteoma).

Ultrasonography. Ultrasound may be used to diagnose myositis ossificans and bursitis and to demonstrate the localization and extent of scar tissue formation following muscle injuries.

Common Injuries

Adductor Tendinosis

The most common cause of chronic adductor tendinosis is overly aggressive rehabilitation after an acute proximal adductor strain, including premature return to sports activity. The disorder may occur with or without a muscle tear: simple overload of the adductor longus muscle-tendon junction or of the tendon at its insertion can result in chronic pain and functional limitation (figure 10.1, page 267). This type of overuse is relatively common among horseback riders, skaters (particularly ice hockey), and cross-country skiers who ski freestyle.

• Symptoms and signs: The initial symptoms are often spread diffusely through the inguinal region. Alternatively, the athlete may have well-localized pain over the adductor longus tendon. As the disorder gradually becomes more chronic and the pain more pervasive, it may radiate inferiorly on the inside of the thigh and superiorly toward the rectus abdominis. The origin of the adductor longus and the insertion of the rectus abdominis on the pubic bone are in close proximity, and the chronic granulomatous changes may on occasion affect both tendons. Other muscles in the area may also become painful because they will be subjected to improper loading when the patient unconsciously attempts to protect and unload the injured area. Pain is often accompanied by stiffness, particularly in the morning and at the start of a training session. As the athlete gradually warms up, the stiffness disappears but the pain increases. When the musculature cools off after training, the stiffness will return. The risk that the athlete will enter a vicious cycle of pain is great. If no attempt is made to break this cycle by unloading the affected areas and by adopting proper training techniques, the symptoms will gradually increase, so that the athlete will eventually be unable to train and even regular walking may be painfully limited.

- Diagnosis: The examination of a patient with chronic groin pain must be very thorough. The differential diagnosis for pain in this region is lengthy, and the diagnosis can be made with any certainty only by means of a good history and careful physical examination. When the tendon of the adductor longus is affected at its insertion, muscle flexibility is often reduced in comparison to the opposite side, and stretching against resistance triggers pain corresponding to the area of injury. Passive hip abduction will also trigger pain in this area, and the patient will often indicate significant pain upon palpation. The remainder of the groin area must also be palpated carefully, particularly the lymph nodes, the scrotum, and the symphysis pubis. A neuromuscular exam of the lower extremities should be completed, and a rectal examination should also be performed if the patient has a long history of groin pain. Supplemental examinations are usually necessary. X rays of the pelvis and hips should be done first and may reveal evidence of calcific tendinopathy in chronic cases. MRI may demonstrate changes proximally in the adductor muscles themselves. Practically, radiographic imaging is requested and often most useful to "rule out" conditions from the differential diagnosis. Bone scan and cross sectional imaging, combined with serological testing, are useful to exclude infection or tumor and are often employed as screening tests to eliminate various diagnostic considerations when the diagnosis remains in doubt (e.g., when the exam is unrevealing or treatment does not yield the anticipated effects).
- Treatment by physician: From the outset, the patient must be clearly informed immediately that conservative treatment of adductor tendinosis is a lengthy process, often taking 4 to 6 months or longer. Treatment primarily consists of various types of exercise. Steroid injections usually provide only temporary relief. If conservative treatment does not produce satisfactory results within 6 to 12 months, the patient should be given the option of surgery. Usually performed under local anesthesia, surgical intervention generally consists of tenotomy, where either the adductor longus tendon or all adductor tendons in the area are released from the periosteum. This procedure normally causes mild bleeding and small reactive changes in the area of the surgery. Postoperatively, the patient avoids weight bearing by using crutches for a few days until full loading can be tolerated. Active and passive stretching and strength training of the adductors begins early, and after 2 to 3 weeks the patient may bicycle with some weight bearing. Running is allowed after about 6 weeks, and the athlete can normally return to full sport activity after 10 to 12 weeks. In some cases, the patient may have persistent mild pain in the area of the surgery, but the pain is usually not so intense that it hinders full activity. A good surgical outcome depends on a proper initial diagnosis, good surgical technique, and optimal postoperative rehabilitation.
- Treatment by physical therapist: The physical therapist should begin treatment by instructing the patient in a program of careful stretching and exercising. As soon as the patient can tolerate it, strength training of the adductors may begin. Both stretching and strength training must be done with minimum provocation of pain! Eccentric strength training should gradually assume a greater role in the exercise program as the athlete progresses. Neuromuscular training of the inguinal and hip musculature is incorporated into the training program as soon as pain allows. There is no definite documented effect from ultrasound, laser therapy, electrotherapy, or similar passive modalities. Once the patient has achieved full pain-free mobility that is symmetric on both sides with normal strength of the adductor muscle group, controlled functional training relevant to the athlete's sport may begin. The return to full sport activity must be gradual and must take place under the supervision of physical therapists, trainers, or coaches.

Rectus Femoris Tendinosis

This disorder may occur as a result of intense shooting drills in soccer and is common among sprinters who begin training with long sessions. It may also be caused by returning to sport activity too early after a proximal partial tear of the muscle (figure 10.2).

- Symptoms and signs: Weight bearing exercise typically results in central groin pain. Attempting to accelerate quickly may be particularly painful.
- Diagnosis: Flexion of the hip or extension of the knee against resistance causes pain to radiate toward the anterior inferior iliac spine. Palpation also causes significant tenderness over the proximal portion of the muscle, about 8 cm distal to the anterior superior iliac spine. Intramuscular bleeding may cause calcium deposition that can be demonstrated on subsequent X rays of the area.
- Treatment: The mainstay of treatment is strength and flexibility training (with gradually increasing loads) as was discussed for the treatment of adductor tendinosis. In treatment-resistant cases marked by pain-limited effort to rehabilitate the injury, an injection of cortisone and local anesthetic can be administered. Surgical treatment to remove granulation tissue from the tendon is rarely indicated. Tenotomy must not be performed on the rectus femoris tendon.
- Prognosis: The prognosis is good with adequate conservative treatment. Rectus femoris tendinosis tends to be significantly easier to treat than chronic adductor tendinosis.

Iliopsoas Tendinosis

Overly aggressive rehabilitation of a partial tear of the distal iliopsoas tendon, or long-term overuse with overloaded hip flexion may cause a chronic, painful tendinosis at the insertion of the iliopsoas on the lesser trochanter.

- Symptoms and signs: The patient typically reports centralized groin pain, often directly over the inguinal ligament and directly lateral to the rectus abdominis that is aggravated by loading (such as running uphill).
- Diagnosis: The Ludloff sign and Thomas test (p. 280) are both positive. Bimanual palpation of the tendon insertion at the lesser trochanter may also trigger significant pain, particularly in thin patients.
- Treatment: The mainstay of treatment is strength and flexibility training (with gradually increasing loads) as was discussed for the treatment of adductor tendinosis. In cases that are resistant to treatment, or if the patient cannot start training because of pain, an injection of cortisone and local anesthetic can be administered under fluoroscopic guidance, 2 to 3 cm proximal to the lesser trochanter. After 1 to 2 weeks of rest, the patient can resume rehabilitation with systematic stretching and strength training of the iliopsoas. Occasionally, all attempts at conservative treatment fail. When that is the case, the patient may be offered surgical treatment (extension tenotomy of the iliopsoas tendon). However, this is a major intervention with somewhat indefinite results. Surgery should therefore be attempted only if the patient has had a favorable response to diagnostic injection of local anesthetic and if he is prepared to embark upon a long-term rehabilitation regimen.

Rectus Abdominis Tendinosis

Long-term overload of the distal tendon of the rectus abdominis, such as in rowing and tennis, may precipitate a chronic painful tendinosis in this area. Premature return to play after an injury to the distal rectus abdominis may also contribute to the development of chronic tendinopathy. The distance between the tendinous insertion of the rectus abdominis and the origin of the adductor longus is short, which in chronic, longstanding cases often results in pain when the adductors are loaded.

- Symptoms and signs: The patient complains of pain radiating inferiorly towards the symphysis upon loading and with activation of the rectus abdominis. The pain may become quite disabling, and in some cases the adductors may also be affected, particularly the adductor longus, due to the anatomical relationship described above.
- Treatment: The mainstay of treatment is the same strength and motion training (with gradually increasing loads) as described for treatment of adductor tendinosis. In treatment-resistant cases, or when the patient cannot start training because of pain, a mixture of cortisone and local anesthetic can be injected around the tendon at its insertion on the pubic bone, followed by 1 to 2 weeks of rest before resuming active rehabilitation. If the patient does not make progress with conservative treatment, surgical resection/debridement of the granulation tissue from the tendon may be indicated.
- Prognosis: The prognosis is generally good with early and adequate treatment. However, some chronic injuries do not heal regardless of what is attempted and have resulted in the end of the sports career of a number of top athletes.

Other Injuries

Injuries to Other Muscles and Tendons in the Inguinal and Hip Region

Other muscles, such as the gracilis, the sartorius, the tensor fascia lata, and the gluteal muscles (particularly the gluteus medius), may also be subjected to strain injury or tendinosis. A thorough examination, including palpation and specific testing of the relevant muscle, is key in determining what has been injured. The guidelines for treatment and prevention are the same as for an adductor longus strain or tendinosis.

Myositis Ossificans—Heterotopic Ossification in the Injured Muscle !

Myositis ossificans refers to a process of calcification and eventual ossification of a deep intramuscular hematoma. It occurs most commonly as the result of distal strains of the adductor group. The etiology is unclear. Some authors believe that calcification results from avulsed periosteal cells, whereas others maintain that fibroblasts in the hematoma differentiate into osteoblasts. In any case, it is typical for the disorder to appear when activity is advanced too quickly following an injury, resulting in local recurrent microinjury, re-bleeding, and a chronic inflammatory reaction in the affected area.

- Symptoms and signs: Symptoms include pain and reduced function corresponding to the affected muscle group.
- Diagnosis: Sometimes a solid tumor can be palpated in the muscle belly. Ultrasound and X rays demonstrate calcium deposition. A supplemental MRI examination is often indicated to exclude a malignant tumor.
- Treatment: The primary treatments are prophylactic, in the form of adequate unloading and gradual, careful rehabilitation after a muscle strain injury. NSAIDs administered over a long period may have a favorable effect. In cases marked by chronic symptoms, it may be necessary to surgically excise the new bone formation. However, this must not be performed before the process of calcification in the area is complete (generally at the earliest, about 1 year after injury). The risk of recurrent ossification within the affected muscle is high if surgical excision is performed too early.

Trochanteric Tendinosis

This is a chronic, painful condition at the insertion of the gluteus medius and minimus on the posterior margin of the greater trochanter (figure 10.10). The

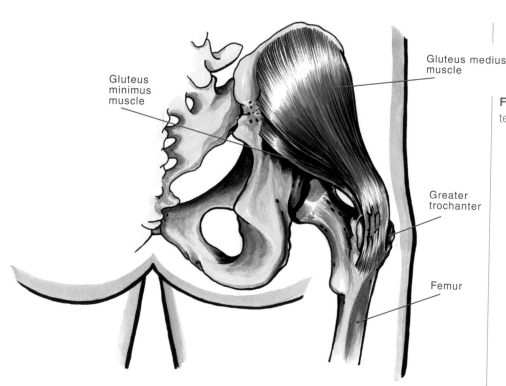

Gluteus minimus muscle

Gluteus medius muscle

Greater trochanter

Femur

Figure 10.10 Trochanter tendinosis.

cause is often simple overloading, and it is most frequently diagnosed in long-distance runners and orienteering runners. Repeatedly running on the same side of the road (usually the left), which effectively causes a functional leg-length discrepancy due to the consistent incline of the asphalt, may trigger the conditions. Endogenous causes, such as true leg-length discrepancy, increased femoral neck anteversion, genu valgum, and foot over-pronation, are important intrinsic risk factors.

- Symptoms and signs: The patient complains of pain over and behind the greater trochanter, frequently both during and after loading. The pain may become so severe that running becomes intolerable.
- Diagnosis: Examination findings include distinct tenderness to pressure over the tendinous insertion of the gluteus medius and minimus at the superior-posterior aspect of the greater trochanter. Abduction in the hip against resistance triggers pain. If the problem has been chronic, X ray may demonstrate calcium deposition in the affected area. The physician must look for triggering reversible causes—both exogenous and endogenous to the patient. The most important differential diagnostic consideration is trochanteric bursitis.
- Treatment: The essential elements of treatment are the strength and flexibility training (while gradually increasing exercise loads) as discussed for the treatment of adductor tendinosis. In treatment-resistant cases, or when the patient cannot start training because of pain, an injection of cortisone and local anesthetic can be performed around the tendon's insertion. To prevent recurrence, the modifiable risk factors must be identified and corrected. Both the training and the training surface must be varied, and any leg-length discrepancy misalignment of the foot must be corrected using specially adapted orthoses or shoes. In cases that are particularly resistant to treatment, surgery may be indicated to remove granulation tissue and calcium deposits from the inserting tendon.
- Prognosis: The symptoms have a tendency to recur if the underlying causes are not corrected.

Stress Fractures

Stress fractures of the femoral neck are relatively common, while stress fractures of the proximal femur or the pubic rami are much less common (figure 10.11). Stress fractures of the femoral neck constitute 7% of all stress fractures sustained by long-distance runners. The most common etiologies include excessively rapid increases in the amount and intensity of training, or switching from a soft to a hard training surface. Running only on asphalt may also predispose the athlete to this injury. Anatomic malalignment such as that caused by leg-length discrepancy is also considered a risk factor for stress fractures of the pelvis and hips.

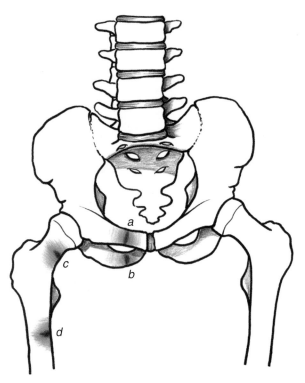

Figure 10.11 Stress fracture. Location of the most commonly occurring stress fractures in the pelvic and hip area: superior pubic ramus *(a)*, inferior pubic ramus *(b)*, femoral neck *(c)*, and proximal femoral shaft *(d)*.

- Symptoms and signs: The patient reports pain in the hip region (usually in the groin), precipitated by weight bearing. The pain disappears at rest, but recurs as soon as weight-bearing training is resumed.
- Diagnosis: The patient's history will typically reveal several risk factors for stress fracture formation. The hop test is a useful diagnostic test. The patient hops on the affected leg, and if this provokes their usual pain, the diagnosis of stress fracture becomes more likely. Forceful passive range of motion of the hip joint often triggers pain as well. Plain film radiography often does not reveal the fracture until 3 to 4 weeks after the fracture recurred, when callus begins to form in the area. However, skeletal scintigraphy will demonstrate intense uptake corresponding to the fracture after only 2 or 3 days. If scintigraphy demonstrates that the patient has numerous stress fractures, the clinician should consider the possibility that the athlete may have an eating disorder (e.g., anorexia). MRI will also clearly demonstrate the lesion and the surrounding edema in the affected bone.
- Treatment by physician: Treatment consists of unloading the involved limb with crutches for 4 to 6 weeks. Fractures of the pubic bone usually heal quickly and without complications. If the femoral neck is fractured, follow-up evaluation must include several radiographs to assess bone healing. If there is evidence of delayed healing, nonunion, or if signs of dislocation are present, the fracture must be surgically fixed.
- Treatment by physical therapist: During the non-weight bearing period, the patient must be prescribed an alternative exercise program, including activities such as swimming, running in water, bicycling, and general strength training. Running must be resumed gradually, with a careful progression that avoids recurrent pain. Modifiable risk factors for stress injury, such as malalignment or excessive training on hard surfaces, must also be corrected if possible.
- Prophylaxis: The use of appropriate equipment, good running shoes, training on soft or varied surfaces, and a well-monitored training program should make it possible to avoid stress fractures of the proximal femur or the pubic rami.
- Prognosis: In general, the prognosis is good for fractures of the pelvis and femur. Displaced fracture of the femoral neck carry a less definite prognosis, including some risk for osteonecrosis of the femoral head and segmental collapse.

Osteitis Pubis

Former theories as to the etiology of osteitis pubis suggested it was associated with chronic urinary tract or prostate infection. However, more recent studies have demonstrated that the disorder is rarely infectious in origin. Even though individual studies have shown a high correlation between osteitis pubis and disorders of the

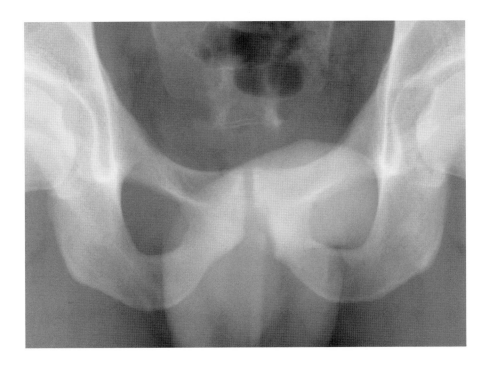

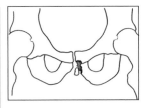

Figure 10.12 Osteitis pubis. The "moth eaten" appearance of the medial aspect of the inferior pubic ramus of the pubis on the left should be noted.

back, the sacroiliac joint, and the hips (increased femoral anteversion, coxa vara), among athletes the condition is almost exclusively related to overuse, particularly due to repetitive traction by the rectus abdominis. Reduced hip joint range of motion (itself usually the result of inflexibility of the short, strong muscles in the area), is commonly found in patients with osteitis pubis. The disorder is three to five times more common in men than in women. It is most common in long-distance runners and in soccer, ice hockey, and tennis players, but may be found in athletes in all sports that require running associated with rapid changes of direction. In a group of professional soccer players, 76% were found to have radiographic changes that are consistent with osteitis pubis (figure 10.12).

- Symptoms and signs: The main symptom is pain localized to the lower abdomen and the inside of the thighs both during and after loading. The pain gradually increases with activity and may become so intense that running may be virtually impossible.
- Diagnosis: A thorough history, including a review of the patient's training program is key, particularly with respect to loading of the abdominal musculature. Clinical examination findings include tenderness when both the insertion of the rectus abdominis and the origin of the hip adductors on the pubic bone are palpated. However, maximal tenderness is usually found over the symphysis pubis. Activation of the abdominal and adductor musculature against resistance reproduces the athlete's pain, and the mobility of the hip joints is often reduced. In chronic cases in which the patient has had pain for a long time, the pubic bone in the region of the symphysis has a typically moth-eaten and partially sclerotic appearance on X ray that is often asymmetric to one side (figure 10.12). Shortly after the onset of symptoms, the X ray may be unrevealing. Isotope scintigraphy, however, will demonstrate intensive uptake, usually in both pubic bones (figure 10.13). Radiographic changes remain for a long time after the symptoms disappear, and in some cases the X ray can demonstrate the typical changes without the athlete having experienced characterisic symptoms. MRI examination during the early phase will demonstrate bone marrow edema in the involved pubic bone (figure 10.14), a finding that should resolve as the athlete's symptoms disappear.

- Treatment: The only effective treatment is avoidance of symptom-provoking activities that cause pain for at least 6 to 8 weeks. NSAID therapy should be attempted during the early phase, and the patient may benefit from a cortisone injection in chronic cases. One or two injections may be given in the direction of the upper portion of the symphysis near the insertion of the rectus abdominis. Abdominal and hip muscle stretching is recommended, especially for patients with reduced hip joint range of motion. The athlete needs an

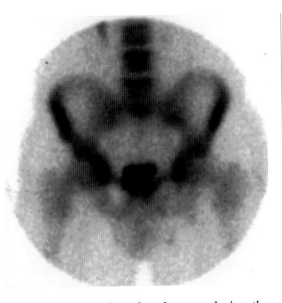

Figure 10.13 Positive scintigraphy findings in osteitis pubis.

alternative training program for maintaining strength and endurance during the unloading period. Treatment in a high-pressure chamber (hyperbaric therapy) may decrease the time needed for healing.

- Prognosis: The prognosis is good with adequate unloading, but 6 to 12 months often elapse before the patient becomes completely asymptomatic.

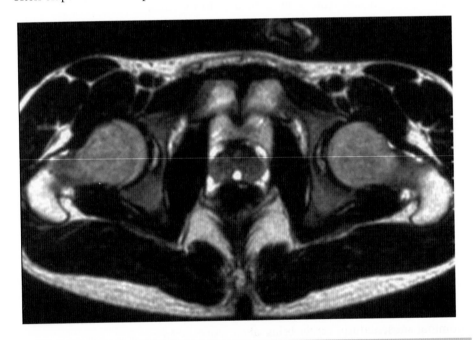

Figure 10.14 Positive MRI findings in osteitis pubis. The image shows bone marrow edema of the pubic bone bilaterally.

Groin Insufficiency–Gilmore's Groin

Groin insufficiency is the end result of chronic overuse of the inferior abdominal musculature, particularly the lower fibers of the external oblique and the aponeurosis of the transverses abdominis (figure 10.15). Chronic overload may result in weakness, a defect, or a tear in the posterior wall of the inguinal canal. The disorder is most common among soccer players but may also occur in athletes in other sports, such as long-distance running, American football, and rugby.

• Symptoms and signs: Loading causes steadily increasing pain in the inguinal region that has the character of a toothache, and the symptoms often persist for a while after the activity has ended. Pain worsens significantly from quick spurts, hitting balls hard, or coughing and sneezing. Eventually, the pain begins earlier and earlier during activity and ultimately, both training and competition may become impossible. It may be difficult for the patient to localize the pain, and if the disorder becomes chronic, secondary pain often develops at the origin of the hip adductors and at the insertion of the rectus abdominis on the pubic bone. Pain frequently radiates to the scrotum, the perineum, and the lumbar area of the back.

• Diagnosis: The physician must take a thorough history and perform a careful physical examination, particularly with respect to differential diagnostic conditions including adductor tendinosis, osteitis pubis, rectus abdominis tendinosis, and iliopsoas tendinosis. Many patients with chronic symptoms will complain of discomfort when the hip adductors and rectus abdominis are palpated along the pubic bone. Loading of these muscles against resistance will also trigger pain. The external inguinal opening is examined via the scrotum as the patient stands and coughs. This, as well as palpation over the middle portion of the inguinal canal, should reproduce the patient's typical pain. The external inguinal opening may be slightly expanded in contrast with the unaffected side. Herniography (with radiographic contrast in the abdominal cavity) and ultrasound examinations are infrequently recommended, as both radiographic and ultrasound images may be difficult to interpret and are often negative during the early stage when changes are minimal.

• Treatment: Attempts at conservative treatment, including unloading and careful strength training of the abdominal musculature, rarely bring about long-term improvement. Several studies have shown that surgical treatment using hernioplasty to reinforce the posterior wall in the inguinal canal has a very good success rate. Most reports indicate that more than 90% of patients return to sport activity after adequate postoperative training. This training consists of unloading the muscles of the abdominal wall for 4 to 6 weeks, after which strength training is initiated and carefully and gradually increased.

• Prognosis: Normally, with appropriate care, the athlete may resume full sport activity after about 3 months.

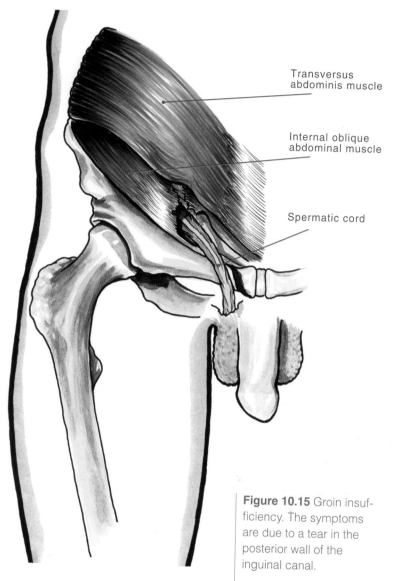

Transversus abdominis muscle

Internal oblique abdominal muscle

Spermatic cord

Figure 10.15 Groin insufficiency. The symptoms are due to a tear in the posterior wall of the inguinal canal.

Bursitis

There are several bursae in the pelvic, inguinal, and hip region. The most important ones clinically are the trochanteric, iliopectineal, and gluteal bursae (figure 10.16). An inflammatory reaction (bursitis) may occur at any of these sites due to (1) mechanical friction, (2) chemical irritation, or (3) infection. In athletes, bursitis is almost exclusively caused by mechanical irritation, usually from a muscle or tendon that glides repetitively back and forth over the bursa. A superficial bursa, such as the trochanteric bursa, may also be subjected to direct trauma that may result in both bleeding and inflammation (page 275). The blood may coagulate and form fibrin deposits in the bursa, which in turn may cause chronic irritation. Eventually, these fibrin lumps calcify, and when the bursa is palpated the calcification may feel like small movable rice bodies.

The *iliopectineal bursa* is situated between the anterior aspect of the hip joint and the iliopsoas muscle (figure 10.16). It is the largest bursa in the body, and in 15% of adults, communication between the bursa and the hip joint is present. Inflammation in this bursa may occur in isolation or in combination with a disorder (strain injury or tendinosis) of the iliopsoas muscle. The most common triggering cause is intense periods of running training, particularly in hurdlers and marathon runners.

- Symptoms and signs: Pain and possibly swelling in the groin anteriorly are reasonably common. Sitting with the hip in flexion for a long time may be provocative of symptoms.
- Diagnosis: Passive flexion and rotation of the hip causes pain, but activation of the iliopsoas in extension against resistance is pain free. If iliopsoas bursitis is suspected, ultrasound or MRI examinations will demonstrate the thickened and possibly fluid-filled bursa.
- Treatment: Treatments include needle aspiration of as much fluid as possible, followed by injection of cortisone if the bursitis is not felt to be purulent. Modification of the training regimen and stretching of the iliopsoas are also recommended.

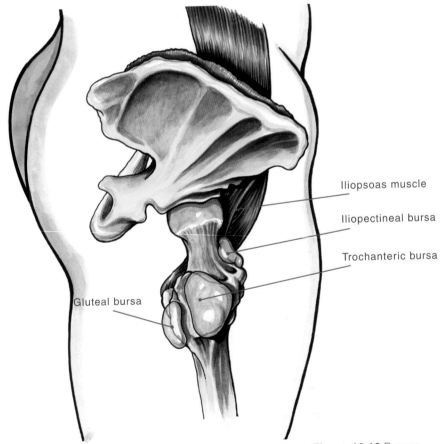

Iliopsoas muscle

Iliopectineal bursa

Trochanteric bursa

Gluteal bursa

Figure 10.16 Bursae in the hip area. Bursitis may occur in several of the bursae of the hip girdle, including the iliopectineal bursa, the trochanteric bursa, and the gluteal bursa.

The *trochanteric bursa* is located between the iliotibial band/tensor fascia lata and the greater trochanter (figure 10.16). Because of its relatively superficial location over the bone, it is subject to direct trauma that may result in bleeding and acute inflammation. Key triggering causes of chronic friction bursitis are anatomic malalignment, such as leg-length discrepancy, increased collum anteversion, a broad pelvis, an inflexible iliotibial tract, and overpronation foot with compensatory internal rotation of the tibia. Another common cause is frequent running on one side of the road (usually the left). This causes a functional leg-length discrepancy, and consequent overuse of the iliotibial tract and the tensor fascia lata on the leg that is closest to the edge of the road, thereby increasing the risk of developing trochanteric bursitis on that side.

- Symptoms and signs: Pain and possibly swelling occur over the greater trochanter. The pain occasionally radiates inferiorly along the lateral side of the thigh. At times, such symptoms may be mistakenly attributed to sciatica.
- Diagnosis: The diagnosis is made on the basis of tenderness, swelling, and possibly crepitation over the greater trochanter. In chronic cases, the examiner may detect small rice like calcifications locally upon exam. Adduction and rotation of the hip with an extended knee will also trigger pain. It is possible to demonstrate the thickening of the wall and an increased amount of fluid in the bursa by using ultrasound and MRI.
- Treatment: Unloading, NSAIDs, and modified training are the recommended treatments for acute cases. If symptoms are chronic or recurring, treatment options include aspiration with removal of fluid, and possibly steroid injection, as well as concentrated stretching of the iliotibial tract and the tensor fascia lata. At the same time, any malalignment and identifiable training errors are corrected if possible. The use of hip protectors may be helpful to athletes who may be prone to falling on their hip (e.g., handball players and goalies). Occasionally, a patient requires surgery with excision of the bursa and removal of an oval "window" in the fascia lata over the greater trochanter. This "window" must be large enough to allow the trochanter to move freely during hip flexion and extension, without "pinching" the edges of the fascia lata.

The *gluteal bursa* is located between the tendon of the gluteus medius and the tensor fascia lata, posterior to the greater trochanter (figure 10.16). Inflammation of this bursa is usually caused by overuse and is most commonly diagnosed in long-distance runners. Malalignment is another important contributing factor in this case.

- Symptoms and signs: The patient experiences pain in the gluteal region that may radiate inferiorly into the posterior thigh. Sitting for a prolonged period may cause significant pain.
- Diagnosis: The diagnosis is made on the basis of the exam findings of pain upon palpation of the bursa and pain upon passive flexion of the involved hip. It is difficult to clinically differentiate these symptoms from those of trochanteric tendinosis, but ultrasound or MRI examination will demonstrate the inflamed bursa.
- Treatment: The treatment is essentially the same as for iliopsoas bursitis but also includes stretching of the gluteal musculature and the tensor fascia lata.

Snapping Hip !

Typical Snapping Hip. The most common cause of snapping hip is irritation of the posterior margin of the iliotibial band, which passes over the top of the greater trochanter (figure 10.17). A fibrous mound-shaped prominence may eventually form at the site of irritation, and secondary trochanteric bursitis also tends to develop concurrently. When the hip is flexed and stretched, the mound-shaped prominence glides back and forth over the trochanter, often with an audible click and visible and palpable "snapping." The disorder is most common among thin, flexible women, such as ballet dancers and gymnasts.

- Symptoms and signs: Aching pain is felt over the greater trochanter during loading with flexion and extension of the hip. Discomfort accompanies the often very audible click of the snapping fascia.
- Treatment: Recommended treatment includes stretching of the iliotibial band and the tensor fascia lata possibly combined with steroid injection of the trochanteric

PELVIS, GROIN, AND HIP

bursa. Persistent pain often results in the need for surgical treatment that is technically similar to the procedure performed for patients with refractory chronic trochanteric bursitis.

Atypical Snapping Hip. This disorder occurs when the iliopsoas tendon glides back and forth over the iliopectineal eminence of the pubic bone or over an osseous prominence near the lesser trochanter (figure 10.17).

- Symptoms and signs: Deep groin pain is accompanied by a click when the hip is extended from a flexed, externally rotated, and abducted position.
- Treatment: The standard treatment includes stretching of the iliopsoas muscle. Occasionally it is necessary to surgically lengthen the iliopsoas tendon.

Nerve Entrapment

The following nerves in the inguinal and hip region may be subject to entrapment or to pressure injuries: the sciatic, lateral femoral cutaneous, ilioinguinal, genitofemoral, and obturator nerves (figure 10.18, a and b). The ilioinguinal, genitofemoral, and lateral femoral cutaneous nerves may become entrapped in scar tissue resulting from local trauma or surgery. They may also be susceptible to pressure from long-term, intense training of the abdominal musculature. Tight belts or tight-fitting jeans may also irritate the lateral femoral cutaneous nerve, a condition known as meralgia paresthetica. Piriformis syndrome occurs when the sciatic nerve is irritated as it exits the pelvis anterior to the piriformis muscle. This disorder occurs most commonly in well-trained people with short, strong, and inflexible musculature. Athletes, particularly those in strength sports and bodybuilding, may develop irritation of the obturator nerve as it passes through the obturator canal.

- Symptoms and signs: The ilioinguinal nerve innervates the base of the penis and scrotum and of the labia majora, as well as the medial side of the proximal thigh. The genitofemoral nerve also innervates the scrotum and the labia majora, as well as the anterior side of the thigh immediately inferior to the inguinal ligament. The lateral femoral cutaneous nerve supplies the skin of the anterior and lateral thigh, and the obturator nerve innervates the adductor muscles and an area of skin that corresponds to the distal portion of the medial thigh approaching the popliteal space (figure 10.18). Irritation of these nerves may cause paresthesias and pain in a distribution corresponding to their area of innervation. Vigorous use of the musculature surrounding the nerve involved may aggravate the symptoms of entrapment. When the piriformis muscle irritates the sciatic nerve, aching pain emanates from the ischial tuberosity, possibly radiating inferiorly into the posterior thigh. Patients with piriformis syndrome often have the sensation that the hamstring muscles are too short, and they may complain of an inability to reach maximum speed during sprints because of the disorder. Typically, pain related to piriformis syndrome also

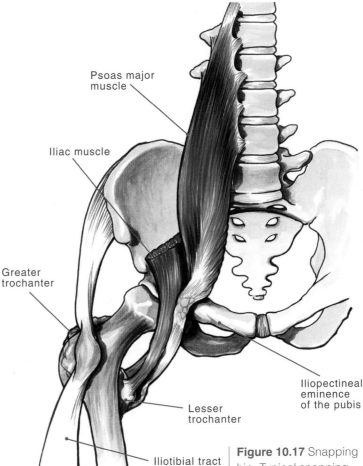

Psoas major muscle

Iliac muscle

Greater trochanter

Lesser trochanter

Iliotibial tract

Iliopectineal eminence of the pubis

Figure 10.17 Snapping hip. Typical snapping hip is caused by the iliotibial tract gliding over the greater trochanter, whereas atypical snapping hip is caused by the psoas major tendon gliding over the iliopectineal eminence of the pubis proximally or a bony eminence at the lesser trochanter distally.

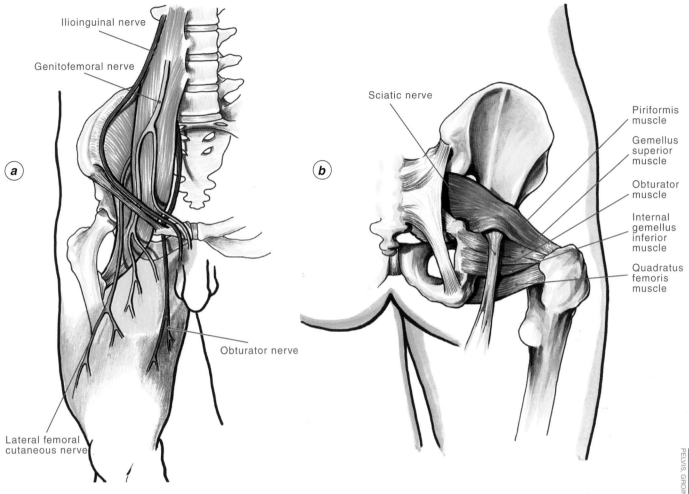

a

b

Ilioinguinal nerve

Genitofemoral nerve

Sciatic nerve

Piriformis muscle

Gemellus superior muscle

Obturator muscle

Internal gemellus inferior muscle

Quadratus femoris muscle

Obturator nerve

Lateral femoral cutaneous nerve

worsens when the patient sits with their hips slightly hyperflexed for a long time, such as when driving a car. Consequently, these individuals often have to stop the car, get out, and stretch their hips before continuing to drive.

- Diagnosis: The patient often indicates reduced sensation, pain, and paresthesias in the cutaneous area supplied by the affected nerve. A peripheral nerve block with local anesthetic confirms the diagnosis. Piriformis syndrome is a diagnosis of exclusion. All other possible causes of pain in the affected region must be ruled out before this diagnosis can be made with certainty. When the piriformis muscle is loaded, the patient typically complains of pain radiating from the ischial tuberosity inferiorly to the posterior thigh. In a few cases, the patient may report pain extending into the calf.
- Treatment: Modification of training routines, particularly reduction of intense strength training combined with required flexibility training, may resolve the patient's complaints related to nerve compression. NSAIDs may also be effective if administered early in the course of the disorder. In some cases, particularly if the patient has meralgia paresthetica, the nerve must be surgically released in the affected area. Piriformis syndrome should be treated conservatively, by emphasizing stretching of the piriformis muscle. Optimal stretching of the piriformis can be performed independently by placing the hip joint through maximum flexion, adduction, and external rotation. Conservative treatment is not, however, universally successful, and for those patients with persistent symptoms, surgical release of the piriformis tendon may be indicated.

Figure 10.18 Nerve entrapment syndromes. The distribution of symptoms is shown when various nerves in the inguinal area *(a)* become entrapped, including the sciatic nerve *(b)*.

Rehabilitation of Injuries to the Pelvis, Groin, and Hip

Hilde Fredriksen and Torbjørn Grøntvedt

Goals and Principles for Treating Acute Injuries

The goals of rehabilitation of acute injuries of the pelvic, inguinal, and hip region are listed in table 10.3.

As soon as the muscle can be activated without pain, the patient may initiate a program of mild dynamic exercise. If pain limits weight bearing, it is possible to begin active range of motion therapy without weight bearing by suspending the affected limb in a sling (see figure 10.2). The patient should begin with mild weight bearing and numerous repetitions. The exercises may be repeated several times during the day. The muscle should be completely relaxed between contractions. The goal is to improve circulation and improve relaxation in the portion of the musculature that is not injured, thereby accelerating the healing process.

Active stretching of the muscles begins as soon as tolerated. Stretching should be performed within the limits of pain, avoiding over-stretching the injured tissue and emphasizing maintenance of the available pain-free range of motion. The exercises must always be done without, or with only minimal, pain.

Exercises are of primary importance during the rehabilitation phase, but other physical therapy treatment may be useful in mobilizing bleeding residue and avoiding excessive scar tissue formation in the injured area. Massage, stretching, and various types of electrotherapy may be indicated. Eventually, the patient will have to train actively through the entire range of motion to regain flexibility comparable to that of the healthy side. It

	Goals	Measures
Acute phase	Reduce swelling	PRICE principle
Rehabilitation phase	Reduce pain	Dynamic exercises with gradually increasing intensity
	Normalize movement, strength, and sensory motor function	Neuromuscular motor training
Training phase	As a minimum, achieve the same sensory motor function, strength, and mobility as before the injury	Functional training
		Sport-specific training
	Reduce the risk of reinjury	Recuperate fully before returning to maximum activity

Table 10.3 Goals and measures for rehabilitation of acute injuries.

294

is important for the patient to achieve an elastic functional scar tissue, thereby preventing recurrence. He must always follow up increased flexibility with improved neuromuscular control and strength training. He must also preserve the stabilizing function of the muscles through exercises that stabilize the pelvis. Various neuromuscular exercises are important for this purpose. The progression of exercise intensity and level of difficulty is controlled by pain and the functional ability of the patient. If the progression proceeds too rapidly, chronic painful conditions can easily develop.

Good alternatives for maintaining general conditioning during the non-weight bearing period of treatment of acute injuries include bicycling, running in water (while wearing a buoyancy vest), and swimming (although the breast stroke should be avoided in adductor injuries).

Rehabilitation of Chronic Painful Conditions

The main elements of rehabilitation of muscle injuries and tendinopathies in the groin, inguinal, and hip region are strength and stability training. Training initially begins with light loading and numerous repetitions (usually 30 repetitions in each series), performed several times a day (assuming that the patient's pain does not worsen). Thereafter, the load is gradually increased while the number of repetitions is correspondingly reduced.

If the pain in an area has become chronic, it may result in altered movement patterns, which can in turn easily result in overload of other tissues or structures. Therefore, when the patient is being rehabilitated for injuries in the hip and pelvic region, he must also train the relevant stabilizing musculature. The quadriceps coxae (external rotators), adductors, and abductors balance and stabilize the pelvis on the femoral head. Therefore, neuromuscular training in this area should be emphasized, in addition to knee and ankle stabilization exercises. Weight transfer and training on a balance or wobble board should be encouraged. The transversus abdominis and the multifidus muscles contribute to stabilization of the lumbar region and the pelvis as a whole and should therefore be activated before doing the exercises outlined in this chapter. The significance of the pelvic floor must also be remembered.

If the patient has chronic pain in this area, malalignment or imbalance (such as leg-length discrepancy and overpronation) may be present, and it may be possible to correct this by using orthoses, both as a basis for rehabilitation and to prevent new injuries.

Return to Sport

Athletes in explosive sports must not exercise at maximal loads before the injury is completely healed, which may take 3 to 6 months (e.g., in the case of an acute groin injury). Injured athletes should not compete before they have trained at maximum intensity, and athletes in team sports must have trained in controlled game-like situations before they should play in a competitive game.

Preventing Reinjury

Because injuries in the pelvic and inguinal region have a tendency to become chronic or to recur, secondary prevention is of paramount importance. Athletes should continue with some of the neuromuscular exercises and stabilization exercises once or twice a week for at least 1 year after they have been fully rehabilitated and have returned to their sport. Any muscular imbalance or structural asymmetry must also be evaluated and corrected if possible.

Exercise Program

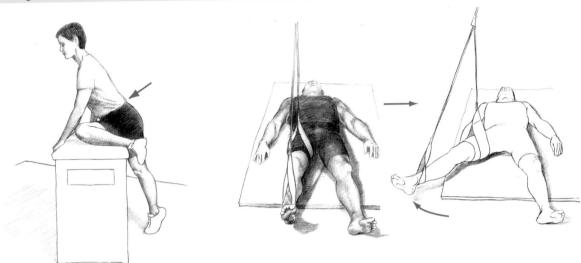

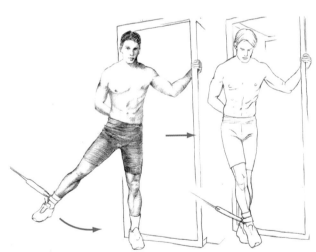

Exercise 10.1 Stretching the deep gluteal muscle (quadriceps coxae)

- Position yourself with one hip and leg on a bench and the other back far enough to cause your pelvis to tilt forward.
- Vary the degrees of adduction, rotation, and flexion in the hip joint to stretch various parts of the muscle.

Exercise 10.2 Sling exercises in adduction and abduction

- Your hip joint must be perpendicular under the sling attachment to the roof.
- Lie on your side to do the same exercise in flexion and extension.

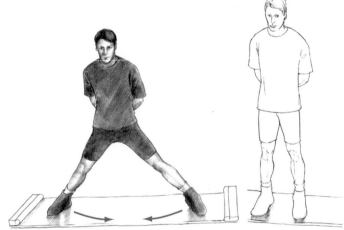

Exercise 10.3 Adductor muscle training

- Use the pulley apparatus or a tension band.
- Stabilize your back.
- Progression: Stand on a balance pad or wobble board.

Exercise 10.4 Adductor muscle training

- Wear wool socks outside your shoes. Stand on a slide board and slide into abduction gently and press gently together again. You can also stand on a smooth floor with a piece of carpet under one foot or both feet.
- Do this with your hip in various degrees of rotation.
- Progression: First increase the degree of abduction, then do the exercise while holding dumbbells in your hands.

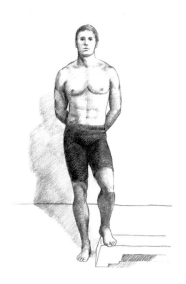
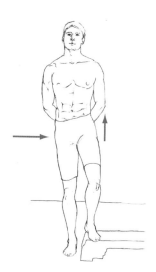

Exercise 10.5 Abductor muscle training

- Stand in a positive Trendelenburg position with one foot on a step. Push your hip in so that your other hip is raised slightly.
- Initially, use a swinging bar to support your weight.
- Do this exercise with varying degrees of hip flexion to train the quadriceps coxae.

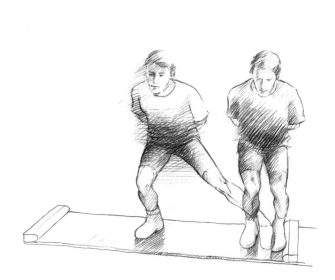
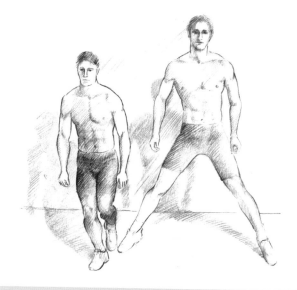

Exercise 10.6 Functional abductor muscle training

- Wear wool socks outside your shoes. Stand on a slide board and push from side to side.
- Make sure that your weight is over the leg that will stop the movement.
- Use slight hip flexion to train the abductor muscles and greater hip flexion (more of a proper skating position) to train your quadriceps coxae.
- Progression: Increase speed.

Exercise 10.7 Functional abductor muscle training

- Hop from side to side. Make sure your landings are balanced, and control the position of your hip so that your hips are on the same level.
- Progression: Increase the height or length of the hops and increase speed.

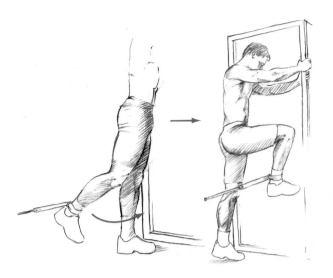
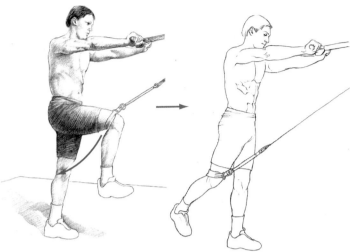

Exercise 10.8 Hip flexor training

- Stabilize your abdomen and back so that movement occurs in your hips and not in your lumbar region.
- This exercise works the iliopsoas more when you pull in flexion with slight adduction and external rotation.

Exercise 10.9 Hip extensor training

- Stabilize your abdomen and back so that movement occurs in the hip and not in your lumbar region.

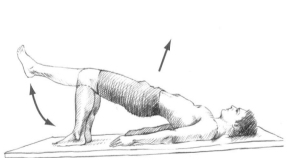
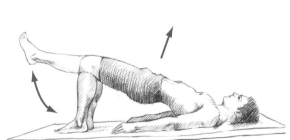

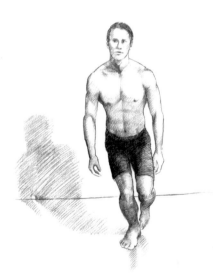

Exercise 10.10 Hip lifts while lying on your back

- Stabilize your back by activating your lower abdomen and lower back. Lift your buttocks until your hip is fully extended. Maintain this position and extend one knee. Make sure that your knee and hip are at the same height on both sides. Switch legs.
- Progression: Place legs on a balance pad.

Exercise 10.11 Single-leg knee bends

- Make sure that your hips and shoulders are at the same height on both sides and that your knee points over your toes.
- Progression: Use a wobble board or a balance board.

Acute Thigh Injuries

Lars Engebretsen

Occurrence

Muscle injuries occur frequently in contact sports such as soccer, handball, bandy, and ice hockey. Studies show that up to 30% of all soccer injuries are thigh injuries. Muscles may be injured by direct contact (contusions) and by being acutely stretched beyond the limits of tolerance of the muscle-tendon apparatus (strains). Both strain injuries and contusions result in tissue damage, bleeding, and pain. Other structures within the thigh, including the nerves, vessels, and bone, may be acutely injured, usually by high-energy trauma, such as a fall during ski jumping or downhill skiing.

Differential Diagnosis

Table 11.1 provides an overview of the differential diagnosis. The biggest problem is hamstring muscle strains, but contusions also occur frequently in contact sports like soccer. In rare cases, pediatric hamstring avulsions may result in long-term absence from sport activity.

Diagnostic Thinking

Thigh injuries are usually not serious and generally should not require surgical intervention. In most cases, they can be treated at the primary-care level. The clinical challenge is to distinguish between intramuscular and intermuscular injuries (figures 11.1 and 11.4), as well as between partial hamstring strain, hamstring avulsions, and total hamstring ruptures. It is difficult to make a diagnosis during the initial on-field examination. Therefore, PRICE treatment should be administered, and the patient should be seen again after 48 hours. At that time it is significantly easier to make a definite diagnosis and to offer a prognosis regarding outcome. Occasionally, a contusion may be so severe that a femur fracture is suspected, or pressure in the anterior thigh muscle compartment becomes so great that acute compartment syndrome becomes a concern. In such cases, the patient must be sent to a hospital for additional examination and definitive management.

Most common	Less common	Must not be overlooked ⚠
Thigh contusion (p. 304)	Avulsion or total rupture of the hamstrings or quadriceps (p. 305)	Acute compartment syndrome (p. 306)
Partial hamstring tear (p. 305)		Femur fracture (p. 301)
Hamstring cramps (p. 305)		

Table 11.1 Overview of the differential diagnosis of acute thigh injuries.

Clinical History

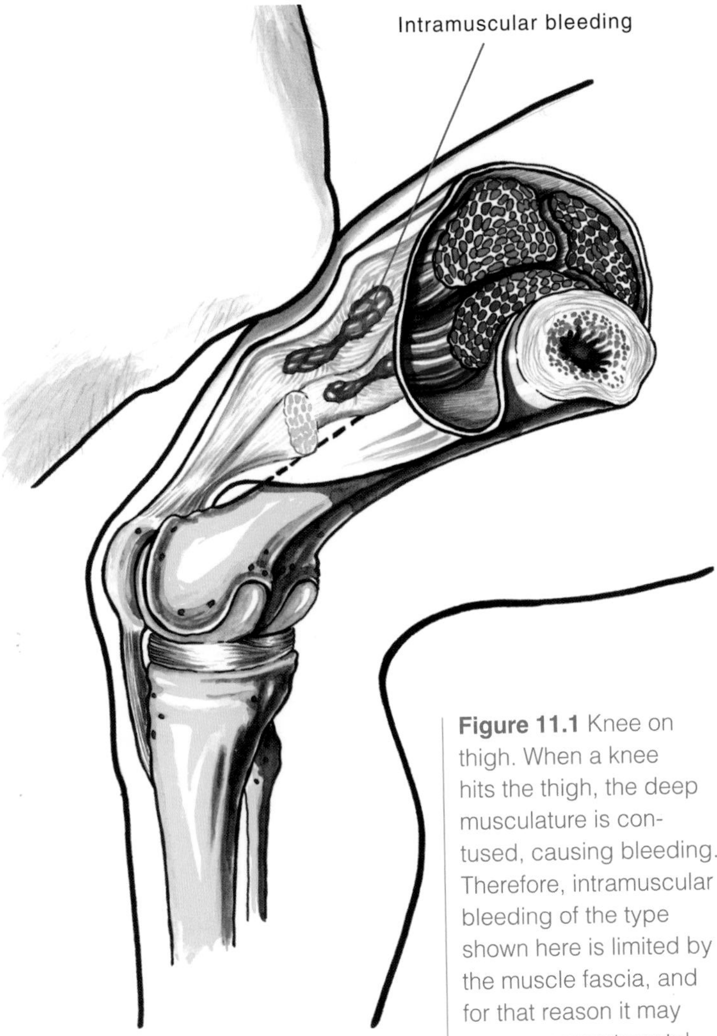

If a thigh contusion is present, the patient usually can recall sustaining a direct blow to the site of injury (figure 11.1). This causes immediate pain, and the diagnosis is therefore usually simple. If the patient's thigh is deformed, the diagnosis of fracture (which is confirmed by X ray) is normally obvious. The anterior compartments of the thigh may be affected by acute compartment syndrome after forceful direct trauma. The pain gradually becomes intense, and the thigh becomes rigid on palpation. In such cases, compartmental pressures of 80 mm Hg or greater have been measured. Unlike in the lower leg (where the upper limit for increased pressure before surgery becomes mandatory is 30 to 40 mm Hg), compartment syndrome in the thigh rarely causes nerve damage. Opening the compartment is indicated in very rare cases—generally, only after high-energy trauma, such as from a motor vehicle accident or a fall from a great height.

Hamstring ruptures are normally located at the muscle-tendon junction—that is, deep in the muscle belly. When a rupture occurs, the patient experiences sudden, stabbing pain, usually on the posterior side of the thigh. The diagnostic challenge is whether to classify the rupture as partial or total and to ascertain if an avulsion has occurred or if the injury is limited to the substance of the tendon. In such cases, a magnetic resonance imaging (MRI) study is indicated. It is often difficult to distinguish between ruptures and cramps. A few athletes, especially sprinters and athletes in contact sports, are bothered by sudden anterior or posterior thigh muscle cramps. The cause is unknown.

Intramuscular bleeding

Figure 11.1 Knee on thigh. When a knee hits the thigh, the deep musculature is contused, causing bleeding. Therefore, intramuscular bleeding of the type shown here is limited by the muscle fascia, and for that reason it may cause compartmental pressure to rise and severe pain to develop after a few hours.

Clinical Examination

Inspection. If a significant injury has occurred, the involved thigh will be swollen compared to the normal side on inspection (figure 11.2). Measuring the circumference of the thigh with a tape measure and comparing it to the healthy side can quantify the degree of swelling. A major contusion may leave a mark on the thigh, leaving no doubt whether the patient sustained high-energy trauma or not. If the patient has a completely ruptured muscle or tendon (figure 11.6), a depression may be visible at the site of the injury, and ecchymosis will gradually appear distal to the location of the rupture. A couple of days after the patient sustains an intermuscular injury, bruises will usually be visible in the skin (often distal to the location of the injury). This does not occur after an intramuscular injury.

Palpation. The anterior and posterior aspects of the thigh are palpated for defects of the tendon or muscle indicative of ruptures. The thigh will feel rigid if the patient has compartment syndrome.

Functional tests. Evaluating the degree of reduced knee flexion can help distinguish between an intramuscular and an intermuscular injury, thus making it easier to predict when the athlete can return to sport. If the compartments are intact, bleeding (usually in the vastus intermedius or rectus) is limited by the fascia. Therefore, an intramuscular hematoma forms, leading to increased intramuscular volume and increased pressure, which reduces muscular flexibility. This in turn reduces flexion in the knee joint (figure 11.3). It is often easier to conduct the necessary functional tests and make an assessment 2 to 3 days after the injury occurs. Less than 90° flexion in the knee joint after a thigh contusion indicates intramuscular bleeding and portends a long period of convalescence. An intermuscular hematoma causes less restriction of range of motion than does intramuscular hemorrhage, and consequently the rehabilitation period tends to be shorter than for injuries resulting in intramuscular bleeding. Functional muscle tests are performed to distinguish between partial and total tendon or muscle ruptures. Both the quadriceps and the hamstring apparatus can be tested isometrically and dynamically to obtain information about the degree of the injury.

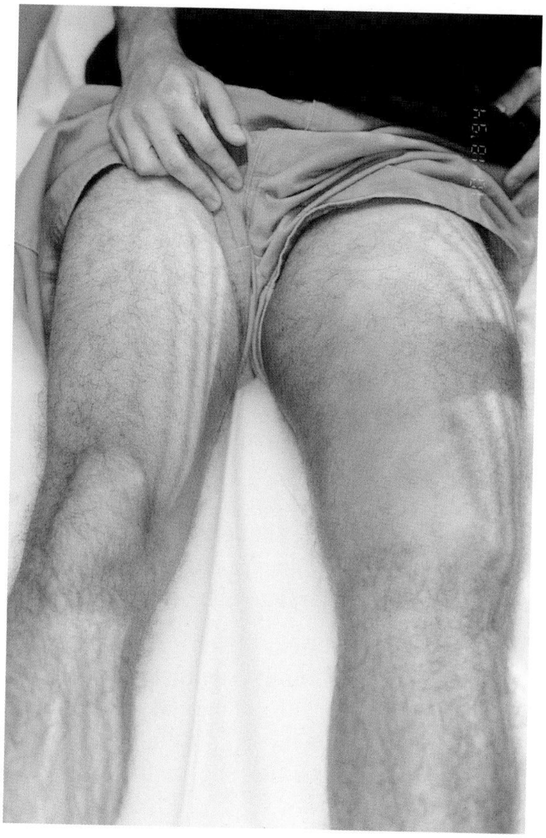

Supplemental Examinations

A plain X ray will rule out a fracture and may reveal gradual deposition of intramuscular calcium if the patient begins to develop posttraumatic myositis ossificans (figure 11.9). MRI is a useful examination for determining whether or not a total rupture of the hamstring or quadriceps musculature has occurred. If compartment syndrome is suspected, the patient must have pressure measurements taken at the hospital.

Figure 11.2 Muscle contusion, with the resultant obvious swelling on the left side. A contusion often causes bleeding and increases anterior thigh intracompartmental pressure.

Figure 11.3 Functional tests. Intramuscular bleeding increases intramuscular volume and pressure, thus reducing knee range of motion. The test can be used to distinguish between intramuscular and intermuscular bleeding and is of prognostic significance. If performed 24 to 48 hours after the injury occurred, knee flexion of less than 90° suggests intramuscular bleeding is likely to have occurred.

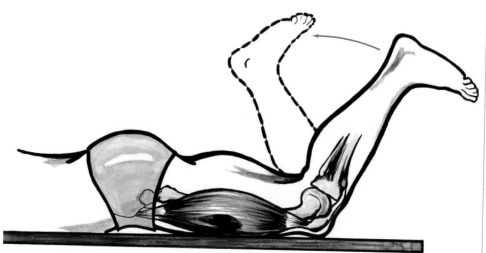

Common Injuries

Thigh Contusion

Thigh contusion (figure 11.1) is the most common acute thigh injury in sport. In a large Swedish study, 14% of all soccer injuries were thigh contusions. The prognosis depends on whether bleeding is intramuscular or intermuscular (figure 11.4). If there is substantial intramuscular bleeding, the muscle compartment fills up with blood and pressure correspondingly increases. An intramuscular hematoma may become organized and eventually calcify. If the patient has intermuscular bleeding, the blood can escape through the fascia (usually in a distal direction) and is distributed between the compartments of the anterior thigh. Consequently, pain and the risk of compartment syndrome are reduced, and the patient retains greater knee range of motion.

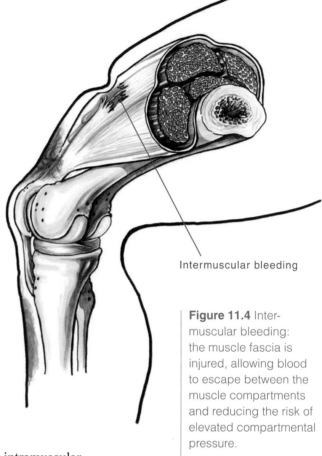

Intermuscular bleeding

Figure 11.4 Intermuscular bleeding: the muscle fascia is injured, allowing blood to escape between the muscle compartments and reducing the risk of elevated compartmental pressure.

- Symptoms and signs: The patient experiences acute pain, eventually significant swelling, and impaired function. If the patient has an intermuscular injury, ecchymosis is usually visible subcutaneously distal to the site of the injury after a couple of days.
- Diagnosis: The diagnosis is based on the clinical history. The practitioner should be aware that compartment syndrome may develop. If the knee cannot be flexed more than 90°, the injury is usually intramuscular.
- Treatment by physician: Treatment is based on the PRICE principle and nonsteroidal anti-inflammatory drugs (NSAIDs). If an anterior thigh contusion is present, PRICE treatment should be administered, keeping the hip and knee in flexion (figure 11.5). This position increases counterpressure inside the injured muscle and contributes to hemostatis. This in turn makes it easier to achieve normal movement when the patient is ready to begin active mobilization. If the patient

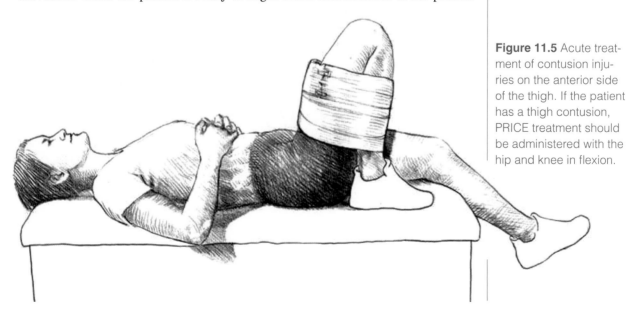

Figure 11.5 Acute treatment of contusion injuries on the anterior side of the thigh. If the patient has a thigh contusion, PRICE treatment should be administered with the hip and knee in flexion.

has a major injury, it may be worthwhile to wait 4 or 5 days before beginning active exercises, but rehabilitation of minor injuries may begin after 2 or 3 days.

- Treatment my therapist: The physical therapist should initiate exercises that promote circulation, such as bicycling, as soon as possible. Stretching exercises are also introduced early but should always be done within the limits of pain. Massage may be used to further improve circulation, but not during the acute phase (the first 2 to 3 days).
- Prognosis: Healing often takes as long as 6 to 12 weeks in the case of intramuscular bleeding. However, an injury with intermuscular bleeding can heal within a couple of weeks. If the injury is minor, strength will normalize within a week. About 50% of the strength is regained in 24 hours. After 7 days, 90% of the strength returns.

Other Injuries

Hamstring Strains

Hamstring strains are common among athletes, particularly among soccer players and sprinters (figure 11.6). The injury results in a tear at the muscle-tendon junction and is usually located in the semimembranosus, semitendinosus, or biceps femoris muscles. All of these muscles have long muscle-tendon junctions, and an injury may occur at any location in this region.

It is likely that reduced flexibility makes an athlete more vulnerable to hamstring injuries, particularly if that athlete has sustained a similar injury in the past. It is also assumed that an athlete who is relatively weaker on the posterior aspect compared to the anterior side of the thigh (reduced hamstring/quadriceps ratio) is at a greater risk of sustaining a hamstring injury. The athlete may have a history of chronic intermittent low back pain without nerve damage but with evidence of mild nerve root irritation. Low back pain may cause the hamstring muscles to become tight, and occasional cramping makes the thigh muscles more vulnerable to injury. The hamstring muscles have a rich blood supply, and circulation is often maximal at the time of injury. Therefore, the injury causes significant bleeding. This may increase pressure in the muscle compartments and/or result in heterotopic calcification and myositis ossificans.

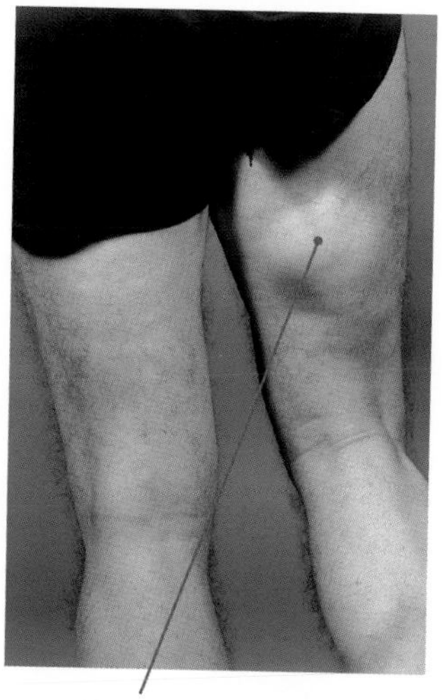

Hamstring rupture

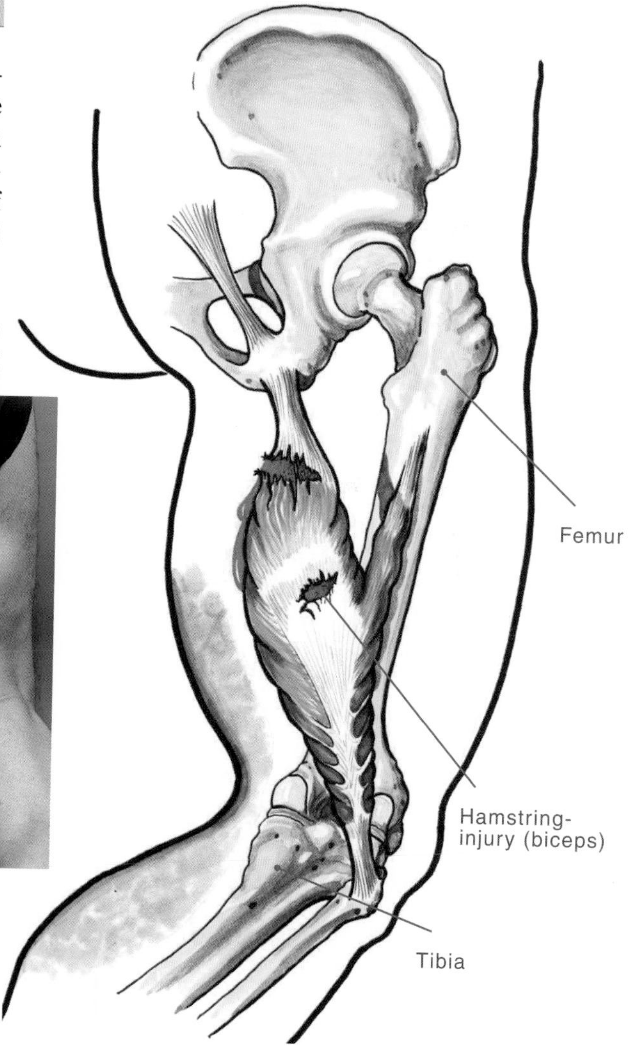

Femur

Hamstring-injury (biceps)

Tibia

Figure 11.6 Hamstring strains.

- Symptoms and signs: A hamstring strain causes immediate intense pain (often described as if someone had struck the athlete in the back of the thigh), forcing the athlete to stop activity. Strength is significantly reduced. The athlete can no longer run at maximal speed.

- Diagnosis: Isometric and dynamic strength are typically reduced. Sometimes a torn tendon or muscle can be palpated. MRI will confirm the diagnosis and determine whether the patient has a total tendon rupture or an avulsion.
- Treatment by physician: Treatment follows the PRICE principle and the standard rehabilitation process for muscle injuries. If an acute tendon rupture from the ischial tuberosity has occurred, it can be surgically repaired with good results. The surgery should be performed within 2 weeks of the injury.
- Treatment by physical therapist: The patient begins exercises to promote circulation 2 days after the injury. The therapist should wait 4 to 5 days before beginning more strenuous exercise therapy. This is followed by more intense exercise therapy, transverse massage, and possibly electrotherapy. The progression of training should be carefully monitored, preferably in cooperation with the coach.
- Prognosis: The prognosis is generally good; in the best case, the athlete can return to training after a couple of weeks, but the injury often results in a long absence from sports that require explosive use of the muscles. If the athlete returns to sport activity too soon, the danger of recurrence is great.

Acute Compartment Syndrome !

Acute compartment syndrome is uncommon; nevertheless, it occurs regularly in sports such as soccer and ice hockey. It is most commonly diagnosed in the quadriceps area, because a strong contusion in this vessel-rich area causes considerable bleeding (sometimes more than 2 L of blood). Bleeding inside an intact muscle compartment increases pressure within the compartment. Whereas normal pressure in a muscle compartment is less than 20 mm Hg, pressure in the rectus femoris muscle compartment may increase to between 80 and 100 mm Hg. If there is no associated femur fracture, the pressure will decrease after a short time so that fasciotomy will be unnecessary. However, the increased pressure causes intense pain for a couple of days following the injury.

- Symptoms and signs: Symptoms include a rigid, inflexible muscle and pain on attempted knee flexion or extension.
- Diagnosis: The patient can be monitored by measuring the circumference of the thigh in comparison to the opposite side. If the circumference of the thigh increases gradually, compartment syndrome may develop, and the patient must be closely monitored clinically. Hospitals that frequently admit multitrauma patients are capable of monitoring the patient's intracompartmental pressure. Pressure measurements often exceed 80 mm Hg.
- Treatment by physician: Beginning PRICE treatment early presumably reduces the likelihood of compartment syndrome. Experience also indicates that thigh compartments can tolerate pressures greater than 30 mm Hg (the upper limit of pressure tolerated by the calf) and thus fasciotomy may be unnecessary. Qualified personnel must closely monitor the patient.
- Prognosis: The prognosis is good, but occasionally myositis ossificans (figure 11.8) develops, resulting in a long absence from sport.

Thigh Pain

Lars Engebretsen

Occurrence

Thigh pain is relatively uncommon in athletes. However, a few athletes experience posterior thigh pain in connection with back problems, and chronic compartment pain has been described in long-distance runners during periods of hard exercise.

Differential Diagnosis

Table 11.2 provides an overview of the differential diagnosis. Myositis ossificans secondary to a muscle contusion in a soccer player is probably the most common diagnosis. Stress fractures of both the superior and inferior pubic rami, as well as in the femur, have been reported in female cross-country skiers. Osteogenic sarcoma has a predilection for the distal femur. Vascular anomalies may also occur.

Diagnostic Thinking

Patients with long-term thigh pain present a diagnostic challenge. Generally, before the diagnosis is made, the athlete has reduced their activity level for a considerable period of time. Previous injuries in the hamstrings and quadriceps are the most common causes of thigh pain. However, the less common conditions listed in table 11.2 are more difficult to diagnose and treat. In athletes older than 50 years, coxarthrosis may refer pain into the thigh, whereas younger athletes may have radiating pain from the pelvis and back. The physician should also remember that young, active athletes are more prone to rare vascular and malignant diseases. It is always necessary to X ray the pelvis, the hips, and the involved thigh to rule out stress fracture, myositis ossificans, or tumor as the etiology of the patient's pain.

Most common	Less common	Must not be overlooked !
Sequelae from hamstring strains (p. 308)	Femoral stress fracture (p. 309)	Bone and soft-tissue tumors
Sciatica (p. 126)	Myositis ossificans (p. 309)	
	Chronic compartment syndrome (p. 310)	
	Vascular anomalies (p. 311)	
	Nerve entrapment (p. 311)	

Table 11.2 Overview of the differential diagnosis of thigh pain.

Clinical History

The clinical history must include any acute trauma that may have occurred. Pain may be caused by the development of myositis ossificans following a previous contusion injury of the thigh. Stress fractures and compartment problems generally result from a process of gradual tissue overload that eventually exceeds the tissue's ability to accommodate and adapt to the chronic loading.

Clinical Examination

Examination findings may include atrophy (e.g., nerve entrapment at the vastus lateralis), swelling (e.g., myositis ossificans or tumors), or sequelae from a tendon rupture in the hamstring or extensor apparatus. Palpation may help confirm the findings. Testing individual muscle groups will help to localize the injury. Neurological status must be evaluated during the exam because thigh pain often originates from a back problem. Although circulatory disorders that cause thigh pain in young athletes are rare and difficult to diagnose by clinical examination alone, the pulses in the lower limbs should be checked routinely.

Supplemental Examinations

Radiographic examination. Frontal and lateral X rays of the thigh and pelvis (including the hips) must always be taken to exclude stress fractures, myositis ossificans, or tumors.

Other examinations. An MRI may be indicated to rule out suspected stress fractures, myositis ossificans, myotendinous ruptures, or tumors. Ultrasonography may demonstrate ruptures of the knee extensor apparatus, but the utility of this imaging modality depends on the skill of the operator. Scintigraphy is highly sensitive for stress fractures, but it is a nonspecific modality, and (in general) positive studies should be followed up with an MRI examination.

Common Painful Conditions

Sequelae From Hamstring Strains

This is usually a problem in sprinters, soccer players, and others involved in intense, hard, eccentric muscle work. A pulled muscle causes scar tissue to form at the muscle tendon junction. Muscle flexibility (and associated joint range of motion) is reduced, and the athlete is unable to train at full capacity because maximum effort causes pain. In some athletes thigh pain may be due to pressure on the sciatic nerve in the lumbar region or more distally.

- Diagnosis: The diagnosis is based on pain on palpation, occasional restricted range of motion, and pain with isometric and dynamic testing. During isokinetic testing, strength is reduced compared to the healthy side. The spine should be examined carefully; and, if there is evidence of lumbar nerve root irritation, radiography—possibly including MRI or computed tomography (CT)—should be considered.
- Treatment by physician: An accurate examination is the key to making the diagnosis. There is no evidence that NSAIDs or cortisone injections have a lasting effect. Surgery may also be useful in the late phase after an avulsion injury, although surgical treatment of muscle injuries is controversial.
- Treatment by physical therapist: The physical therapist should instruct the patient in a strength training and stretching program. Gradual return to sport is advised.
- Prognosis: The prognosis for muscle injuries is good, but the patient should plan on a prolonged period of rehabilitation (often as long as 6 months).

Other Conditions

Femoral Stress Fracture

A stress fracture (figure 11.7) is a rare problem; therefore, the diagnosis is often delayed. The injury is typical of athletes in endurance sports who either increase their running distance or who begin training on a new and harder surface. Occasionally, the patient may have a femoral neck stress fracture, which reduces range of motion and causes pain in the hip joint. Stress fractures occur most frequently in female athletes and may be related to eating disorders and irregular menses.

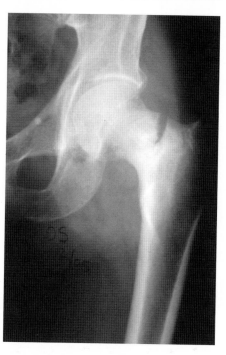

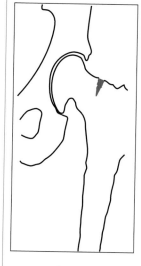

Figure 11.7 Femoral stress fracture. Long-term overloading, often in combination with reduced bone mineral density, may cause stress fractures of the femoral neck.

- Symptoms and signs: Throbbing pain, which steadily worsens the longer training lasts, is the primary symptom. The athlete may eventually complain of pain during normal weight bearing activities, and not just during exercise.
- Diagnosis: The diagnosis is made on the basis of scintigraphy or, preferably, MRI. X rays are often negative. Athletes with stress fractures should be evaluated for eating disorders and irregular menses.
- Treatment: The patient should be restricted from bearing weight on the affected limb for at least 6 weeks. Surgery is indicated if the patient has a femoral neck fracture.
- Prognosis: The prognosis is good, but the athlete will often miss the season due to the time required to heal and rehabilitate the injury.

Myositis Ossificans

Myositis ossificans (i.e., heterotopic bone formation in the thigh muscles) is a consequence of major bleeding in the deep thigh muscles (figure 11.8). The process often begins with an innocent thigh contusion that causes swelling and pain. However, a thigh contusion may result in considerable muscle injury and often causes a significant hematoma either inside or between the muscle compartments. Usually, the hematoma is absorbed after a few weeks, but occasionally it calcifies. At the beginning of the calcification process, the area is still swollen and often very tender (warm phase). Pain and swelling result in long-term inflexibility, which usually restricts knee joint flexion. The calcification eventually stabilizes (cold phase).

- Symptoms and signs: Symptoms include swelling and pain, followed by reduced knee joint range of motion, particularly in flexion.
- Diagnosis: X rays, MRI, or ultrasound confirm the clinical diagnosis.
- Treatment: The patient can engage in stretching and exercise therapy to the extent that pain allows. Usually, the calcification and hematoma are resorbed without surgical treatment, but if more than 6 months pass without evidence of resorption, the patient should be referred to a surgeon for consideration of possible surgery.
- Prognosis: The prognosis is good, but it often takes a long time before the calcification is resorbed.

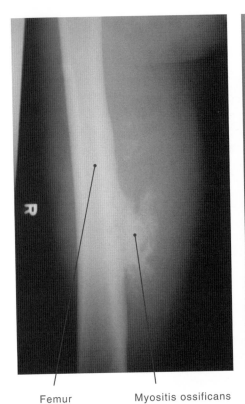 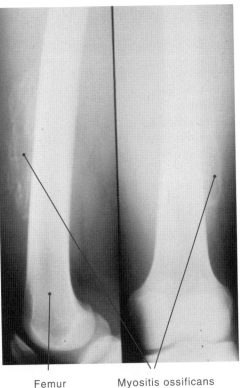

Figure 11.8 Myositis ossificans. X ray views of two femurs that show major calcification after intramuscular bleeding. This patient had a large contusion that caused a great deal of bleeding. The hematoma has become organized and calcified.

| Femur | Myositis ossificans | Femur | Myositis ossificans |

Chronic Compartment Syndrome

Chronic compartment syndrome in the thigh is rare. Usually, acute compartment syndrome is caused by high-energy trauma resulting from a motor vehicle accident or a fall from a great height. However, the same type of syndrome has been reported to occur chronically. This usually occurs in athletes after chronic overuse, and therefore the syndrome is thought to occur as a result of overload of the involved musculature. We have seen the syndrome in the lateral compartment of long-distance runners, bicyclists, and skaters.

- Symptoms and signs: Patients experience thigh pain after strenuous exercise such as after a long run on skis or after a long bicycle ride. Pain eventually makes it impossible to continue the activity and to train at a high level of intensity.
- Diagnosis: Patients suspected of having compartment syndrome are referred to a specialist for evaluation. The diagnosis can be made by measuring thigh pressure in connection with physical activity. However, the method is controversial, because no standard pressure values have been established for the thigh. Therefore, it may be necessary to compare the injured thigh with the healthy thigh.
- Treatment: The patient should reduce the intensity and amount of training so that their training routine does not cause pain. Fasciotomy may be necessary in some cases.
- Prognosis: The prognosis is usually good, and the condition typically resolves spontaneously. Resolution of symptoms may take as long as one year.

Vascular Anomalies

Vascular anomalies are rare but may lead to reduced circulation in the lower extremities and produce symptoms similar to the symptoms of intermittent vascular claudication. Unfortunately, routine diagnostic examination of the lower limb vessels are often unrevealing, so the diagnosis is delayed. In the majority of cases, the flow disturbance will be identified within the popliteal artery as it passes between the lateral and medial gastrocnemius tendons at the knee. The artery may follow an irregular course and undergo compression by the medial gastrocnemius tendon.

- Symptoms and signs: Pain occurs during activity, although the athlete remains asymptomatic if at rest, or if he does not train or compete.
- Diagnosis: Patients suspected of having vascular anomalies should be referred to a vascular surgeon for evaluation. Patients often have a normal pulse and normal Doppler measurements immediately after activity. The diagnosis is made by dynamic angiography and often requires competence in interventional radiology.
- Treatment: The treatment options include interventional radiology or surgery.
- Prognosis: The prognosis is good if the correct diagnosis is made.

Nerve Entrapment

Some athletes may experience sudden atrophy of the vastus lateralis in the course of a few weeks. The athlete may on occasion relate this to a puncture wound or to extremely hard training. Generally, however, no definite explanation is found. On physical examination, the involved vastus lateralis is distinctly smaller than the one on the healthy side. Anatomical studies show that the femoral nerve has several small nerve branches that extend to the distal portion of the vastus lateralis. There are several small fibrous areas along the main nerve where the nerve may become compressed as a result of muscle hypertrophy from intense strength training or from trauma to the area.

- Symptoms and signs: The patient experiences painless atrophy and gradual weakness of the vastus lateralis.
- Treatment: Normalization of vastus lateralis muscle bulk and strength usually occurs within 12 months. Surgery is unnecessary.
- Prognosis: The prognosis is good, but it often takes 12 months before muscle function returns to normal.

THIGH

Rehabilitation of Thigh Injuries

Grethe Myklebust and Lars Engebretsen

Goals and Principles

The goals for the rehabilitation of acute thigh injuries are listed in table 11.3.

The rehabilitation of most minor thigh injuries should begin with active mobilization 2 or 3 days after the injury. However, it may be worthwhile to wait 4 or 5 days before beginning active exercises after a major injury. The patient should start with gentle stretching of the relevant joints and should let pain guide exercise intensity. External force should not be applied during the initial phase. Use of a bicycle ergometer is a gentle and effective method of increasing function. The seat should be adjusted so that it is high, and the foot should be placed further forward on the pedal than normal. This position reduces the demand on knee flexion and makes it easier to pedal. If knee joint range of motion is so restricted that the patient still can't pedal, then the patient should oscillate gently as far as possible in both directions on the bicycle. For major muscle strain injuries and contusions, it is advisable to allow the area to rest for up to 5 days before beginning active mobilization.

Exercises are of primary importance during the rehabilitation phase, but other physical therapy interventions may promote hematoma resorption and minimize scar tissue formation in the injured area. Massage, stretching, and various types of electrotherapy may be indicated.

	Goals	Measures
Acute phase	Minimize or reduce swelling	PRICE principles with emphasis on effective compression
Rehabilitation phase	Normalize range of motion and reduce pain so that the patient can achieve normal function	Exercises, massage, stretching
Training phase	At a minimum, regain previous strength and range of motion Reduce the risk of injury	Functional exercises–sport-specific training Recover fully before engaging in maximum activity

Table 11.3 Goals and measures for rehabilitation of acute thigh injuries.

The exercise program should include various strengthening exercises, flexibility exercises, neuromuscular exercises, and sport-specific functional exercises. Exercise progression of the exercises is controlled by pain and return of function. In general, numerous repetitions and light loads (such as four series repeated 20 to 30 times) are emphasized early in the rehabilitation phase. Loads will be gradually increased, and the number of repetitions decreased as function improves. Exercises are performed lightly during the start-up phase, and then the tempo and degree of explosiveness gradually increase.

Athletes in explosive sports with muscle strain injuries must not run at their maximum pace during training until the injury is completely healed. It often takes as long as 6 to 8 weeks before the muscles will tolerate maximum sprints or turns. Light running in a relaxed style may begin as soon as pain allows. A neoprene sleeve is useful during the retraining phase to help keep the muscles warm. A good warm-up including stretching should be routine. The athlete should train without symptoms at a competitive intensity level before participating in games or returning to competition.

Rehabilitation of Painful Conditions in the Thigh

Athletes with chronic thigh pain who have been referred to a physical therapist often come to the sports medicine specialist because of sequelae from a strain injury or because they are bothered by cramps during exercise and competition. If there is a muscle strain, the goal is to loosen up any scar tissue and achieve maximum range of motion and strength in the affected area. The athlete should be informed that these injuries may take a long time to heal, so that he has realistic expectations from the outset of the rehabilitation program.

The patient who struggles with cramp-like pain in the thigh should be examined for trigger points in the muscles and within the painful area. The practitioner must also examine the lumbar spine, because spine disorders may result in cramp-like sensations in the thigh musculature, among other symptoms.

Preventing Reinjury

Athletes with muscle strain injuries often experience recurrent injuries. The most common reason for recurrent injury is inadequate recovery from a prior injury before resuming maximum training and competition.

The practitioner should convey the following points of emphasis to the patient about reducing the risk of reinjury:

- Allow injured tissue time to heal.
- Keep the injured area warm with the help of a warming orthosis.
- Achieve sufficient strength, emphasizing eccentric training.
- Regain, and possibly improve, range of motion through stretching.
- Work on neuromuscular function, coordination, and balance.
- Train specifically for your sport and for explosiveness, if your sport requires it.
- Make full recovery between exercise sessions a high priority.
- Listen to your body, and be aware of mild symptoms and cramping in the injured area.

THIGH

Exercise Program

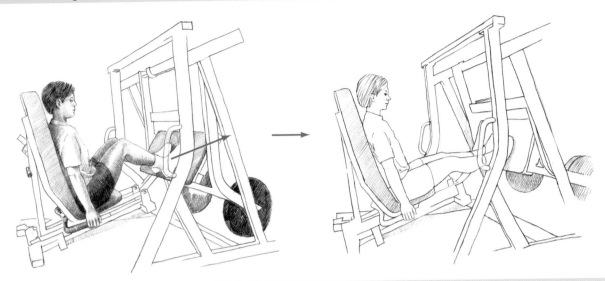

Exercise 11.1 Leg press

- Use mild resistance.
- Begin with very light loads and move within the limits of pain.
- Exercise with both legs or with the injured leg alone.
- Use light loads and numerous repetitions (e.g., four series of 20 to 30 repetitions).

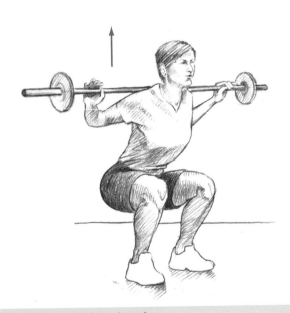

Exercise 11.2 Knee bends

- Use mild resistance.
- Begin the knee bends by using your own body weight, then add loads on your shoulders.
- Keep equal weight on both legs.
- Keep hips level.
- Avoid having your weight too far forward.
- Use a mirror to make yourself aware of weight distribution during the start-up stage.

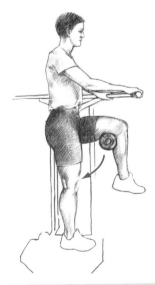

Exercise 11.3 Hamstring strength while standing using apparatus

- Use mild resistance.
- Stand on your healthy leg and work with your affected leg.
- Press backward until you have extended your hip, then gently return to the starting point.

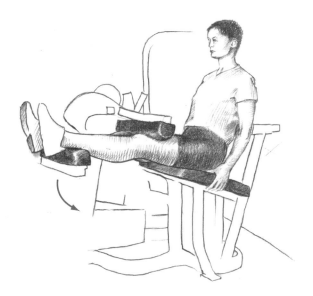
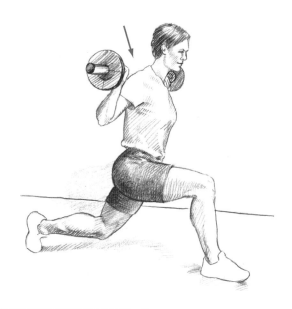

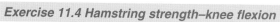

Exercise 11.4 Hamstring strength–knee flexion

- Press both legs down gently as far as you can without pain.
- Work with both legs or with the injured leg alone.
- Gradually increase knee flexion.

Exercise 11.5 Hamstring strength–lunges

- Begin by lowering yourself a short distance, then gradually lower yourself longer and deeper (as shown in the figure).
- Keep knee over toes.
- Keep hips level.
- The same movement may be done straight, or at an angle, out to the side.

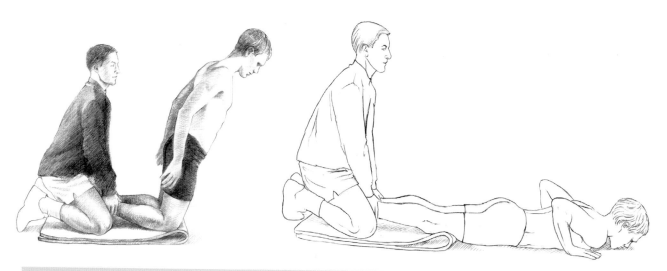

Exercise 11.6 Hamstring strength–eccentric training

- Perform partner exercise with your partner stabilizing your legs.
- Lean forward in a smooth movement; work on holding the hamstrings as long as possible until you must use your hands.
- Go all the way down so that your chest is on the floor. Push up with your arms immediately until your hamstring musculature can take over and you can straighten up all the way into a kneeling position again.
- Keep your back and hips straight.

THIGH

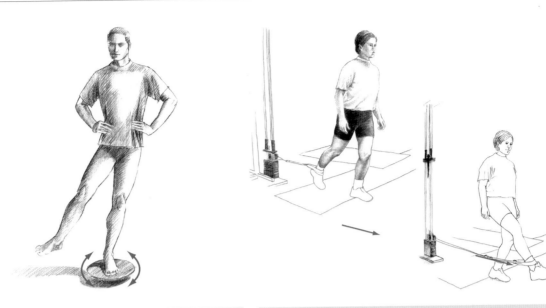

Exercise 11.7 Balance board

- Stand on one leg on a balance board or balance pad.
- Stand as still as possible for 15 to 20 seconds.
- Keep knee over toes.
- Stabilize the hip of the leg you are standing on.
- Increase the degree of difficulty by using a ball or by closing your eyes.

Exercise 11.8 Balance using a pulley apparatus

- Stand on the affected leg. Swing the other leg back and forth with mild resistance.
- May be repeated in several directions.
- Increase the degree of difficulty by standing on a board or by closing your eyes.

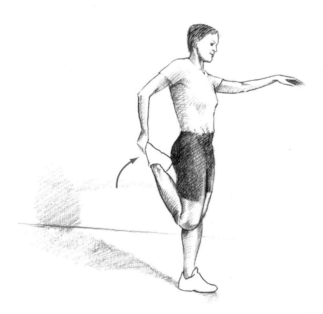

Exercise 11.9 Stretching the anterior side of the thigh

- Stand on one leg. Support yourself so that you can maintain your balance. Hold your ankle using your hand on the same side, then press your hip forward and your knee backward. Your knee should point straight down. Do not allow your thigh to slide out to the side. Feel to make sure that you are stretching the anterior side of your thigh. Do not use much force. Hold about 30 seconds, release gently, and then go a little farther in the path of motion. Repeat this stretch two or three times.
- Early in the rehabilitation stage, knee flexion can be reduced so much that you cannot hold your ankle. In that case, put your leg on a bench or low stool at a height that allows you to stretch the anterior side of your thigh.

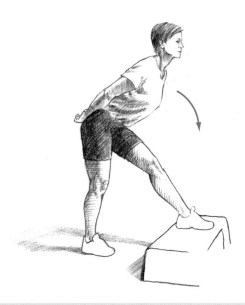

THIGH

Exercise 11.10 Stretching the posterior side of the thigh

- Place your leg at a low height, with your hands on your back. Bend at your hips and bring your upper body forward gently with your back straight until you stretch out the back side of your thigh. Hold about 30 seconds, release gently, and then go a little farther in the path of motion. Stretch two to three times.
- First stretch with your knee extended, then slightly bent.

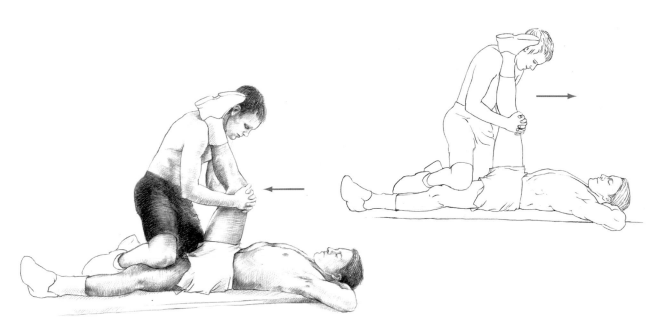

Exercise 11.11 Stretching the posterior side of the thigh

- Partner exercise: Partner lifts your leg with your knee bent slightly until you feel the posterior side of your thigh stretch.
- Hold this position a while before actively pressing your leg against your partner's shoulder so that your knee straightens out completely. Hold 10 seconds.
- Relax completely while your partner definitely, but carefully, stretches by leaning forward. Hold that position for at least 45 seconds.
- Keep your ankle relaxed so that you stretch the posterior side of your thigh and not your lower leg.

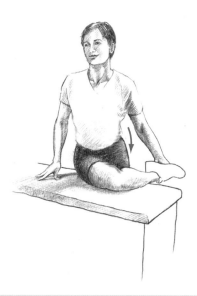

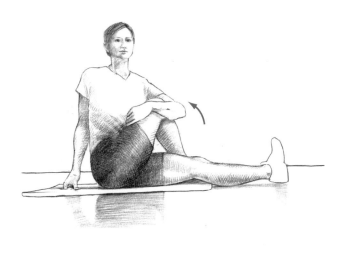

Exercise 11.12 Stretching the deep gluteal muscle

- Place your leg on a table or similar object. Lean your upper body forward gently until you feel it stretch deep in your bottom. Hold about 30 seconds, then release gently, and go a little farther in the path of motion. Repeat this stretch two or three times.

Exercise 11.13 Stretching the gluteal muscles

- Hold your knee and thigh, and pull your knee toward the opposite shoulder until you feel it stretching the back. Keep your lumbar region straight. Hold for about 30 seconds, release gently, and then go a little farther in the path of motion. Repeat this stretch two or three times.

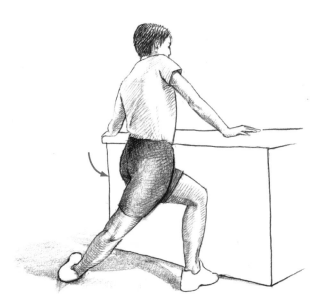

Exercise 11.14 Stretching the iliotibial tract

- Bring the leg that needs to be stretched across the back of your other leg. Ease your hip out on the same side and twist your upper body slightly toward the other side, so that you feel stretching on the outside of your hip. Hold about 30 seconds, release gently, and then go slightly farther in the path of motion. Repeat this stretch two or three times.

Acute Knee Injuries

Lars Engebretsen and Roald Bahr

Occurrence

Knee injuries constitute almost 5% of all acute injuries treated in physicians' offices, emergency rooms, and outpatient clinics. However, only 10% of these acute knee injuries represent severe soft-tissue injuries, such as torn menisci or torn anterior cruciate ligaments (the two most common soft-tissue injuries of the knee). Half of all knee meniscus and ligament injuries represent sports injuries. The annual incidence of anterior cruciate ligament injuries and meniscus injuries is 2 to 5/10,000 and 1/1,000, respectively.

Acute knee injuries may be very severe. The largest annual payment of insurance benefits in Scandinavia is awarded for this sport-related knee trauma. In Norway, there has been a special focus on team handball as the major cause of most cruciate ligament injuries, but soccer players and skiers also sustain numerous severe knee injuries. Three-fourths of all anterior cruciate ligament injuries in Norway are sport related. Of all insurance losses from Norwegian handball, more than 10% were due to cruciate ligament injuries, most of which were sustained by women. The incidence of cruciate ligament injuries among Norwegian female elite handball players is 4% to 8%. Hence, every team loses one to two players per year to this injury.

Most common	Less common	Must not be overlooked ❗
Injuries that usually cause hemarthrosis		
Anterior cruciate ligament rupture (p. 330)	Lateral collateral ligament rupture (p. 328)	Knee dislocation (p. 335)
Peripheral meniscus rupture (p. 331)	Cruciate ligament avulsion in children (p. 338)	Extensor apparatus rupture (p. 328)
Tibial plateau fracture (p. 333)	Quadriceps/patellar tendon rupture (p. 336)	
Dislocated patella (p. 332)	Osteochondral fracture (p. 336)	
	Femoral condyle fracture (p. 333)	
	Patellar fracture (p. 337)	
Injuries that usually do not cause hemarthrosis		
Central meniscus rupture (p. 331)	Cartilage injury (p. 336)	Epiphyseal injuries (children) (p. 338)
Medial collateral ligament rupture (p. 328)	Posterior cruciate ligament rupture (p. 334)	Total rupture in the lateral ligament apparatus (p. 328)

Table 12.1 Overview of the differential diagnosis of acute knee injuries.

Diagnostic Thinking

Knee injuries that result in a hemarthrosis must be evaluated by an orthopedic surgeon and are usually treated surgically. By contrast, injuries without hemarthrosis generally do not require acute surgery and can be evaluated and treated at the primary-care level. Therefore, it is important to detect injuries that cause hemarthrosis (table 12.1).

Intra-articular bleeding will usually occur within 12 hours, so that if a patient has a swollen knee within 12 hours of an accident, it may be assumed that the knee joint contains a bloody effusion. Of course, it is possible to "tap" the joint if the presence of hemarthrosis is in doubt, but the aspiration must be done in a sterile manner. Female team handball athletes with a hemarthrosis of the affected knee will, in more than 85% of the cases, be found to have an ACL injury.

A peripheral bucket-handle meniscus injury can be repaired if the diagnosis is made within 1 to 2 weeks. An osteochondral injury can also be repaired during the acute phase. In addition, a major injury on the lateral side of the knee is much easier to repair during the first 2 weeks following the injury than it is later. However, the only injury that requires acute treatment is a fracture or a major knee injury (such as a dislocation) with possible vascular and nerve injury. It is worth noting that, in Scandinavia, surgery will not be performed on an anterior cruciate ligament injury until 4 to 8 weeks have elapsed, unless there are other simultaneous injuries that require acute surgery.

The goal of the clinical examination during the acute phase should be to determine whether a reparable meniscus or cartilage injury exists or whether a fracture exists. A routine X ray will usually reveal a regular fracture, whereas the patient's clinical status and magnetic resonance imaging (MRI) will reveal a meniscus injury or an osteochondral injury. Because many patients do not have access to MRI, it is comforting to know that there is plenty of time to triage (and treat) this type of injury. Acute cruciate ligament injuries and patellar dislocations may be demonstrated clinically without the help of MRI. If the patient has a dislocated knee, the clinical examination will reveal such extensive instability that there will be no doubt that the patient has a severe knee injury. These patients must be transported to an orthopedic surgery department for immediate assistance.

Clinical History

Information about the mechanism of injury often proves diagnostic even before the patient is examined. Therefore, a thorough case history is extremely important and should include comparative information from trainers, coaches, and teammates, whenever possible. Performing a "plant-and-cut" fake or landing on a nearly extended and slightly valgus (or varus) knee after a jump is typical of a basketball- or handball-related anterior cruciate ligament injury (figure 12.1). This mechanical injury often results in a concomitant partial lateral meniscus injury, in addition to subchondral knee bruising of the lateral femoral condyle and tibial plateau. Meniscal injury occurs in more than 70% of ACL trauma, while bone bruising occurs in more than 80% of cases. Hyperextension trauma is not uncommon (figure 12.2) in soccer. The anterior cruciate ligament is vulnerable to tearing when an opponent falls over the athlete's knee, extending the joint backward. Trauma to the lateral aspect of the knee often injures the medial structures and may, in addition, cause an injury to the anterior cruciate ligament (figure 12.2).

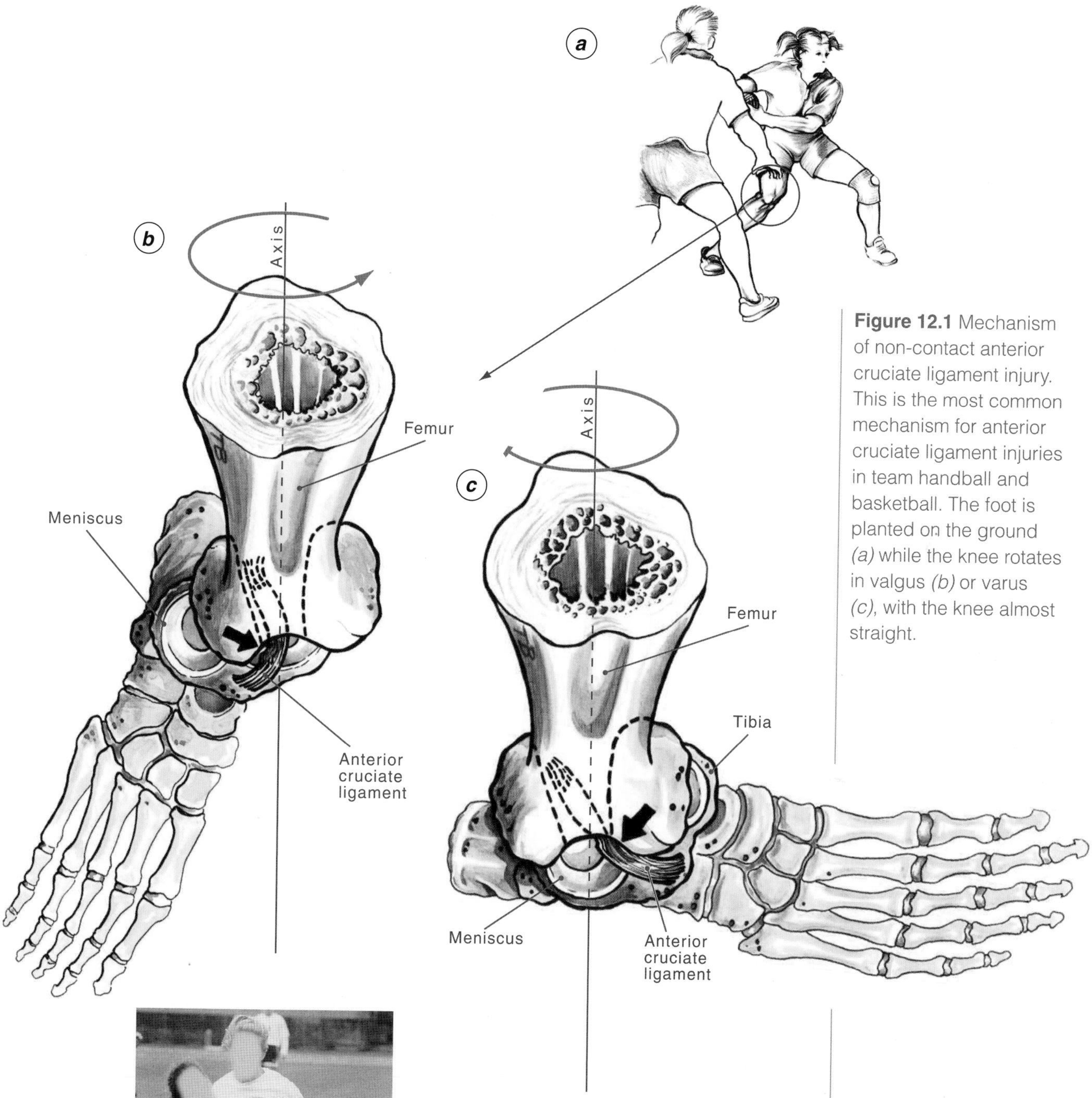

Figure 12.1 Mechanism of non-contact anterior cruciate ligament injury. This is the most common mechanism for anterior cruciate ligament injuries in team handball and basketball. The foot is planted on the ground (a) while the knee rotates in valgus (b) or varus (c), with the knee almost straight.

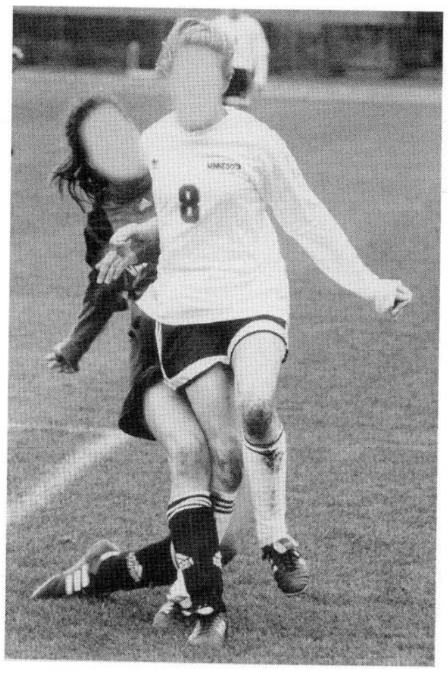

Figure 12.2 Mechanism of contact-related anterior cruciate ligament injury. This is unfortunately a common contact injury. In this case, both players injured the anterior cruciate ligament. The anterior cruciate ligament of the player on the left was injured by hyperextension. The player on the right suffered a valgus trauma that caused injuries to the following structures, in the order listed: the medial collateral ligament, the anterior cruciate ligament, the lateral meniscus, and the lateral femoral cartilage.

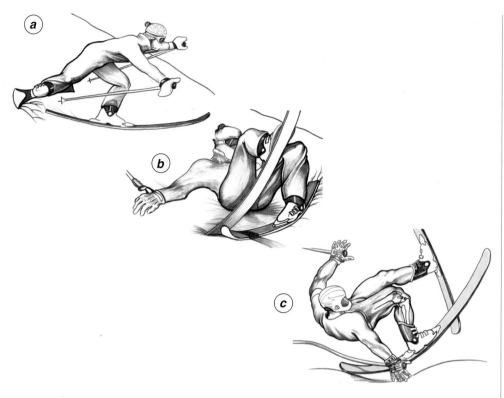

Figure 12.3 Injury mechanisms in downhill skiing. Valgus-rotation injury caused by the tip of the ski, getting a ski stuck in the snow or a slalom gate *(a)*. Phantom-foot injury: This is a typical mechanism for anterior cruciate ligament injuries in recreational skiers *(b)*. Top-level downhill skiers may sustain this injury when they jump and land with their weight too far to the rear *(c)*.

Recreational skiers are usually injured when the tip of their ski gets stuck in the snow, causing valgus external rotational trauma to the knee (figure 12.3a). This results primarily in tearing of the medial collateral ligament, followed by the medial meniscus, and occasionally by the anterior cruciate ligament as well. In addition, these patients often have bone bruises. The anterior cruciate ligament may also tear if a downhill skier falls backward, putting all his weight on the outer ski–even at low speed (figure 12.3b). This causes the ski to cut inward, producing internal rotational trauma to the knee. In the same situation, the ski can also cut outward, causing external rotational trauma, which will also injure the anterior cruciate ligament.

Top professional skiers may sustain anterior cruciate ligament injuries as a result of a combined blow to the rear ski, concentric use of the quadriceps, and slight varus or valgus angulation of the knee if the athlete lands with his weight too far back after a jump (figure 12.3c). This is likely to cause bone contusion in the medial compartment as well. Instead of a ligament injury, the same injury mechanism may cause a tibial plateau fracture to the athlete (especially women).

Posterior cruciate ligament injuries usually occur as a result of a direct anterior blow to the tibia. Half of these injuries result from traffic accidents (such as when the knee hits the dashboard), and the other half are sport-related injuries, caused, for example, by falling to the floor in handball or crashing into the sideboard in bandy. Half the posterior cruciate ligament injuries are isolated (i.e., only the posterior cruciate ligament is injured), whereas the other half are injuries in which both the lateral collateral ligament and the popliteus tendon are also injured.

Patellar dislocations usually occur because of a direct blow to the medial patellar margin, with the knee slightly flexed (a typical example is an injury caused by running into a slalom gate). However, valgus trauma sustained during handball play may also cause the patella to sublux or dislocate and immediately slip back into place again. Patients with patellar dislocations will have hemarthrosis and will complain of pain along the medial patellar retinaculum.

Clinical Examination

Inspection. With the patient's knee at rest on a pillow at 15° to 20° flexion, the practitioner inspects both knees from the foot of the examination table. Usually, there is no doubt that the knee contains intra-articular fluid (figure 12.4). If at least 3 of the 4 main ligaments (anterior cruciate ligament, posterior cruciate ligament, medial collateral ligament, and/or the lateral collateral ligament) are torn, the knee is effectively dislocated. This is a major injury, and when it is examined, there will be no doubt that something serious happened. However, several hours often elapse between the time the injury occurs and the time the patient is examined, and after several hours, swelling and pain will make an examination difficult. It is often possible to see that the patella is laterally dislocated or possibly that the patella is high or low, indicating that a patellar dislocation, a rupture of the patellar tendon or of the quadriceps tendon, respectively, has occurred.

Palpation. The patellar tendon, the patellar retinaculum, and the quadriceps tendon should be palpated for pain or discontinuity. The medial ligaments cannot be felt directly, but painful points on the origin of the femoral condyle and on the tibia are typical. However, the lateral collateral ligaments can easily be palpated, and the practitioner should compare them with the healthy side. The biceps tendon can be similarly palpated. If major lateral injuries have occurred, the collateral ligament and the biceps tendon are often less easily recognized than the ones on the healthy side. The joint spaces can be palpated and a meniscus injury will usually cause pain along the joint line.

Movement. Normal range of motion in the knee joint is 0° to 10° extension and more than 140° flexion. If the patient has an acute knee injury, both flexion and extension will typically be reduced. The challenge is to determine whether there is "real" locking or "pseudo" locking. Real locking suggests that the meniscus has usually become impinged, due to a rupture such as a "bucket handle tear", but there may be pieces of the anterior cruciate ligament or a piece of cartilage between the femur and the tibia, causing the injured knee to intermittently "lock" as well. However, pseudo locking (caused by intense pain but where no structural or mechanical block exists) is diagnosed as frequently as true meniscal pathology with locking is diagnosed.

Neuromuscular function. The practitioner palpates the pulse on the dorsum of the foot and behind the medial malleolus, and then compares it with the healthy side. Strength and sensation should be checked; the musculature innervated by the peroneal nerve is frequently weak. This nerve is particularly vulnerable to varus trauma and to knee dislocation. In such cases, the patient will have demonstrable and reproducible weakness of great toe extension and possibly of ankle dorsiflexors and toe extensors, and loss of sensation between the first and second toes in the involved side.

Special Tests

If the patient has an acute knee injury, a series of special tests are administered to evaluate the integrity of the cruciate ligaments, the collateral ligaments, and the menisci. It is always necessary to compare the injured side with the healthy side.

Varus or valgus stress test at 30°. The test (figure 12.5) is used to determine whether the patient has a collateral ligament injury. The knee is held at 30° flexion and loaded

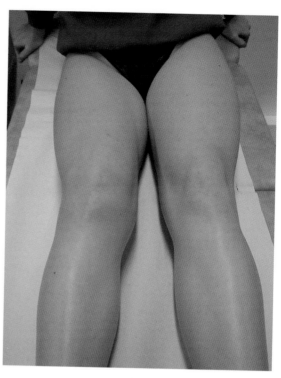

Figure 12.4 Hemarthrosis of the right knee. When the patient sustains an intra-articular injury, the joint promptly fills with 60 ml to 70 ml of fresh blood (usually within a few hours [<12]). The blood comes from the cruciate ligament, the meniscus, the capsule, or the bone. The best way to evaluate hemarthrosis is by comparing the patient's legs by viewing them from the foot end of the examina-

KNEE

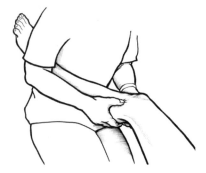

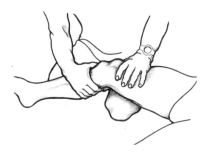

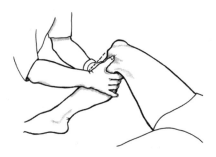

Figure 12.5 Varus/valgus stress. Hold the knee at 30° flexion and load in varus or valgus, so that the collateral ligaments are stretched. Place your thumbs in the joint line to detect gapping (opening) of the joint space.

Figure 12.6 Lachman test. With the knee joint flexed 30°, stabilize the femur and apply an anteriorly directed force on the tibia in relation to the femur.

Figure 12.7 Posterior drawer test. With the knee flexed 90°, push the tibia posteriorly.

in varus or valgus so that the collateral ligaments are stretched. The practitioner places a finger in the joint space and feels to see whether it "gaps" open. Medial and lateral collateral ligament injuries are graded according to how large the opening of the joint space is, as follows: grade I, less than 5 mm difference between sides; grade II, 5 to 10 mm difference between sides; and grade III, more than 10 mm difference between sides. The test may also be positive for physeal injuries in children and tibial plateau fractures in adults.

Lachman test at 30°. The test (figure 12.6) is used to evaluate the integrity of the anterior cruciate ligament. At 30° knee flexion the examiner stabilizes the femur and applies an anteriorly directed force on the tibia. In an ACL deficient knee, the tibia will "slip" forward in relation to the femur, resulting in an absent or soft end point.

Posterior drawer test at 90°. The test (figure 12.7) is used to evaluate the integrity of the posterior cruciate ligament. With the knee flexed to 90°, the tibia is pushed straight backward. If the posterior cruciate ligament is torn, the tibia will slip backward in relation to the femur.

Sag test. The test (figure 12.8) is used to evaluate the posterior cruciate ligament. The patient is placed in a supine position with the hip and knee flexed. When a posterior cruciate ligament injury exists, the tibia will sag backward compared with the healthy side.

Posterolateral Lachman at 30°. The test (figure 12.9) is used to evaluate whether the structures in the posterolateral corner of the knee are injured (i.e., the lateral collateral ligament, the popliteus tendon, and the popliteofibular ligament). The test is administered like a reversed Lachman, with the knee flexed to about 30°, and a posteriorly directed force placed on the tibia with the leg in an externally rotated position.

Recurvatum test. This test (figure 12.10) is also used to evaluate a potential posterolateral ligament injury. With the patient supine, both feet are lifted up from the surface. If a major injury to the posterolateral corner or other posterior structures has occurred, the injured knee passively hyperextends.

McMurray meniscus test. This test (figure 12.11) is used to evaluate the lateral and medial meniscus. The knee is flexed to 90°, after which it is gradually and passively

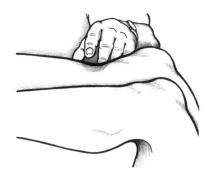

Figure 12.8 Sag test. In this position, the tibia will sag posteriorly if the posterior cruciate ligament is torn.

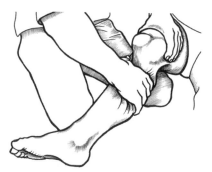

Figure 12.9 Posterolateral Lachman. A "reversed Lachman," where the tibia is pushed posteriorly with the leg in an externally rotated position.

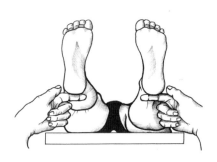

Figure 12.10 Recurvatum test. With the patient in a supine position, lift both feet off the surface.

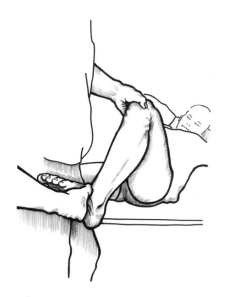

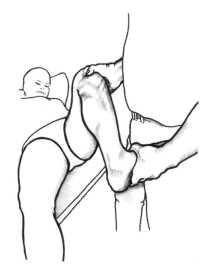

Figure 12.11 McMurray test. The knee is passively extended with the thumb over the joint line while the tibia is internally/externally rotated and varus/valgus stress is applied.

extended. To test the medial meniscus, the practitioner palpates the medial joint line while the tibia is externally rotated and slight valgus pressure is applied to the knee. The lateral meniscus is tested by palpating the lateral joint line with simultaneous internal rotation and varus stress. The test is positive if the patient feels pain in the joint space. If a medial meniscus injury has occurred, a click can sometimes also be palpated over the medial joint line.

Supplemental Examinations

Routine X rays should always be ordered for acute knee injuries, but more specialized diagnostic tests should be reserved for the specialist to request.

Radiographic examination. Fractures can be identified on frontal and lateral X rays. If a tibial plateau fracture is suspected, oblique X rays can also be requested. The practitioner should be aware that if an anterior cruciate ligament injury is suspected, avulsion of the intercondylar eminence may have occurred.

Other examinations. If an epiphyseal injury is suspected, routine X rays should be taken first. If these are negative, but palpation causes severe pain in the growth zone, it is necessary to stress the knee joint under fluoroscopy. MRI is an accurate method

KNEE

of demonstrating cruciate ligament, meniscus, and collateral ligament injuries. Note that when the extremities are examined by MRI, the entire extensor apparatus is not routinely included, so quadriceps tears may be overlooked. Injuries of the extensor apparatus may also be revealed by ultrasound, but the utility of this method depends a great deal on the skill of the operator.

Common Injuries

Medial and Lateral Collateral Ligament Injuries

About 40% of all severe knee injuries involve the medial collateral ligament (MCL), making the MCL the most frequently injured knee structure. The most common mechanism of injury involves an opponent falling over the patient's slightly flexed knee, forcing it into valgus. MCL sprains often occur in isolation, and the pathology is typically limited to the proximal (figure 12.12) or the distal ends of the ligament. Lateral collateral ligament injuries are less common but are usually more complicated, because the lateral aspect of the knee consists of a series of ligaments and tendons (figure 12.13). A lateral knee injury may involve the iliotibial tract, the lateral collateral ligament, the biceps apparatus, the popliteus apparatus, or the lateral gastrocnemius tendon, whereas a medial knee injury usually involves only the medial collateral ligament. Lateral ligament injuries are generally caused by external trauma to the medial side or by hyperextension trauma. Ligament injuries are traditionally categorized into grades I, II, and III, based on the extent of the opening of the joint space during stress tests compared to the normal knee (0 to 5 mm = grade I; 6 to 10 mm = grade II; >10 mm = grade III). Grades II and III are often combined injuries that may involve the cruciate ligaments and the menisci.

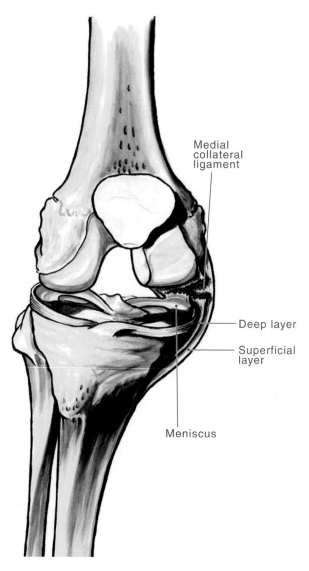

Figure 12.12 Medial ligament injury. If valgus stress is present, the medial structures will be stretched, then torn.

- Symptoms and signs: The patient complains of intense pain medially or laterally. The most common injury is a medial ligament injury. Collateral ligament injuries do not cause swelling in the joint, but reduced flexion and extension are typical of the acute phase. After a lateral ligament injury there is usually hemarthrosis.

- Diagnosis: Valgus stress testing is usually positive (most often grade I) if the patient has experienced a medial collateral ligament injury. A positive varus test suggests that the athlete has a major lateral injury. The practitioner should compare it with the healthy side first. Then the lateral collateral ligament should be palpated. If it cannot be palpated, the patient probably has suffered a major injury that involves the popliteus tendon, the biceps, and other structures on the lateral aspect of the knee. If a major injury with significant varus malalignment has occurred, the recurvatum test is also often positive. A complete tear of the lateral collateral ligament often causes less pain than does a minor sprain injury. The practitioner should always obtain a routine X ray to exclude a fracture.

- Treatment by physician: Acute treatment of grade I injuries is administered according to the PRICE principle. Many patients benefit from special orthotic devices

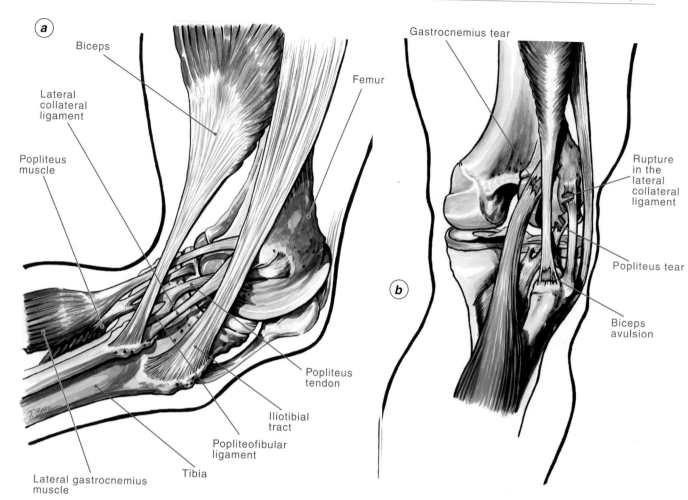

(a)

Biceps

Lateral
collateral
ligament

Popliteus
muscle

Femur

Gastrocnemius tear

Rupture
in the
lateral
collateral
ligament

(b)

Popliteus tear

Biceps
avulsion

Popliteus
tendon

Iliotibial
tract

Popliteofibular
ligament

Tibia

Lateral gastrocnemius
muscle

Figure 12.13 Lateral
structures. The anatomy
of the lateral knee is
more complicated than
that of the medial side.
Therefore, the injuries
on the lateral side are
greatly more compli-
cated and require sur-
gery more often than do
injuries on the medial
side of the knee. Normal
anatomy *(a)*; common
injuries *(b)*.

that contain ice water and apply compression. Nonsteroidal anti-inflammatory drugs (NSAIDs) will reduce pain and swelling and are useful for 3 to 5 days. Subsequently, the active rehabilitation process begins, emphasizing restoration of strength, range of motion, and neuromuscular function. Grade II and III injuries on the medial side are treated for 6 weeks with an orthosis that allows full range of motion. An orthopedic surgeon must evaluate higher grade (II, III) injuries on the lateral side, often with the assistance of MRI. Grade III laterally are often surgically repaired. The main point is that major (grade II and III) medial and lateral knee ligament injuries, combined with cruciate ligament injuries, will result in a very unstable knee if the central stabilizer of the knee (the anterior cruciate ligament) is not repaired. In some cases, the cruciate ligament is reconstructed while the collateral ligament is treated with a brace. In other cases, the lateral side will be repaired concurrently with the anterior cruciate ligament reconstruction. Collateral ligament injuries should never be surgically treated as the sole pain generator of knee pain if the anterior cruciate ligament is also torn.

- Treatment by physical therapist: Rehabilitation exercises may begin as soon as pain allows, usually after 2 to 4 days. The patient should avoid exercises with valgus stress. When swimming, the athlete should avoid the breaststroke.
- Prognosis: Grade I and II collateral ligament injuries often normalize after 6 to 12 weeks. The prognosis for grade III injuries depends on accompanying injuries, and they therefore usually take significantly longer. With the exception of major lateral ligamentous injuries, the athlete can usually return to sport activity without problems.

KNEE

Anterior Cruciate Ligament Rupture

In Scandinavia, the annual incidence of anterior cruciate ligament injuries is 5 to 10 injuries per 10,000 inhabitants. This injury is definitely most common in team handball, where 4% to 8% of the players are injured annually, and where women are injured three to five times more often than men. The anterior cruciate ligament usually tears completely if injured (figure 12.14), but because the ACL consists of two parts, there are cases in which only the posterolateral or the anteromedial portion of the ligament is torn. Of the patients with anterior cruciate ligament injuries, about 75% sustain simultaneous meniscal injuries, 80% have concurrent bone contusion, and 10% have accompanying cartilaginous injuries that require treatment. Some also have accompanying injury to the medial or lateral collateral ligament. The most common injury mechanisms are shown in figures 12.1-12.3.

- Symptoms and signs: Anterior cruciate ligament injuries usually cause rapid swelling, producing a prominent hemarthrosis within 12 hours and severe pain. The patient often states that her knee gave way when she attempted to bear weight on her leg immediately after the injury occurred. It is often difficult to complete an adequate examination immediately after the injury occurs. The usual tests can be administered as described after a few days (usually a week). The Lachman test is considered positive if the end point is soft. It is unnecessary, and generally impossible, to perform pivot shift tests during the acute phase. With injuries in basketball and team handball, the athlete usually also has a lateral meniscus injury in addition to a lateral bone contusion with a corresponding pattern of pain.

- Diagnosis: A positive Lachman test is considered diagnostic for ACL tears. The clinical diagnosis is highly accurate when made by a trained specialist, with greater than 90% accuracy when compared to arthroscopic findings. Greatly restricted range of motion in the joint may be due to a bucket-handled meniscal tear or an osteochondral injury, and an MRI should be requested. The practitioner should also obtain X rays to rule out a fracture or avulsion of the intercondylar eminence. Arthroscopy should not, therefore, be necessary to diagnose this injury; the diagnosis is made clinically.

- Treatment by physician: For acute injuries, the PRICE principle is recommended. The patient often needs crutches, and NSAIDs reduce swelling and pain. If it is not possible to make a definite diagnosis during the acute phase, the primary-care physician should re-examine the patient after 5 to 7 days. Only patients with fractured or dislocated knees need to be admitted to the hospital within the first few hours. A specialist should evaluate patients with suspected anterior cruciate ligament injuries. The determination of whether the anterior cruciate ligament needs to be reconstructed surgically depends on the patient's requirements for future knee function: one-third will manage well without the cruciate ligament, one-third must significantly reduce their activity level to avoid surgery, and the

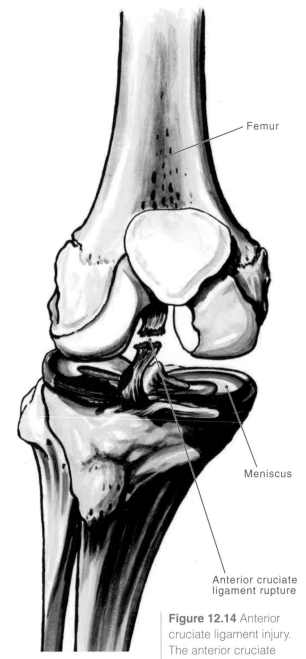

Femur

Meniscus

Anterior cruciate
ligament rupture

Figure 12.14 Anterior cruciate ligament injury. The anterior cruciate ligament, if injured, usually tears completely in the midsubstances of the ligament. Such injuries do not typically heal spontaneously.

remaining third are so loose that they may require surgery to stabilize the knee in any case. If a patient with an anterior cruciate ligament injury requires surgery, repair should occur within 4 to 8 weeks after the injury, whereas the other groups often train for 6 months and are reevaluated for surgery at that time. The indication for surgery also depends on what additional injuries the patient has sustained.

- Treatment by physical therapist: Physical therapy in which strength, range of motion, and neuromuscular function are emphasized is the cornerstone of the rehabilitation phase of care. The same type of program is used for conservative and surgically treated cruciate ligament injuries, but the progression is more rapid if treatment is conservative. Rehabilitation is long and often tough for patients, and close follow-up of the training program is essential to taking care of all aspects of the rehabilitation phase of care. Patient follow-up should occur regularly for the first 6 months.

- Prognosis: If the athlete functions at a high level, an ACL injury will make the patient feel like the injured knee is unstable or prone to giving way. The risk of secondary meniscus or cartilage injuries is high without surgical repair. After surgery, more than 80% of patients have a stable knee. In Scandinavia, studies show that up to 90% of soccer players and about 60% of handball players return to their former level of function. About 70% of untreated patients develop radiographic evidence of arthrosis 10 years after the injury. No similar follow-up outcome study of contemporary surgical repair has been published. The athlete can choose surgery to prevent chronic instability in the knee joint but cannot be guaranteed a reduced risk of arthrosis in the long run.

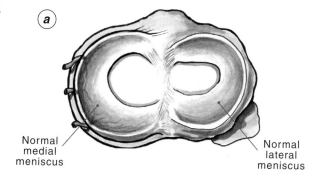

Normal medial meniscus   Normal lateral meniscus

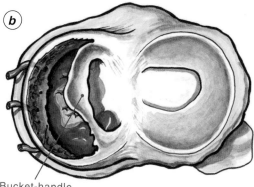

Bucket-handle rupture

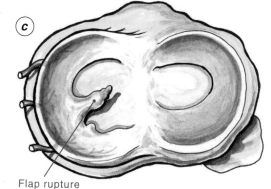

Flap rupture

Meniscus Injuries

The meniscus is the knee's shock absorber. The meniscal ligaments also help to stabilize the knee joint. Meniscal injuries may occur in isolation or in combination with ligament injuries. About 75% of patients with anterior cruciate ligament injuries sustain a simultaneous meniscus injury. A medial meniscus injury increases loading of the cartilage in the medial joint compartment and increases the risk of arthrosis. Nevertheless, a lateral meniscal injury is more serious than a medial one, because the lateral meniscus is of greater functional significance to knee joint stability. Therefore, lateral meniscal injuries increase the risk of future instability and of "wear and tear" in time. The risk of developing arthrosis depends on how much of the meniscus is injured. Figure 12.15 shows the most common types of mensical injuries. The most important factors are whether the injury is located peripherally in the so-called red zone (where there is a good blood supply) and therefore can be repaired, or whether the injury occurs more centrally in the white zone (an area with no direct blood supply) thereby necessitating resection of the injured portion of the meniscus.

- Symptoms and signs: Meniscus injuries that result in hemarthrosis are peripheral and generally reparable because the blood supply to the periphery of the meniscus is good. However, peripheral injuries are less common than centrally located injuries. Radial and horizontal tears are the most common kind of central meniscal

Figure 12.15 Meniscal injuries. Normal *(a)*. Bucket-handle tears *(b)* cause locking and pain; flap ruptures *(c)* usually cause only pain.

KNEE

pathology. These injuries usually result in less bleeding than peripheral injuries but do cause pain and eventually edema due to accompanying local synovitis. A peripheral rift may cause a bucket handle tear, which often causes locking in extension but is well suited to operative repair.

- Diagnosis: The diagnosis is based on pain along the joint line and a positive McMurray test. If a hemarthrosis exists, joint range or motion is often reduced. In contrast with a knee joint that is filled with blood, in which pain limits range of motion, a bucket-handled meniscal tear will often cause elastic resistance to knee extension. An MRI is accurate in demonstrating meniscus injuries but is not always necessary for establishing the diagnosis. On MRI meniscal injuries can be divided into four categories, in which grade I represents a slightly increased signal; grade II reflects an increased signal within the entire meniscal substance without penetrating to the surface; and grades III and IV are descriptive of superficial tears with a dislocated meniscus. In children and adolescents, grade I and II injuries can heal spontaneously, whereas grades III and IV usually require surgery.
- Treatment by physician: It is preferable to perform arthroscopic repair of a peripheral meniscal tear within the first 2 weeks following the injury. If the tear is minor, a partial arthroscopic resection may be performed. Small tears that do not transverse the entire meniscus may heal without surgery.
- Treatment by physical therapist: Treatment consists of general strength training and neuromuscular training following surgical resection of the meniscus. The practitioner should be particularly aware that there may be significant muscle atrophy in patients who have suffered chronic knee pain before the injury was discovered. Rehabilitation continues until muscle strength and volume are restored.
- Prognosis: The prognosis is generally good. A sutured meniscal injury requires a period of at least 4 to 6 months rest before the athlete returns to any sport activity which torsionally loads the repaired knee. The athlete may return to sport activity within 4 weeks of a minor resection. The long-term prognosis is not precisely known. Total resection of a medial meniscus puts the patient at high risk for developing radiographically evident joint arthrosis within 10 years, whereas a partial resection appears to result in only a moderately increased risk of arthrosis.

Dislocated Patella

The most common cause of hemarthrosis after anterior cruciate ligament and meniscus injuries is patellar dislocation (figure 12.16). Normal patella function is necessary for achieving good knee extensor strength. Some athletes have poor patellar stability, and the patella may be dislocated laterally—either spontaneously or because of a blow to the medial aspect of the patella (e.g., from a slalom gate).

- Symptoms and signs: While a patellar or quadriceps tendon rupture causes significant local swelling, a dislocated patella always causes hemarthrosis. The patella always dislocates laterally and therefore usually causes the knee to lock. If the patella is reduced before the physician arrives, the diagnosis may be more difficult to make. This may occur spontaneously and almost immediately, and often the patient may not fully realize what has happened. However, palpation along the medial patellar edge and along the associated ligaments will always cause intense pain, although the patient's knee is otherwise stable.
- Diagnosis: The diagnosis is based on reduced range of motion, particularly in flexion, and on the finding of pain along the medial patellar border. Patients usually have a significant hemarthrosis. The practitioner should always obtain X rays, because a dislocation may result in an avulsion or an osteochondral fracture of the patella or lateral femoral condyle.
- Treatment by physician: The patella must always be reduced; often reduction is performed under anesthesia. Extending the knee and pushing the patella medially

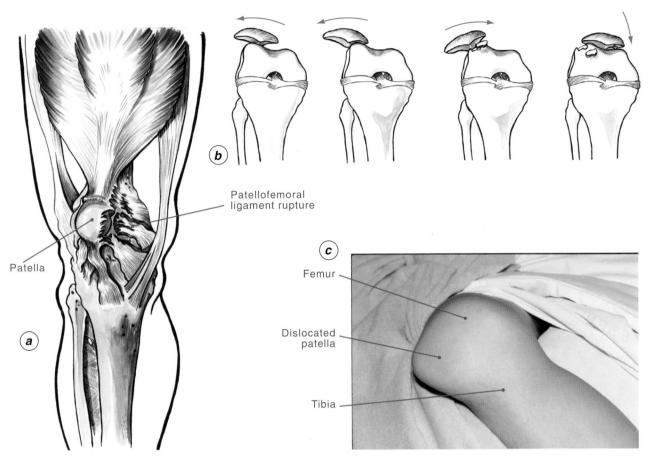

Patellofemoral
ligament rupture

Patella

Femur

Dislocated
patella

Tibia

reduces the dislocation. After repositioning, the patella is stabilized with a cast, brace, orthosis, elastic bandage, or tape for a couple of weeks. There is good evidence that after early surgical repair of the patellar retinaculum, recurrence is rare. Nonsurgical treatment of younger active patients, such as with a cast or orthosis for 6 to 8 weeks, results in recurrent dislocation in more than 50% of patients. If there is an avulsion fracture, the indications for surgery increase.

- Treatment by physical therapist: Exercise therapy is recommended.
- Prognosis: The prognosis is very good. The athlete is almost always back in sport activity within 3 or 4 months.

Femoral Condyle/Tibial Plateau Fracture

Femoral condylar or tibial plateau fractures occur more often as the result of traffic accidents and falls than sport activities. However, tibial plateau fractures are relatively common in girls, most commonly in connection with skiing. The same injury mechanisms that cause anterior cruciate ligament and collateral ligament injuries may also result in fractures, most frequently of the tibial plateau (figure 12.17) and less commonly of the femur or the patella. Such fractures are more common in older recreational skiers than in younger athletes. A tibial plateau fracture may cause a step-off in the joint surface, and blood may enter into the joint space from the bone marrow. If the defect is more than 2 to 3 mm, the patient must undergo surgery to avoid subsequent knee joint arthrosis and instability.

- Symptoms and signs: The patient will complain of pain upon loading the knee, and hemarthrosis will be present. Tibial plateau fractures must be suspected when

Figure 12.16 Patellar dislocation. The patella dislocates laterally. The patellofemoral ligaments tear on the medial side, and severe bleeding occurs into the joint (a). Often a small fracture occurs in the femur when the patella relocates (b). Typical clinical appearance (c).

KNEE

the patient has sustained high-energy trauma, especially among elderly patients and patients with osteoporosis.

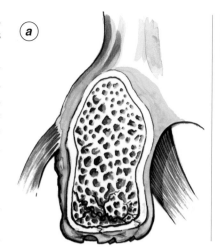

- Diagnosis: X rays will demonstrate the diagnosis, but occasionally the depression of the tibial plateau will be so minor that only MRI can demonstrate the relevant anatomy and make the diagnosis. Oblique views may also help produce the diagnosis. The practitioner should be alert for epiphyseal injuries in children. They may be difficult to find; therefore, if the patient is younger than 15 years, the physician should always request X rays of the healthy side for comparison.

- Treatment by physician: Patients who may have a fracture or who have a fracture verified by X ray must be referred to an orthopedic surgeon for evaluation. Most of these injuries require surgery.

- Prognosis: The prognosis depends entirely on the nature of the fracture, which may vary from major crushing of the tibia in ski jumpers to minimal depression fractures in recreational slalom skiers. The normal healing period for minor injuries is 6 to 12 weeks, and the athlete will be away from sport activity for at least 3 months.

Other Injuries

Posterior Cruciate Ligament Ruptures

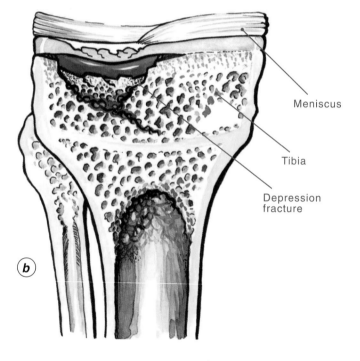

Figure 12.17 Femur fracture *(a)*; tibial plateau fracture *(b)*.

Meniscus

Tibia

Depression fracture

Only one of 10 cruciate ligament injuries involves the posterior cruciate ligament (figure 12.18), with more than half of the PCL injuries occurring in combination with injuries to other knee structures (figure 12.18c). The majority of PCL injuries are sport-related; the remainder are caused by motor vehicle accidents. The most common cause of posterior cruciate ligament injury is a direct blow to the upper portion of the tibia, such as colliding with a hockey sideboard or when an opponent falls directly on the tibia so that it is forced posteriorly. This posteriorly directed force will push the tibia backward in relation to the femur, often causing an isolated posterior cruciate ligament injury. If the force is applied anteromedially or anterolaterally to the tibia, the posterior cruciate ligament may tear in combination with other structures (laterally or medially, respectively).

- Symptoms and signs: The patient often recalls absorbing a direct blow to the tibial tuberosity during sporting activity. Generally, the patient experiences acute onset of severe pain after such trauma. Patients with posterior cruciate ligament injuries do not necessarily develop knee hemarthrosis with early onset swelling, but swelling does eventually occur in some patients.

- Diagnosis: The diagnosis is made clinically, based on a positive posterior drawer test and a positive sag test. Patients often sustain combined injuries and must be carefully examined for such pathology. If a combined injury is suspected clinically, an MRI of the knee should be obtained to confirm the clinical diagnosis.

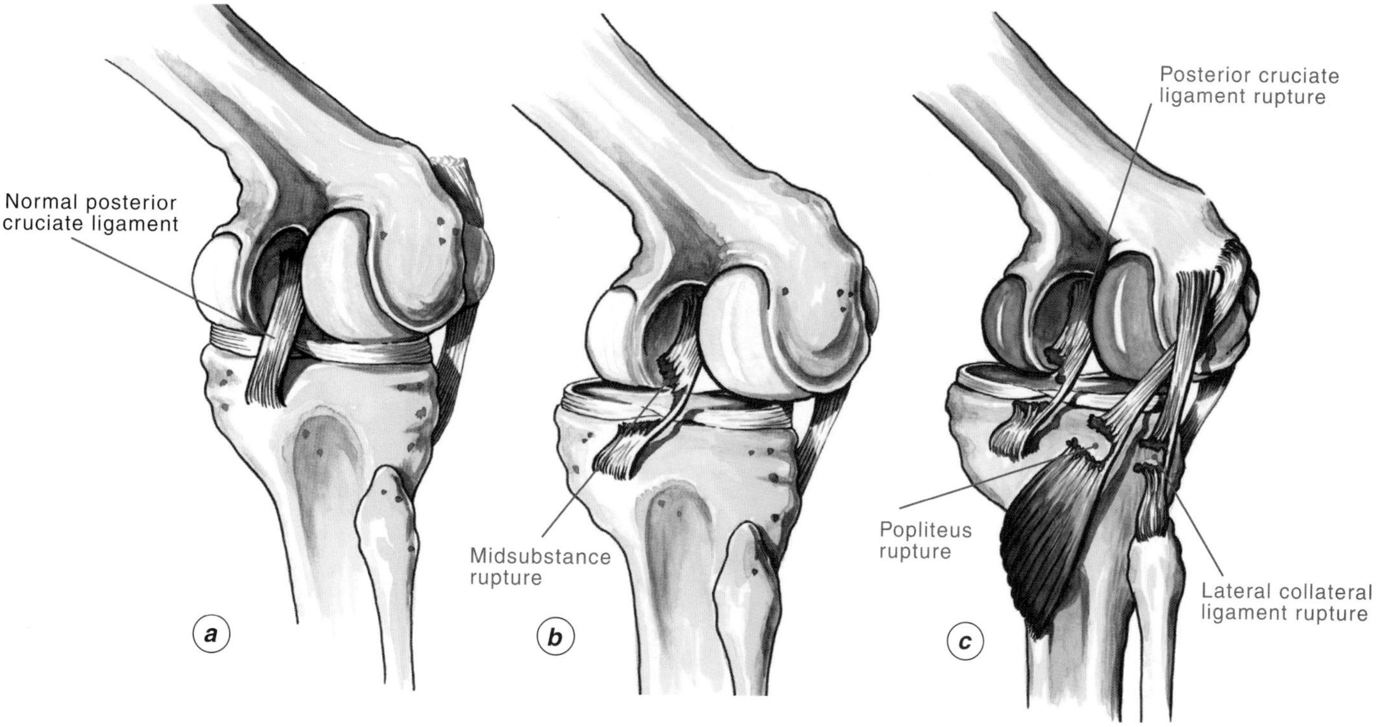

Normal posterior cruciate ligament

Midsubstance rupture

Posterior cruciate ligament rupture

Popliteus rupture

Lateral collateral ligament rupture

Figure 12.18 Posterior cruciate ligament injury. The injury may be isolated or part of a more extensive combined injury.

• Treatment by physician: Isolated PCL injuries may be treated by active rehabilitation and need not be referred to an orthopedic surgeon. Patients with combined injuries, especially those with major lateral injuries or dislocated knees, require surgical intervention, preferably within 2 weeks of being injured. As is the case for anterior cruciate ligament injuries, orthoses do not have any documented effect on posterior ligamentous injuries.

• Treatment by physical therapist: Patients often require several months of rehabilitation that includes both strength and neuromuscular training. It is particularly important to train the quadriceps muscle after a posterior cruciate ligament injury, because it may limit translation of the tibia in relation to the femur.

• Prognosis: Isolated posterior cruciate injuries seldom cause symptoms during sport activity. However, the knee may gradually become less stable, as the secondary stabilizers become stretched out and overloaded. Thus, a few of these patients will eventually require surgery.

Knee Dislocation ❗

Knee dislocations (figure 12.19) are rare, but because they are often accompanied by vascular and nerve injury, it is extremely important that these injuries not be overlooked. In sport, knee dislocations typically result from a major fall–for example, during ski jumping or when riding motorcycles–but dislocations also occur in soccer and team handball. A dislocated knee is defined as damage to at least three of the knee's four main ligaments–the medial and the lateral collateral ligaments, and the anterior and posterior cruciate ligaments.

• Symptoms and signs: The patient usually is in severe pain. About one of three patients has evidence of concomitant injury to the peroneal nerve. The practitioner should always check for a pulse at the dorsum of the foot: 10% of patients with knee dislocation have associated vascular injury. If the vessel is torn at the knee level, circulation must be restored within a few hours to avoid irreparable ischemic injury to the leg. If more than 8 hours elapse, the amputation rate is 80%.

KNEE

- Diagnosis: The diagnosis is based on evidence of knee instability in at least three directions. There will be no doubt about the presence of a major injury. The Lachman test and posterior drawer test are usually positive, as are the varus and/or valgus tests at 30° knee flexion.
- Treatment by physician: On site reduction of the dislocated knee may on occasion prove difficult. The physician must longitudinally distract carefully the involved extremity and simultaneously reduce both the tibia and the femur. If transport to the hospital is delayed or will take a long time, the knee should be stabilized with an orthosis, cast, or brace. Further orthopedic evaluation of this type of injury must occur immediately. At the hospital, the patient should undergo an MRI in addition to accurate neurological and vascular diagnostic tests to demonstrate the extent of the injury. Associated vascular injury should be immediately repaired, while the ligamentous injuries can be attended to a few weeks later. If no vascular injury has occurred, the cruciate ligaments will be reconstructed initially, and the collateral ligaments will be repaired thereafter. The goal is to stabilize the patient so that he may begin exercises to avoid knee joint contraction.
- Treatment by physical therapist: Recovery from a knee dislocation is a prolonged process. Patients often require intensive therapy to initially mobilize the knee joint, in addition to strength and neuromuscular training.
- Prognosis: This is such a severe injury that only rarely do patients return to sport activity.

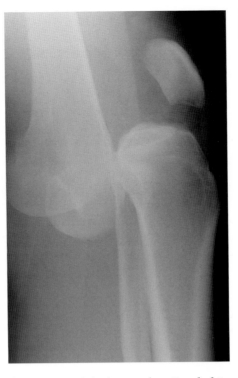

Figure 12.19 Knee dislocation. The injury is defined by complete tears of at least three of the four most important passive knee joint stabilizers: the medial and lateral collateral ligaments and the anterior and posterior cruciate ligaments.

Quadriceps/Patellar Tendon Rupture

Total rupture of the patella or quadriceps tendon occurs infrequently. The mechanism of injury is generally a fall on a flexed knee. Medications, such as the use of corticosteroids by rheumatic patients, may contribute to weakening of the tendon. However, this type of injury has also been related to anabolic steroid abuse.

- Symptoms and signs: The main symptoms include pain and limited knee extension. If the patient's extensor apparatus is ruptured, he will be unable to keep the knee extended when the limb is lifted off the table. Patients may also sustain partial tears that leave the ability for extension intact.
- Diagnosis: MRI or ultrasound examinations are helpful in making the diagnosis.
- Treatment by physician: Extensor apparatus ruptures require surgery, generally within 2 weeks of the date of injury.
- Prognosis: The prognosis is good, but the athlete often loses some ability to flex the knee during the first year after the injury.

Chondral and Osteochondral Injuries

In up to 90% of serious knee injuries, the subchondral bone and the underlying marrow are also damaged (figure 12.20). Eventually, the cartilage overlying the bone is also affected. Despite this, the cartilage may look unremarkable. About every 10th patient who is referred for arthroscopy has cartilaginous injury, and about half of those may benefit from surgery that preserves cartilage. Osteochondritis dissecans (OCD) occurs in patients without a history of knee trauma (see page 346).

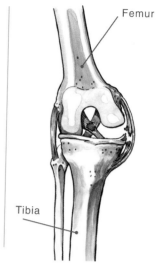

Femur

Tibia

- Symptoms and signs: Patients routinely give a history of torsional trauma, followed by activity-dependent swelling of the knee joint and intermittent pain with occasional locking.
- Diagnosis: It is difficult to make an acurate clinical diagnosis in the absence of locking. Therefore, arthroscopy is often recommended if the patient has recurring swelling or locking. An X ray may reveal OCD, while an MRI may reveal other cartilage disorders. The practitioner should be aware that recently developed smaller MRI scanners, designed specifically for examining the extremities, are in fact poorly suited to high-resolution diagnostic imaging of cartilage.
- Treatment by physician: Usually, a loose piece of cartilage will be discovered and removed during arthroscopy. Occasionally, such fragments may be amenable to pin fixation. A number of possible treatments are available, including the microfracture technique, mosaic plasty, and cartilage transplantation, but the long-term results of these interventions are not known.
- Prognosis: The prognosis is good in the short term. In the long term, lesions more than 2 cm² in area increase the risk of subsequent osteoarthritis and are associated with significantly reduced knee function after 10 years.

Patellar Fracture

Patellar fractures occur as the result of direct trauma to the patella, which may be incurred by a fall from a bicycle or a blow from a puck (if the athlete's knee padding is inadequate). The most common patella fractures due to sport-related trauma are transverse in orientation, but longitudinal fractures also occur.

- Symptoms and signs: The patient experiences the immediate onset of intense pain. Swelling occurs rapidly and the athlete may be unable to stand upright. The fracture cleft can often be palpated.
- Diagnosis: X ray of the patella confirms the diagnosis.
- Treatment by physician: Surgical repair using pins and steel wire is typically indicated, with the goal of making the patella stable for exercising without any step-off of the articular surface. Following surgery, a cast is worn for 1 to 2 weeks before the patient is permitted to move the knee, although he will remain non-weight bearing on the involved limb.
- Treatment by physical therapist: Physical therapy focuses on flexibility training after 1 to 2 weeks of immobilization, with emphasis on restoring range of motion. Isometric strength training may begin after 2 weeks.
- Prognosis: The short-term prognosis is good, in the sense that patellar fractures almost always heal within 6 to 8 weeks. However, patellar fractures often result in a long-term reduction in knee flexion. Restricted knee flexion is particularly common following cartilage injuries, which usually remain asymptomatic until about 3 to 12 months following the injury, when the patient begins full loading of the knee.

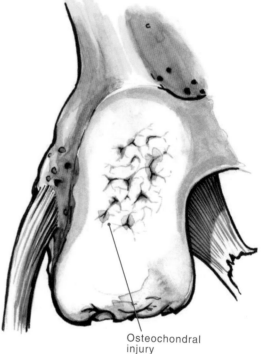

Osteochondral injury

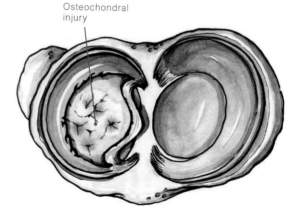

Osteochondral injury

Figure 12.20
Osteochondral injuries.

KNEE

337

Special Injuries in Children

Children have growth zones in both the femur and the tibia and an apophysis at the tibial tuberosity. This makes the knee a particularly vulnerable area. Even if the injury clinically resembles a typical adult ligament injury, X ray may frequently demonstrate an epiphyseal injury or an avulsion injury in children. The anterior cruciate ligament is particularly vulnerable to avulsion from the femur or tibia, whereas collateral ligament injuries may be confused with epiphyseal injuries. Acute pain in the region of the tibial tuberosity is often diagnosed as Osgood-Schlatter disease, but it may also reflect varying grades of avulsion of the patellar tendon from the tuberosity (Ogden grades I to IV). Instead of a ruptured patellar tendon or quadriceps tendon, a child may have what is known as a "sleeve fracture", in which the patellar tendon tears away from its insertion onto the patella like a glove. It is important to remember the differences between the anatomy and physiology of children and that of adults. For example, pediatric knee injuries often must be immobilized, whereas adult patients with knee injuries often require active rehabilitation after only a couple of days. Pediatric meniscal injuries also often differ from those in adults. Some children have tears in what is known as the discoid meniscus (a large meniscus that covers the entire surface of the tibia), while others have partial injuries, and still others have meniscal cysts. Unlike in adults, the entire meniscus of children is vascularized, so that the conditions for healing are good. Therefore, the possibilities for repairing meniscal injuries in children, both by conservative procedures and by surgery, are good. Hence, it is crucial to detect these injuries early.

- Symptoms and signs: Cruciate ligament injuries in children are rare, but they do occur. Avulsions of the cruciate ligament off the tibia or femur occur more commonly than do midsubstance tears in children. In both cases, the child has acute swelling in the knee, significant pain, and restricted joint mobility for stretching and bending. An acute meniscus injury usually also causes the joint to swell. In contrast, grade I epiphyseal injuries of the femur or tibia (which cause instability for valgus or varus testing) or an avulsion fracture of the tibial tuberosity only cause local swelling and tenderness.

- Diagnosis: The Lachman test is positive if the child has a cruciate ligament injury, whereas varus and valgus tests are positive if the patient has an epiphyseal injury. An avulsion fracture of the tibial tuberosity results in pain upon active knee extension; sleeve fractures make it impossible for the child to keep the knee in an extended position. X rays are necessary when looking for an epiphyseal injury, always comparing the injured side with the healthy side. MRI may be helpful in determining whether a meniscus injury is causing locking or if the cruciate ligament injury is due to avulsion or to a midsubstance tear.

- Treatment by physician: The acute treatment of knee injuries is the same for children and adults (in accordance with the PRICE principle). However, although there is plenty of time for treating knee injuries in adults (with the exception of knee dislocations), knee injuries in children require immediate treatment. *A qualified professional must evaluate a knee extension deficit in a child within a few days*. An avulsed anterior cruciate ligament can be reattached within the first 2 weeks following injury. There is currently no consensus on surgical treatment alternatives for midsubstance cruciate ruptures in children. This group of patients should be treated with an orthosis during sports activity until the patient is fully grown, when the ligament can be surgically reconstructed. Orthoses can be used prophylactically for all twisting activity and will help prevent dislocations and new, major injuries while the patient awaits surgery. Separation of the tibial or femoral epiphysis, which causes varus or valgus instability, must be treated by 4 to 5 weeks of immobilization. Grade I and II avulsions from the tibial tubercle can be treated by immobilization for 4 to 5 weeks, whereas grade IV (total separation) must be evaluated for surgery. Sleeve fractures from the patella require surgical treatment.

- Prognosis: Follow-up studies of children who undergo surgery for an avulsed cruciate ligament report very good results with respect to stability and function. Epiphyseal injuries increase the risk of growth disturbances, but this rarely occurs if the patient has the most common (grade I) type of epiphyseal injury. The prognosis is also very good for cartilage and meniscus injuries in children: These injuries seldom cause symptoms as children enter into adulthood.

KNEE

Knee Pain

Lars Engebretsen and Roald Bahr

Definition

Painful conditions affecting the knee are discussed in this section. In most cases, knee pain develops gradually, without known trauma and without an acute mechanism of injury. Once in a while an overuse injury will begin as a result of a single hard or overtaxing training session, but generally, knee pain sets in gradually over the course of several days or weeks. Athletes may also have developed significant symptoms from a previous ligament injury if the knee has since become unstable.

Differential Diagnosis

Table 12.2 provides an overview of the most important diagnoses to consider when evaluating knee pain. Meniscus injuries and overuse injuries, such as jumper's knee and patellofemoral pain syndrome, are the most common painful conditions affecting the knee. However, secondary recurring instability following a major knee injury often prevents athletes from returning to sport activity. Meniscal injuries are discussed in the chapter on acute injuries. In addition, meniscal cysts caused by a chronic injury (usually involving the lateral meniscus) are also discussed here.

Diagnostic Thinking

A main point in evaluating the athlete with knee symptoms is to determine whether the principle problem is pain or instability. Most patients develop anterior knee pain

Most common	Less common	Must not be overlooked
Patellofemoral pain syndrome (p. 342)	Osteochondral injuries (p. 336)	Osteochondritis dissecans (p. 346)
Patellar tendinopathy (p. 343)	Osteochondritis dissecans (OCD)	Posterior and combined instability (p. 345)
Quadriceps tendinopathy (p. 343)	Popliteus tendinopathy (p. 347)	Tumor
Meniscus injuries (p. 331)	Biceps tendinopathy (p. 347)	
Knee instability (p. 345)	Iliotibial band syndrome (p. 348)	
	Bursitis (p. 349)	
	Medial plica syndrome (p. 350)	
	Osgood-Schlatter disease (p. 351)	
	Sinding-Larsen-Johanson disease (p. 351)	
	Knee osteoarthritis (p. 342)	

Table 12.2 Overview of the differential diagnosis of knee pain.

due to overuse rather than trauma. Occasionally, a single hard training session may precipitate chronic knee pain. For example, a patient with symptoms and signs of jumper's knee felt sudden pain in connection with a bout of heavy training. In children and adolescents, it is usually the growth zone that is affected, but osteochondritis dissecans (OCD) must not be overlooked. Therefore, the physician should always obtain X rays of the knee. In addition, the diagnosis is usually based on the athlete's history and the results of the clinical examination. If pain persists despite a period of reduced training, the patient should be referred to a specialist for evaluation. The history of a patient who has suffered previous knee trauma may provide information about the mechanism of injury and may furthermore suggest the type of instability experienced by the athlete in a twisting sport (such as soccer or handball).

Clinical History

A description of the pain is central to the case history. Pain at the start of activity that wears off after warm-up but worsens after the activity ceases indicates a tendinopathy, such as runner's knee. Pain that worsens both with warm-up and with activity indicates a structural injury, such as a meniscal tear.

Clinical Examination

The examination is essentially the same as for acute knee injuries. However, it is much easier to examine an athlete who does not have a joint effusion or severe pain than it is to examine one with swelling and more moderate levels of pain. It is possible to move the knee more and, consequently, to obtain more information. In addition, the patient should be examined for factors that predispose the athlete to overuse injuries, such as malalignment.

Inspection. First, the patient is examined while in a standing position, so that lower limb alignment (including the standing Q [quadriceps] angle (figure 12.21), valgus or varus positioning, and foot mechanics [e.g., flat foot or rigid, cavus foot]) can be evaluated. Atrophy of the quadriceps is noted, if present. The best way to measure this is with a tape measure placed a fixed distance from the upper patellar pole; the healthy side should then be compared. Then the lower extremity is inspected while the patient is sitting down, and the position of the patella on the femoral condyles is noted (e.g., rotated, oblique, high, or low). It is usually evident from inspection whether the knee contains intra-articular fluid. Any bruising of the skin should also be noted.

Palpation. The patellar tendon, the patellar retinaculum, and the quadriceps tendon are palpated for pain or discontinuity. Pressing the patella inferiorly when the knee is slightly flexed makes it possible to palpate the origin of the patellar tendon. The quadriceps insertion to the patella is also palpated, with special emphasis on the vastus medialis obliquus muscle. The jumper's knee (patellar tendinopathy) test is administered by pushing the patella inferiorly, while the proximal origin of the patellar tendon is compressed along the inferior patellar pole). If the patient complains of pain, the test is considered positive. The medial ligaments may not be directly palpated, but pain at the origin of the medial collateral ligament at the femoral condyle and the tibia are typical. By contrast, the lateral collateral ligament can be easily palpated and must be compared with the healthy side. The biceps tendon can be similarly palpated. The joint line can be easily palpated, and a meniscal injury will usually cause pain along the joint line.

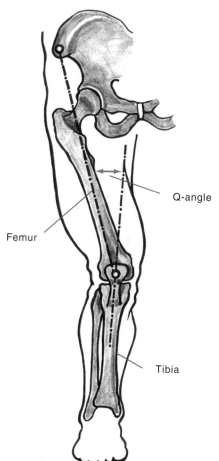

Femur

Q-angle

Tibia

Figure 12.21 Q-angle. The Q angle describes the angle formed by the axes of the femur and tibia. A Q-angle that is greater than 20° increases the risk of instability in the patello-femoral joint.

341

Mobility. Normal range of motion in the knee joint is 0° to 10° hyperextension, and more than 140° flexion. If the patient has a chronic knee injury, both flexion and extension will typically be reduced. This is often due to osteoarthritic changes, including osteophytes and a thicker and less elastic knee capsule. It is often possible to feel hyperextension and patella alta bilaterally in patients with patellofemoral pain syndrome.

Neuromuscular function. The practitioner should palpate the pulse on the dorsum of the foot and behind the medial malleolus and compare it with the healthy side. Functional knee tests (one-leg hop, triple jump, and stair hop tests) are used to detect lower limb dysfunction. For the one-leg hop test the patient stands on the uninvolved leg and jumps as far as possible onto the same leg. The procedure is repeated for the involved leg. For the triple jump test, the patient stands on the uninvolved leg, jumps twice onto the uninvolved leg, followed by a jump onto both legs. The procedure is repeated for the involved leg. The jump distance for the uninvolved and involved leg for the one leg hop and triple jump tests are recorded and compared. For the stair hop test, the patient jumps up and down a staircase on the uninvolved leg, and subsequently on the involved leg. The times are recorded for both legs and compared.

Special tests. The stability of the knee joint is evaluated using the varus or valgus stress tests (figure 12.5), the Lachman test (figure 12.6), the posterior drawer test (figure 12.7), the sag test (figure 12.8), the pivot shift test, the posterolateral Lachman test (figure 12.9), and the recurvatum test (figure 12.10). The menisci are evaluated by the McMurray test (figure 12.11). The jumper's knee test is performed with the knee flexed at 20° and the patella pressed distally. The origin of the patellar tendon at the lower patellar pole is then carefully examined and palpated (figure 12.23).

Supplemental Examinations

Routine X rays are usually included in the evaluation of patients with knee pain. A specialist should order additional examinations (e.g., MRI), depending on the tentative diagnosis. Frontal images must be taken with the patient standing and the knee flexed to 20° in order to evaluate the height of the cartilage and the degree of radiographic osteoarthritis. If OCD is suspected, a tunnel image is also taken. Standing weight-bearing X rays are used to measure the degree of varus or valgus knee alignment (the "Q angle").

Common Injuries

Patellofemoral Pain Syndrome (PFPS)—Anterior Knee Pain

This problem is usually caused by overuse, but it may also be caused by direct trauma to the patella, such as from a fall on the floor. A number of other causes have been suggested. An increased Q angle creates the tendency toward lateralization of the patella, increasing the load on the medial patellofemoral ligaments and resulting in pain (figure 12.22). Pathological nerve endings that may mediate pain have also been found in these structures. Most younger athletes have normal patellar cartilage. Cartilaginous changes involving only the superficial aspect of

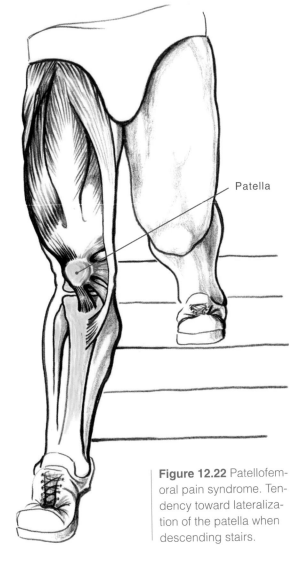

Patella

Figure 12.22 Patellofemoral pain syndrome. Tendency toward lateralization of the patella when descending stairs.

the articular surface of the patella do not cause pain in young patients. However, athletes with established cartilaginous injuries that extend down to the bone may be symptomatic. Some patients who experience sustained trauma to the patella develop subchondral changes (visible on MRI) that may subsequently precipitate changes in the patellar cartilage and bone in addition to increased pressure inside the patella. Thus, the causes of patellofemoral pain syndrome are multifaceted. The practitioner should also remember that at least 30% of all 16-year-olds have such symptoms and that 90% of this group recover without treatment.

- Symptoms and signs: Patients with patellofemoral pain syndrome may have pain in various situations, as shown in table 12.3.
- Diagnosis: If three of the symptoms listed in table 12.3 are present, the patient qualifies for the diagnosis of patellofemoral pain syndrome. The diagnosis is clinical, and no additional information is provided by routine X rays, computed tomography, or MRI.
- Treatment by physician: In most cases, the athlete will be referred to a physical therapist who emphasizes strength and neuromuscular training. Many patients benefit from the McConnell program with taping to correct and support patellar position during the training phase, but the available documentation for the program is not entirely convincing. Surgery is only indicated if there are clearly documented findings of recurring patellar dislocations or subluxations, or a tilted or laterally positioned patella. Researchers are studying the effect of surgical treatment of cartilage, and the results in patients with significant cartilaginous changes are promising.
- Treatment by physical therapist: Patients require guidance for training, particularly strength training of the vastus medialis obliquus and the gluteus medius. Basic strength is often so poor in these areas that several hundred quadriceps contractions will be required daily. The patients require a home program, in addition to supervised training. Many patients benefit from taping or an orthosis to reduce pain.
- Prognosis: The prognosis is good for more than 90% of patients with PFPS. The remainder of the patients should be evaluated to find specific causes for their pain.

Most common	Mechanism	Commentary
Pain when going down stairs	Eccentric use of the extensor apparatus elevates pressure in the patellofemoral joint	Worse in patients with established osteoarthritis of the patellofemoral joint
Pain when squatting	Difficult to get down, and unable to get up without assistance	
Pain when driving	Prolonged pressure within the patellofemoral joint	
Pain when sitting for a long time ("theater sign")	Prolonged pressure within the patellofemoral joint	
Pain when braking	Forceful activation of the knee extensor apparatus	Most common in patients with irritation in the patellar tendon

Table 12.3 Overview of the typical symptoms of patellofemoral pain syndrome.

Patellar Tendinopathy—Jumper's Knee

Patellar tendinopathy (figure 12.23) is a common sport-related diagnosis. The prevalence in volleyball is approximately 40%, and the disorder is also common among top-level basketball and soccer players. Pain is usually localized to the distal patellar pole, but in 10% of patients the pain is localized to the quadriceps insertion to the

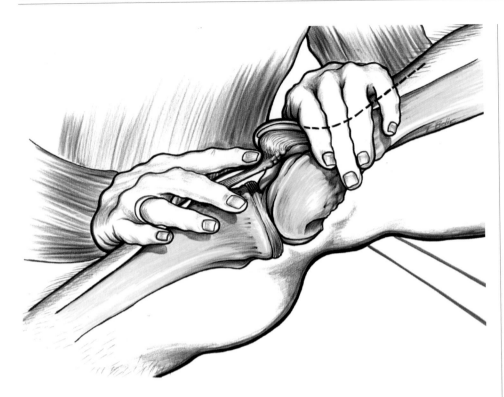

Figure 12.23 Patellar tendinopathy. The injury is usually located in the deeper layers of the patellar tendon proximally.

patella. In some patients, pain begins after a single jump, lift, or landing; in others, it begins after a hard training session or game; in still others, the onset is gradual. The cause of the disorder is unknown. Histologically, there is typically no evidence of inflammation within the affected tendon; instead, degenerative changes are found. In many patients, MRI and ultrasound examination is entirely normal.

• Symptoms and signs: The patient describes activity-dependent pain, which is usually localized to the proximal portion of the patellar tendon and its origin from the inferior patellar pole. In some cases, pain may be localized to the insertion of the quadriceps tendon to the superior patellar pole. The symptoms may be graded according to the criteria listed in table 12.4. Patients often describe symptoms similar to those of patellofemoral pain syndrome—for example, pain when walking down stairs, when driving a car, or when sitting for a long time with a flexed knee ("theater sign").

• Diagnosis: The diagnosis is made on the basis of distinct tenderness to palpation over the affected tendinous insertion, coupled with a history of activity-related pain in the same location. The correlation between ultrasound, MRI, and clinical findings is poor.

Grade	Symptoms
I	Pain after exercise
II	Pain at the start of an activity, which subsides after warm-up but returns after exercise
IIIa	Pain during and after activity, but the athlete may participate in competition and training at their usual level
IIIb	Pain during and after activity, but the athlete cannot participate at their previous level
IV	Total rupture of the tendon

Table 12.4 Classification of patellar tendinopathy according to the grade of symptoms during training.

- Treatment by physician: Eccentric strength training, usually for a minimum of 12 weeks, should be the first intervention attempted for jumper's knee. However, patients who do not benefit from 6 months of faithful eccentric training usually proceed to surgical resection of the injured area. No evidence supports the use of cortisone injections or other local therapy (such as electrotherapy), but NSAIDs often provide temporary pain relief.

- Treatment by physical therapist: Eccentric strength training has a positive effect on some patients with this diagnosis. Eccentric training should be performed twice daily with each session consisting of 3 sets of 15 repetitions. The exercises can be done without warming up, and each training session takes about 5 minutes. The exercises can be prescribed as part of a home program and should be performed on a 25° decline board. The athlete should squat to about 90° of knee flexion. The athlete should squat on the affected lower limb, eccentrically loading the quadriceps on the involved side, then arise by concentrically activating the knee extensors on the asymptomatic leg. If both knees are symptomatic the patient uses her arms to assist during the concentric phase. She should count 2 seconds for the eccentric component of each repetition. The subjects should perform these exercises despite pain provoked by the exercise, unless the pain is disabling, in which case the athlete should stop or reduce the load. At the onset of training there should be no external load. As the athlete's pain improves, weights can be added to a backpack in 5 kilogram increments. The program should be carefully monitored by a therapist, who should also closely track the athlete's activities to ensure that other exercises that may provoke pain are avoided.

- Prognosis: The prognosis is good for grades I to IIIa, for which conservative treatment usually suffices. Surgical treatment works in 60% to 70% of the cases. Other patients do not recover enough to return to sport activity at a high level, but fortunately the condition does not lead to arthrosis or persistent knee problems in later life.

Knee Instability

Knee instability is usually the result of anterior cruciate ligament injury that has not been surgically repaired. If the ACL deficient athlete continues to participate in her sport, her knee may be subjected to new injuries (figure 12.24). Because the anterior cruciate ligament is absent, other ligaments have to assume the load. Eventually, these ligaments become overdistended and the athlete may develop either posterolateral instability or medial instability. These combined instabilities often make it difficult or impossible for the affected athlete to participate in sports that place twisting or torsional loads on the knee.

- Symptoms and signs: An accurate history will always reveal a history of knee injury. Patients complain about instability more than they do about pain. The most bothersome symptom is the nearly constant subluxation caused by twisting sports. Subluxation eventually causes meniscal or cartilaginous injury, and the affected athlete may demonstrate activity-dependent joint swelling.

- Diagnosis: The clinical diagnosis is based on tests of knee stability. The Lachman and pivot shift tests for anterior cruciate ligament injury are positive if the individual is ACL deficient. The posterior drawer test at 90° flexion will be positive in cases of posterior cruciate ligament ruptures; and combined posterior and posterolateral instability will be marked by a positive posterior Lachman at 30°, increased external rotation of the tibia at 30°, and a positive reversed pivot shift. A positive recurvatum test suggests general overstretching out of the posterior and posterolateral structures. Routine X rays are useful in evaluating the degree of osteoarthritis. MRI is not diagnostically useful during the chronic phase with respect to evaluating instability.

KNEE

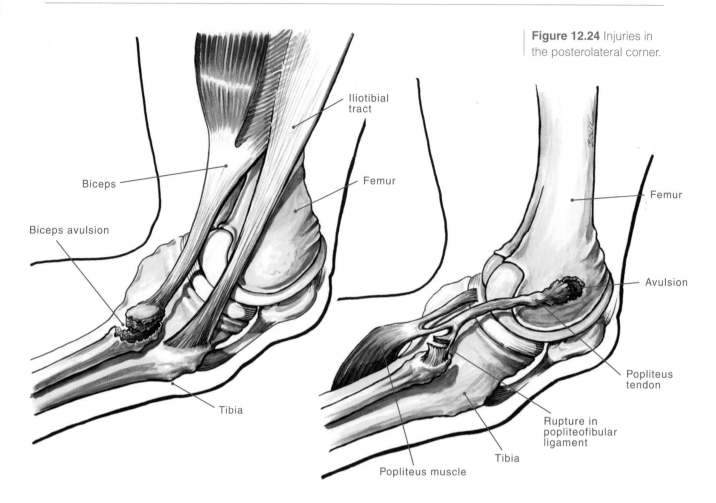

Figure 12.24 Injuries in the posterolateral corner.

- Treatment by physician: If an anterior cruciate ligament injury has occurred, the athlete usually either should stop participating in sports placing torsional loads on the knee or must undergo surgery. Surgery is also indicated for combined instability, but even with surgery the athlete may not be able to return to sport activity. An orthosis is not helpful when the athlete participates in pivoting and twisting sports, nor will functional training alone help an athlete return to pivoting and twisting sports if she has significant instability.
- Treatment by physical therapist: Strength exercises and neuromuscular training will improve the patient's coordination, control, and functioning for activities of daily living.
- Prognosis: A chronic anterior cruciate ligament injury will generally result in at least 1 year's absence from sport. Athletes with significant, combined instability will generally be unable to tolerate pivoting and twisting sports.

Other Causes of Pain and Injuries

Osteochondritis Dissecans (OCD) !

Osteochondritis dissecans is a disorder in which the supply of blood to an area of the bony femoral articular surface is reduced for unknown reasons and without trauma. The end result is the separation of a bone fragment from the femoral condyle (figure 12.25), which in turn causes the overlying cartilage to either become painfully unstable or to come completely loose (also painful). Most patients are young, often less than 16 years of age. Older patients with OCD often state that they have been mildly symptomatic for several years, suggesting that the disorder may be both chronic and progressive.

- Symptoms and signs: Patients with OCD frequently deny any history of trauma to the affected knee, a fact which distinguishes OCD from cartilaginous injuries in general. However, the symptoms of OCD are often similar to traumatic cartilage injuries and include pain from loading, locking, and load-dependent joint swelling.
- Diagnosis: The diagnosis is difficult to make clinically. Plain X rays of the knee with tunnel views often reveal the diagnosis. MRI may also be requested, but the utility of MRI in evaluating cartilaginous injuries is still uncertain. To clarify whether the bone fragment is loose, the magnetic resonance image must be supplemented with arthrography. If contrast fluid leaks in under the osteochondritis fragment, it is a sign that the lesion is loose.
- Treatment by physician: The patient should be referred to an orthopedic surgeon. The preferred treatment for patients who are not fully grown is usually a trial of non-weight bearing (perhaps using crutches) and to perform range of motion exercises for 6 weeks. Treatments often used for adults include arthroscopy with surgical fixation of the bone and cartilage fragments, "microfracture technique", and mosaic plasty, or cartilage transplantation.
- Prognosis: The prognosis is good for children with OCD: more than 90%

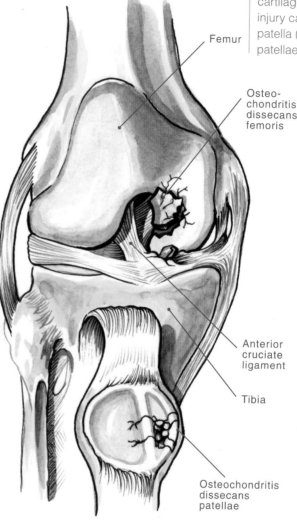

Figure 12.25 Osteochondritis dissecans. Loose bone fragments on the femoral condyle with accompanying cartilage disrepair. The injury can also affect the patella (osteochondritis patellae).

Femur

Osteochondritis dissecans femoris

Anterior cruciate ligament

Tibia

Osteochondritis dissecans patellae

of pediatric patients are asymptomatic 5 years after diagnosis. Unfortunately, the prognosis is not as good for adults, although newer methods of treating cartilage appear promising over the short term. However, long-term results are unknown. It seems probable that OCD increases one's lifetime risk for the early development of osteoarthritis.

Biceps Tendinopathy and Popliteus Tendinopathy

Thick, strong tendons surround the knee joint, and these tendons can become painful with overuse. This is particularly true of the two-headed knee flexor muscle (biceps femoris) and the tendon that is directly anterior to the lateral collateral ligament (the popliteus tendon) (figure 12.26).

- Symptoms and signs: A femoris biceps tendon injury often results in an acute avulsion injury of the fibular insertion of the long and short biceps tendon. Therefore, an early X ray may be useful to rule out avulsion or fracture. If the athlete's symptoms are the result of an overuse injury, the patient should complain of pain during resisted hip flexion. Popliteus tendinopathy is usually found near the muscle-tendon junction of the popliteus muscle, about 18 mm in front of the origin of the lateral collateral ligament on the femur. In both cases, the patient will complain of pain while running or playing ball games.

- Diagnosis: The diagnosis is clinical and depends on the palpating exam in addition to isometric testing of both the biceps femoris and the popliteus. It may be useful to attempt to provoke the athlete's symptoms by having her go for a long run before her reduction. Diagnostic injestion of a small amount of local anaesthesia may be helpful. MRI may reveal increased fluid content as a sign of active tendinopathy.

- Treatment by physician: If the radiographic examination is negative, the use of cortisone may be worth attempting, but there are no studies in the literature to document a definite therapeutic benefit. NSAIDs, possibly in gel form, are an alternative treatment option during the early phase of the condition.

- Treatment by physical therapist: Adjusting the athlete's training is important to alter the loading pattern of this patient group.

- Prognosis: The prognosis is generally good.

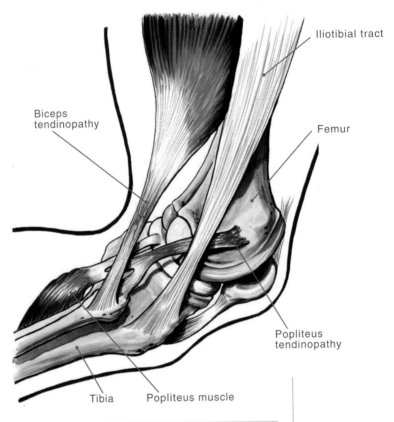

Biceps tendinopathy

Iliotibial tract

Femur

Popliteus tendinopathy

Tibia   Popliteus muscle

Figure 12.26 Biceps tendinopathy and popliteus tendinopathy. Other tendons in the area may also be affected, but these two are the most prone to overuse pathology.

Iliotibial Band Syndrome—Runner's Knee

Iliotibial band syndrome (figure 12.27) has also been called "runner's knee" because the condition is problematic for so many long-distance runners. With overuse, the tendon of the iliotibial tract becomes tender, and the athlete can no longer tolerate long training runs. The distal portion of the iliotibial tract becomes irritated as it slides back and forth over the lateral femoral condyle. There is often a small bursa between the tendon and the bone, and this may become inflamed, as well.

- Symptoms and signs: The main symptom is activity-dependent pain that corresponds to the largest prominence of the lateral femoral condyle. There may be crepitation, but usually the exam is remarkable only for focal tenderness to palpation. Pain often decreases after warm-up and during training, but it increases again the next morning following training.

- Diagnosis: The diagnosis is dependent on clinical findings of focal tenderness to palpation and the appropriate history. A diagnostic injection of a small dose of lidocaine may help to confirm the diagnosis by temporarily relieving symptoms. X rays can be obtained to exclude other conditions.

- Treatment by physician: Alternative training, stretching of the iliotibial tract, and cortisone injections have been documented to be effective in treating ITB syndrome. Surgery is an option if the pain persists for longer than 6 months.

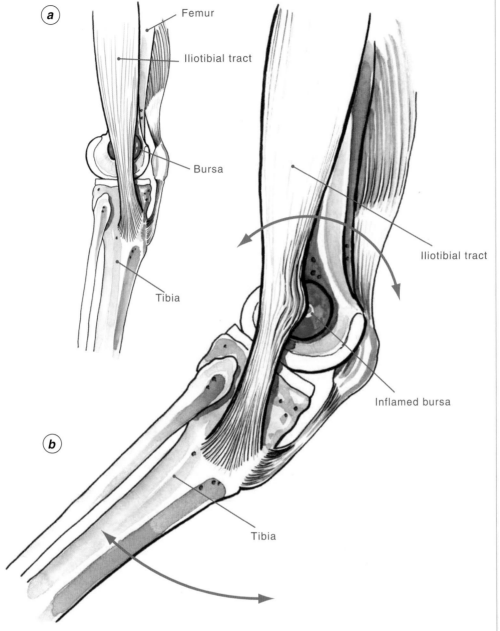

Femur

Iliotibial tract

a

Bursa

Tibia

b

Iliotibial tract

Inflamed bursa

Tibia

Figure 12.27 Runner's knee. The iliotibial band is affected where it glides back and forth over the lateral femoral condyle *(b)*.

KNEE

- Treatment by physical therapist: Stretching of the iliotibial tract (exercise 11.14), in addition to the gluteal and thigh muscles (exercises 11.12 and 11.13), is generally helpful. The physical therapist should also direct training and provide advice about altering the loading pattern.
- Prognosis: The prognosis is good with appropriate treatment, including activity modification.

Bursitis

Several bursae are found around the anterior-lateral aspect of the knee (figure 12.28), all of which, in principle, can become inflamed. Such inflammation is generally due to overuse of the surrounding tendinous structures but can also result from repeated trauma, such as falling on a knee or direct trauma resulting in bleeding into the bursa. Occasionally, the prepatellar bursa may become infected by bacteria, which could possibly result from scraped skin or a small wound over the bursa.

- Symptoms and signs: Usually, the prepatellar bursa is the most commonly affected, usually as a result of falling on the kneecap. Infrequently, the bursa at the pes anserinus becomes irritated, and in rare cases, the patient develops bursitis where the lateral collateral ligament inserts on the proximal fibula. The athlete will complain of pain and swelling, and if the bursitis is infectious, the area becomes erythematous and warm. Occasionally the athlete may develop systemic symptoms that include fever and a general feeling of malaise.
- Diagnosis: The diagnosis is usually made clinically, based on the finding of a tender area of swelling with local fluctuation. MRI or ultrasound confirms the clinical diagnosis. The physician should be aware that MRI may demonstrate several bursae around the knee that may be completely normal. If infection is suspected (red, warm bursa) the bursa should be tapped. If the patient has aseptic bursitis, the fluid contents are clear. If the bursa is infected, the fluid content will be cloudy, and a sample should be sent for a bacterial culture and susceptibility testing. In addition, the patient's rectal temperature should be taken, and the C-reactive protein, white cell count, and erythrocyte sedimentation rate should be tested. If the patient has traumatic bursitis, the contained fluid is sometimes mixed with blood.
- Treatment by physician: If the patient has aseptic bursitis, the bursa can be aspirated and cortisone can subsequently be injected. The affected bursa can also be removed surgically, if necessary, in case of recurrence. If the bursa is infected, antibiotics should be administered and adjusted as needed, based upon the results of the susceptibility tests.
- Prognosis: The prognosis is generally favorable for all types of bursitis.

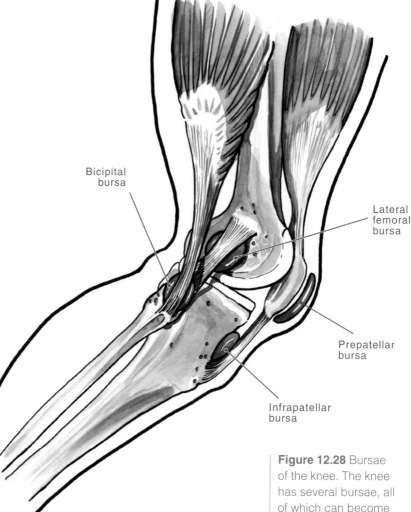

Bicipital bursa

Lateral femoral bursa

Prepatellar bursa

Infrapatellar bursa

Figure 12.28 Bursae of the knee. The knee has several bursae, all of which can become inflamed.

Medial Plica Syndrome

Patients with a thickened plica often have pain medial to the patella. The medial plica is a commonly occurring structure that extends from the suprapatellar fossa along the medial patellar edge and down toward the anteromedial recess (figure 12.29). The plica may become enlarged, thickened, and irritated at the site that slides

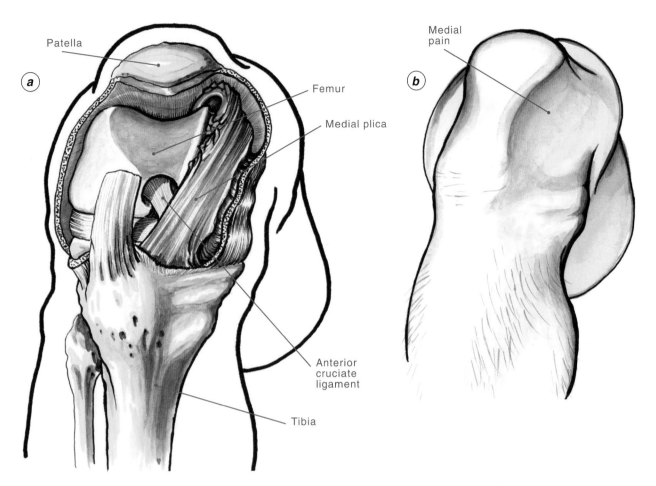

back and forth over the medial femoral condyle during knee flexion. Therefore, medial plica syndrome is often included in the differential diagnosis of patients with anterior-medial knee pain. As shown in figure 12.29, the symptoms appear when the membrane becomes thickened and looks inflamed upon arthroscopy. Medial plica syndrome is thought to occur rarely among athletes.

- Symptoms and signs: Activity-dependent anterior or medial knee pain. Careful palpation may reveal an area of thickening along the medial patellar border.
- Diagnosis: The diagnosis is difficult to make clinically. The medial plica is a difficult structure to find on ultrasonography. Although it is visible on an MRI examination, the radiologist should be asked to look specifically for a medial plica. Arthroscopically, the plica looks like a thickened, reddish sail that spreads out over the medial femoral condyle.
- Treatment by physician: If all other possibilities have been excluded, the plica may be removed arthroscopically. The plica is quite often quite vascular, and as a result there is almost always significant postoperative bleeding, which may prolong rehabilitation.
- Prognosis: Most athletes should be able to return to their sport, but the recovery time is often as much as 3 months (sometimes more).

Figure 12.29 Medial plica syndrome. The medial patellar plica of the knee is a common anatomic finding in the knee but is thought to cause pain only rarely.

Osgood-Schlatter Disease and Sinding-Larsen-Johanson Disease

These two conditions occur exclusively in older children and adolescents. They are caused by overuse of the patellar tendon, either at its origin on the patella (Sinding-Larsen-Johanson disease) or its insertion to the tibial tuberosity (Osgood-Schlatter

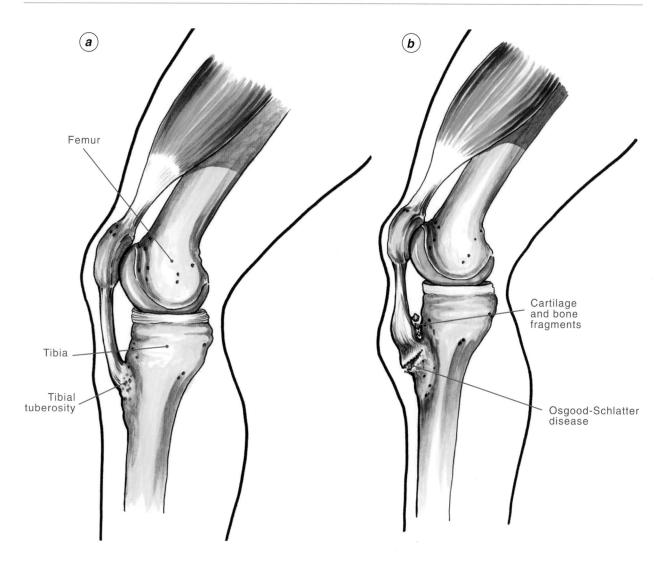

a

Femur

Tibia

Tibial tuberosity

b

Cartilage and bone fragments

Osgood-Schlatter disease

disease) (figure 12.30). When the growth zones of the distal patellar pole and the tibial tuberosity are overloaded (usually as a result of jumping exercises by volleyball and basketball players or repeated kicking drills by soccer players), they can become irritated and painful. The growth zone will be disturbed, resulting in pain from the area around the affected physeal plate.

Figure 12.30 Osgood-Schlatter disease. Normal *(a)*; the tibial tuberosity often becomes enlarged and tender *(b)*.

- Symptoms and signs: The main symptom of Osgood-Schlatter disease is pain with active knee extension. This condition is common among athletes in jumping and sprinting sports, such as track and field, soccer, volleyball, and basketball. The athlete is usually in the middle of a growth spurt (12 to 18 years old). Swelling eventually occurs.
- Diagnosis: The diagnosis is clinical, but the physician should always obtain X rays to exclude any tuberosity epiphysiolysis or tumors.
- Treatment by physician: Affected athletes should modify their activity patterns so as to reduce the load on the extensor apparatus for 6 weeks. Most patients recover in that time, but a few must refrain from jumping and sprinting sports for as long as 6 months. There is no relationship between Osgood-Schlatter disease and the incidence of detachment of the tibial tuberosity, so strict restrictions on the child's activities are unnecessary.
- Prognosis: Everyone recovers. At the latest, recovery occurs when the growth zones close, although there may be minor fragmentation of the tibial tuberosity in a few patients. If this causes symptoms when the patient is fully grown, the small bone fragments can be surgically removed at that time.

Rehabilitation of Knee Injuries

Grethe Myklebust and Lars Engebretsen

Goals and Principles

The goals of acute knee injury rehabilitation are listed in table 12.5.

Healing of the injured structure(s) without loss of mechanical knee joint stability is the principle goal of treatment and rehabilitation of knee injuries. The goals and principles of rehabilitation are similar, whether the athlete has injured the meniscus, ligament, cartilage, or cruciate ligament. The exercises used during the rehabilitation period are basically the same for all types of knee injuries. However, the rate and sequence of functional progression may differ depending on the diagnosis (e.g., when exercises may begin, when resistance training may be introduced, and when the number of repetitions and the speed of certain activities may be advanced).

After surgical intervention, the patient is usually sent home from the hospital with a rehabilitation routine that represents a good starting point for follow-up of the patient. Patients then enter the rehabilitation phase, and it is vital for the patient to begin active exercises. Pain and function are used to guide the progression of activity. If exercising causes pain or swelling, thereby reducing function, the patient's routine needs to be adjusted so that the knee has a chance to recover. The patient should return to the level that was tolerated before the symptoms progressed. It is recommended that thereafter only one exercise be changed at a time, in order to better determine what may be provoking the symptoms. The patient should generously ice the knee after exercising.

	Goals	Interventions
Acute phase	End swelling	PRICE principle with emphasis on good compression
Rehabilitation phase	End pain	Exercises, mobilization, stretching, ice
	Normal range of motion	
Training phase	Normal strength in the quadriceps and hamstring group compared with the healthy side	Strength training
	Normal neuromuscular function: knee injuries may reduce neuromuscular function, resulting in slowed reaction to changes of position, thereby increasing the risk of new injuries caused by cutting and landing	Balance exercises, functional exercises, progressing to controlled sport-specific training
	Reduce the risk of reinjury	The athlete should be fully recovered physically and mentally before resuming competitive activity

Table 12.5 Goals and interventions for rehabilitation of acute knee injuries.

Patients should generally begin a rehabilitation training program with many repetitions (e.g., four series of 20 to 30 repetitions) and light loads, gradually progressing to heavier loads and fewer repetitions (e.g., three series of 12 to 15 repetitions). During the final phase of the rehabilitation period, the athlete should train maximal strength or explosive strength, depending on the type of activity the athlete hopes to return to. Collaboration with coaches regarding this type of training is important, so that the training may be adjusted to the demands of the sport and managed with respect to what the knee can tolerate.

When retraining these patients, the therapist should train neuromuscular function as well as strength and range of motion. Knee injuries usually alter neuromuscular control, and retraining takes time. Therefore, it is important to motivate the patient to perform a daily home exercise program in order to normalize neuromuscular function.

Many of the most severe knee injuries result in a long-term absence from sports, and some athletes never return to sport. This is a traumatic experience for the affected athlete; health care workers must therefore remember the psychological aspect when dealing with patients with serious knee injuries.

Return to Sport

After surgical intervention, the patient is counseled regarding the expected timeline for return to full function. If the patient is recovering from anterior cruciate ligament injury, it is common to plan on 6 to 12 months of recovery and rehabilitation before the athlete can return to sports that demand sudden stops and quick turns. After meniscus resection, the time off varies from 14 days to several months, depending on which sport the athlete is going to return to and how much time elapsed before the original intervention took place. The patient should wait a minimum of 6 to 8 weeks if he sustained a medial ligament injury, since that is generally how long it takes the ligament to heal. These time frames are by no means absolute; above all, an athlete should not be sent back to contact or pivoting and twisting sports without being well prepared both physically and mentally. The patient's knee should be tested and found comparable with the healthy side before declaring the patient fully rehabilitated.

Strength test. Differences in hamstring and quadriceps strength on the injured side compared with the healthy side can be evaluated with the help of isokinetic testing equipment. It is recommended that the athlete's injured side be at least 90% of the strength on the healthy side before she returns to pivoting and twisting sports. A quadriceps bench may be used for testing both maximal strength and strength endurance.

Functional tests. Before an athlete returns to sport from a knee injury, lower limb function should be tested—for example, by using timed running tests that include turns and dead stops or timed stair jumping tests, comparing the injured to the healthy side. The athlete should be tested by approximating, as closely as possible, the sport to which he will return. These types of tests will uncover any deficit of neuromuscular control. The patient should have nearly equal function on both sides before returning to competition. Including such tests during rehabilitation may help to motivate the athlete to do additional training for strength and neuromuscular control. If the patient is away from work or sport activity for a prolonged period because of the injury, it is also important for the athlete to mentally prepare for competition.

Preventing Reinjury

Athletes in pivoting and twisting sports are at risk for reinjuring the rehabilitated knee. Optimal rehabilitation can reduce the risk of a reinjury. Optimal rehabilitation involves healing all structures and achieving symmetric strength, range of motion, and neuromuscular control in both knees.

If the athlete has a major knee injury, she needs to be evaluated with respect to whether she can realistically hope to tolerate the demands of sport participation at all. The physician, the physical therapist, and the athlete (and possibly her parents and trainer or coach), should discuss the problem with respect to the risk of reinjury and the long-term consequences of the injury.

Rehabilitation of Painful Knee Conditions

A large part of the rehabilitation of patients with chronic knee pain will consist of adjusting training and loads to an appropriate level, as well as stretching. The examination must include an evaluation of the patient for possible foot problems. The practitioner should take a thorough history with respect to the amount and type of training. The cause of overuse injuries can usually be understood if the amount and type of training are carefully studied. Symptoms are often triggered by an increase in the amount of training or a change in the training conditions (e.g., temperature, surface, and shoe type).

The most common cause of chronic knee pain among recreational athletes is patellofemoral pain syndrome. Patients with this syndrome may benefit from an orthosis or McConnell taping (which is believed to change the position of the patella). This brings pain relief to many patients, enabling them to train nearly pain free. Electrostimulation (a technique used to help activate the vastus medialis obliquus muscle) may also help (figure 12.31). The exercise can be done from several starting positions–lying, sitting, or standing–or it may be done during functional exercises (such as knee bends). This makes it possible to interrupt a vicious cycle of pain, reduced activity, poor muscle function, and atrophy (particularly in the vastus medialis or vastus medialis obliquus) and to stop further inactivity. When treating this type of patient, the athlete should be counseled to be willing to accept some pain during exercise. Using a visual analog pain scale, where pain can be rated from 0 (no pain) to 10 (intolerable pain), it is common to accept pain up to 3 or even 5 on the scale during exercise and in the immediate post-exercise period.

The muscles of patients who have chronic pain should be examined for possible tender points or trigger points and then treated.

In patients with "runner's knee," it is important to stretch the gluteal muscles and the iliotibial band, in addition to adjusting the demands of the athletic training regimen (see exercises 11.12, 11.13, and 11.14 on page 318).

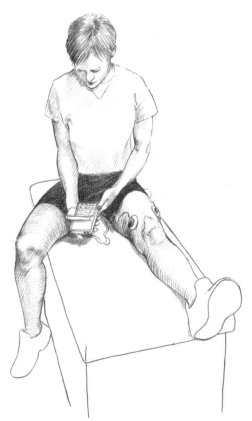

Figure 12.31 Electrostimulation of the vastus medialis muscle.

Training adjustments are also necessary for patients with jumper's knee: the athlete should avoid exercises that push the extensor apparatus beyond the limits of pain. An eccentric strength-training program that lasts at least 12 weeks may work well for many patients, but it must be emphasized that this disorder takes time to heal. In many cases, it is necessary for the practitioner to work together with the athlete's coach to adjust the load to which the athlete is subjected during training.

A training routine that is based on strength and neuromuscular control benefits patients with chronic knee instability. Exercises for knee instability are similar to those used for the rehabilitation of acute knee injuries. If the patient also has a cartilaginous injury of the knee, she can count on mild pain when exercising. The pain must not exceed a value of 3 (out of 10) on a visual analog pain scale. The athlete's pain may disappear when the strength and stability of the knee have improved. The patient should be prepared to accept (at a minimum) a 12-week training program that includes at least three training sessions per week before experiencing any noticeable symptomatic improvement.

Exercise Program

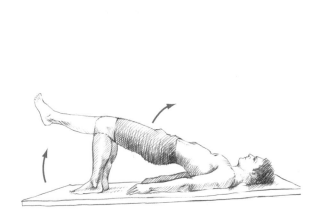

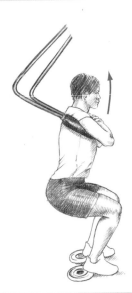

Exercise 12.1 Hip lifts

- Load your affected leg with about 90° flexion in the knee.
- Extend your other leg and hold that position for about 6 seconds.
- Lower your leg gently.
- This is a great exercise for working the muscles around the knee joint and the gluteal muscles.

Exercise 12.2 Knee bends with unloading

- Do this exercise early in rehabilitation.
- Keep knees over toes.
- Keep hips level.
- Determine unloading on the basis of pain and body weight.
- Exercise gently, using controlled movements.
- Do numerous repetitions.
- Consciously use your affected leg.

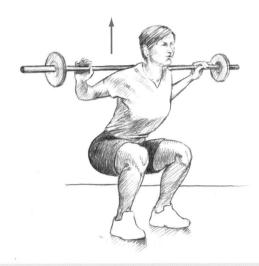

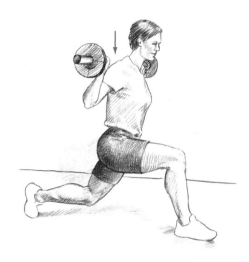

Exercise 12.3 Knee bends with loading

- Initially, use a bar to support your body weight, then use body weight, and eventually a load on your shoulders.
- Keep knees over toes.
- Keep hips level.
- Avoid getting your weight too far forward.
- Look up and straight ahead.
- Use a mirror to make yourself aware of knee position and weight placement during the start-up stage.

Exercise 12.4 Single-knee bend (lunge)

- Lower yourself a short distance at first, gradually longer and deeper (as shown in the figure).
- Keep knee over toes.
- Keep hips level.
- Do the same movement at an angle or straight out to the side.
- Use a mirror during the start-up stage.

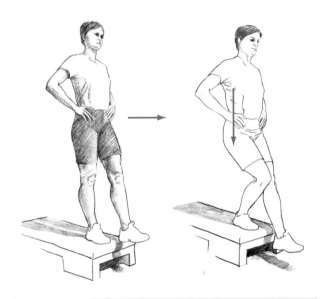

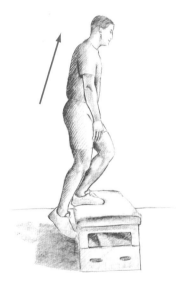

Exercise 12.5 Going down stairs

- Stand on your affected leg and go down gently on your healthy leg.
- Start with a step that is not very high.
- Use a mirror to control movement.

Exercise 12.6 Going up stairs

- Stand on your healthy leg, and ascend the stairs gently on your affected leg.
- Keep knee over toes.
- Use a mirror to monitor movement.
- Avoid lifting your hip.
- Initially, use a bar to support your body weight.

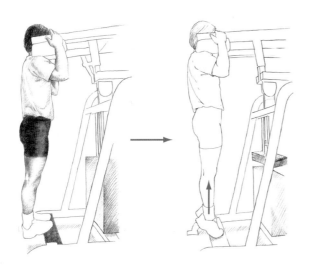

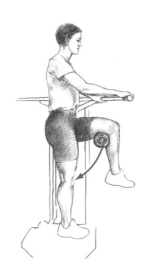

Exercise 12.7 Toe raises

- Do standing toe raises.
- Use equal loading on both legs.
- At first, hold onto something, such as gym-wall stall bars.
- Gradually increase loading.

Exercise 12.8 Hamstrings, standing hip extension

- Stand on your healthy leg; work with your affected leg.
- Stretch until your hip is extended, then return gently to the start position.

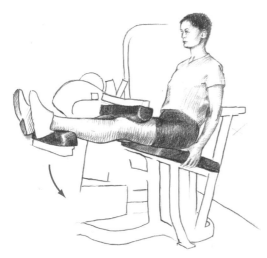

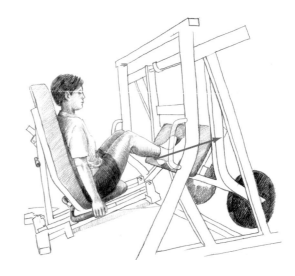

Exercise 12.9 Hamstrings, sitting knee flexion

- Work with both legs or your affected leg alone.
- Gently bend in the direction of the arrow as far as your knee will allow.
- Gradually increase knee flexion.

Exercise 12.10 Leg press

- Start with very light loading and move within the limits of pain.
- Exercise with both legs or with your affected leg alone.
- Make straight and stable movements with the knee.

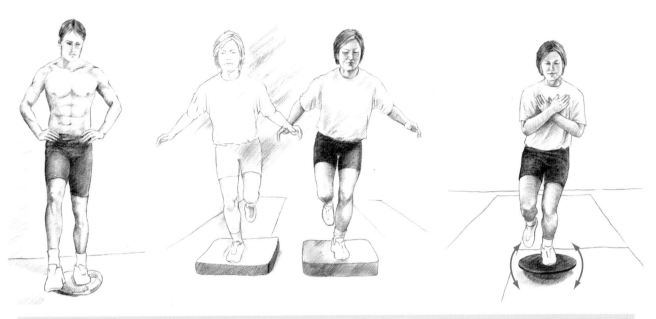

Exercise 12.11 Neuromuscular training

- Stand on one leg on a balance board or balance pad.
- Stand as still as possible for 15 to 20 seconds.
- Keep knees over toes.
- Stabilize your hip over the leg on which you are standing.
- Increase the degree of difficulty by using a ball or by closing your eyes.

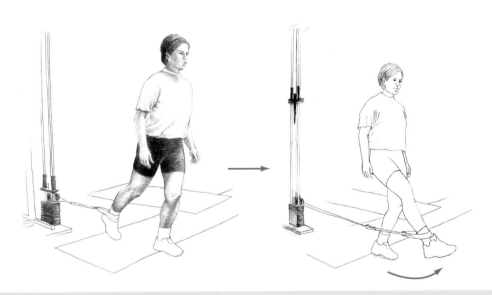

Exercise 12.12 Exercise using a pulley apparatus

- Stand on your affected leg, and swing your other leg back and forth against slight resistance.
- Do the exercise in several directions.
- Increase the degree of difficulty by standing on a board or closing your eyes.

Acute Lower Leg Injuries

Torbjørn Grøntvedt

Occurrence

Acute lower leg injuries are relatively uncommon in athletes, but chronic overuse injuries of the leg are a major problem. Formerly, downhill skiers frequently sustained lower leg fractures (known as boot edge fractures), but because ski boots and bindings have evolved, ligamentous knee injuries are more common now (particularly ruptures of the anterior cruciate ligament). The mandatory use of leg padding (shin guards) in soccer has also significantly reduced the occurrence of fractures and muscle and periosteal contusions.

Differential Diagnosis

The differential diagnosis of acute lower leg pain is fairly limited (table 13.1). Children, particularly adolescent boys in the midst of a growth spurt, are at risk for avulsion fractures of the tibial tuberosity, in addition to epiphysiolysis of the proximal or distal tibia and fibula. Tumors of the bone or soft tissues (usually sarcoma) may also cause acute symptoms, including bleeding or spontaneous pathologic fracture.

Diagnostic Thinking

The diagnosis of acute lower leg injuries is usually made by means of a thorough history and a physical examination. The injury mechanisms are often typical for the most frequently occurring bone, muscle, and tendon injuries. Direct trauma (e.g., being kicked in soccer) may cause a contusion injury of the musculature or

LOWER LEG

Most common	Less common	Must not be overlooked (!)
Muscle strains (p. 366)	Acute compartment syndrome (p. 371)	Epiphysiolysis (p. 374)
Crus fracture (p. 366)	Nerve contusion (p. 372)	Tibialis posterior tendon rupture (p. 417)
Tibial fracture (p. 366)	Subperiosteal hematoma (p. 373)	Peroneus tendon rupture (p. 406)
Fibular fracture (p. 367)		
Complete Achilles tendon rupture (p. 368)		
Partial Achilles tendon rupture (p. 370)		

Table 13.1 Overview of the differential diagnosis of acute lower leg injuries.

a fracture (usually of the tibia). In case of a spontaneous rupture of the Achilles tendon, both the athlete and any bystanders will hear a snap, and the athlete will typically spin around to see who kicked him in the lower leg. Intense pain after a contusion injury or a fracture of the lower leg should always raise the suspicion of acute compartment syndrome.

Clinical History

If the patient has suffered an acute lower leg injury, the history (including the mechanism of injury) will most often provide the best clues leading to the correct diagnosis. Contusion injuries may result in muscle trauma, fracture, nerve injury, or periosteal damage, depending on the location and magnitude of the force. A distention injury can cause a muscle or tendon strain or, in some cases, an avulsion fracture. Indirect trauma, such as strong torque of the lower leg over the edge of a slalom ski boot, may cause a leg fracture or a cruciate ligament injury.

Clinical Examination

Inspection. A malaligned or compound lower leg fracture is easily diagnosed by inspection. Significant muscle tears and total ruptures of the Achilles tendon will typically result in a visible defect in the countour of the skin over the site of injury. This defect will eventually fill with blood and edema fluid and will begin to swell. Subsequent appearance of ecchymosis locally and in gravity dependent adjacent areas suggests an intermuscular injury (in which blood from the muscle belly spreads along the fascial planes and percolates its way to the skin). If the patient has contused the anterior tibia and sustained a periosteal injury, painful local swelling usually develops quickly, and eventually the skin becomes ecchymotic.

Palpation. If the patient has a nondisplaced fracture of the tibia or fibula, the patient will upon palpation localize the pain to the site of the fracture. Minor swelling may be the only result of this type of injury. The patient will also complain of "indirect pain," meaning that pressure applied to the tibia or fibula some distance away from the fracture will trigger pain at the site of the injury.

If the patient is examined immediately after a muscle tear, a tender defect can be palpated in the muscle belly. However, this defect will quickly fill up with blood and edema fluid, causing swelling.

A partial rupture of the Achilles tendon may be difficult to identify on palpation, but pressure over the injured area always triggers pain. A reasonably experienced practitioner should be able to confidantly diagnose a total rupture of the Achilles tendon through physical examination alone. By palpating the tendon with two fingers, the Achilles tendon can be followed provisionally from its insertion onto the calcaneus. Typically, the injured tendon "disappears" within a couple of centimeters of its insertion site. This defect is the newly separated ends of the ruptured tendon. Advancing proximally, the tendon can be "found again" a couple of centimeters closer to musculotendinous junction of the triceps surae muscle.

The Thompson test will be positive if the patient has a total Achilles tendon rupture. This test is conducted with the patient prone and in a position of slight knee flexion. Alternatively, the patient may kneel, resting the involved leg on the examination table (figure 13.1). Squeezing the calf musculature will cause involuntary plantar flexion of the ankle joint if the tendon is intact, but no movement will occur if there is a total rupture.

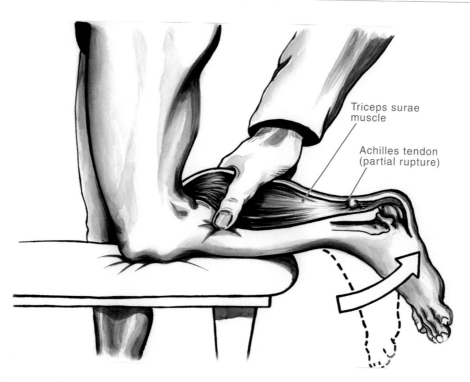

Triceps surae
muscle

Achilles tendon
(partial rupture)

Figure 13.1 The Thompson test is used to demonstrate the integrity of the Achilles tendon. If the patient has a partial rupture (as shown), passive plantar flexion will occur at the ankle joint when the triceps surae is squeezed. If the tendon is completely torn, no motion will result in the ankle joint.

Acute tendinitis, particularly tenosynovitis, will cause the tendon to be tender and possibly somewhat thickened. Crepitation is common, and it can often be appreciated by applying pressure and palpating along the course of the tendon (like squeezing a wet sticky snowball).

Acute compartment syndrome is characterized by severe pain, a tense quality to the affected muscle component, and intense pain with palpation. Passive toe movement also triggers significant pain in the affected musculature, and late in the course the patient will experience a loss of sensation distally in the lower leg and in the foot. The practitioner must remember that even with a fulminant compartment syndrome, the dorsalis pedis and posterior tibial pulses may be virtually unaffected.

Supplemental Examinations

Radiographic examination. A radiographic examination in two planes (frontal and lateral) is necessary to evaluate clinically manifest or suspected fractures. Occasionally, a fracture of the fibula or tibia may be only a thin fissure that may be difficult to detect on X ray. If a fracture is still suspected, the patient should undergo a supplemental skeletal scintigraphic examination. One to two days following the injury, scintigraphy will be positive, with strong radiotracer uptake at the fracture site. Magnetic resonance imaging (MRI) will demonstrate the fracture as well, and it will provide an even clearer image of edema formation in the surrounding cancellous bone. Therefore, if available, MRI should be considered the imaging modality of choice, ahead of scintigraphy.

Measuring compartment pressure. If the athlete is suspected of developing muscle compartment syndrome, she should be taken immediately to a hospital, where the pressure in the affected compartment can be measured. Pressure is often elevated in all four compartments of the lower leg if the patient has a fully developed compartment syndrome. A pressure of 45 to 50 mmHg is an indication for acute surgical intervention with fasciotomy.

LOWER LEG

Common Injuries

Muscle Strains

Muscle injuries are divided into contusion injuries and strain injuries (figure 13.2). Contusion injuries are caused by direct impact (such as a kick in soccer to the posterior or lateral aspect of the lower leg). The musculature gets crushed against the underlying bone, often causing deep injuries. Strain injuries are usually partial tears of the soleus or the gastrocnemius (most often affecting the medial gastrocnemius). Athletes in sports in which jumping ability and speed are important factors (like tennis, badminton, squash, volleyball, basketball, team handball, and soccer), as well as hurdlers and sprinters in track and field, are particularly vulnerable to muscle strains. "Tennis leg" is a partial thickness tear at the junction between the muscle and the distal tendinous fibers of the medial gastrocnemius (figure 13.2).

- Symptoms and signs: The athlete reports pain of sudden onset that corresponds to the location of the injury. The patient has difficulty walking on tiptoe.
- Diagnosis: It may initially be possible to palpate a defect in the muscle belly, but eventually there will be soft tissue swelling locally due to bleeding and edema. Local tenderness to palpation over the site of the rupture is typical. Muscle fasciae in the lower leg are very thick, so bleeding frequently is contained within the muscle belly. If the fascia tears, the skin will become bruised over and distal to the injury after 2 or 3 days.
- Treatment: Acute treatment using RICE and nonsteroidal anti-inflammatory drugs (NSAIDs) should be prescribed for 2 or 3 days. Caution is advised in using NSAIDs if major muscular bleeding has occurred. However, if adequate compression is applied to the affected area, such medication should not unduly increase the risk of additional bleeding. Three days later, the patient should be reexamined. If intermuscular bleeding (indicative of a rupture of the muscle fascia) has recurred, the overlying skin will be ecchymotic. The flexibility of the muscle should be carefully tested. On the 3rd day after injury, the patient starts rehabilitation with strength and flexibility exercises. Tennis leg may cause longlasting pain, despite adequate initial treatment. An injection of local anesthetic and cortisone in and around the area of scar formation, followed by an adequate stretching and strength training regimen, will often provide symptomatic relief.
- Prognosis: The athlete may return to sport activity once he achieves full painless range of motion that is symmetric on both sides, and has fully restored strength in the muscle. If intermuscular bleeding has occurred, this should take 2 to 4 weeks, whereas it likely will take at least 8 to 12 weeks for a patient to fully recover from an injury with intramuscular hemorrhage. If the injured area is allowed to heal with a permanent area of scar tissue that is inflexible and insufficiently stretched, subsequent loading of the area may easily cause a recurrent strain injury.

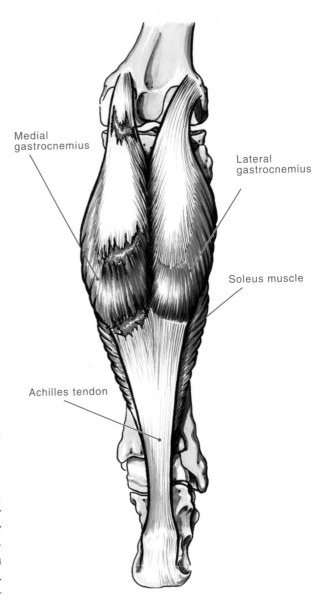

Medial gastrocnemius

Lateral gastrocnemius

Soleus muscle

Achilles tendon

Figure 13.2 Muscle injuries in the lower leg. The muscle tendon junction of the medial gastrocnemius is a commonly injured area (called "tennis leg"). However, strain injuries can occur at several other locations in the leg, most often at the muscle-tendon junction.

Crus Tibial Fracture—Lower Leg Fracture

Lower leg fractures are categorized according to which bones are fractured: crus fractures (both the tibia and fibula are broken) and isolated fractures of the tibia and of the fibula (figure 13.3). These injuries occur most frequently in contact sports (e.g., soccer and ice hockey) and in high-energy sports (e.g., downhill skiing and motor sports). The mechanism of injury may be direct or indirect trauma, and the injury may be from a high- or low-energy activity. Direct trauma, such as a kick, usually causes a transverse fracture, whereas indirect twisting trauma often results in an oblique or spiral fracture. Low-energy injuries are usually simple transverse, oblique, or spiral fractures, whereas high-energy trauma often causes a multi-fragmented injury or compression fracture and may also result in an open fracture with associated soft-tissue injuries. The practitioner should classify these injuries for treatment purposes and to evaluate the healing potential of the fracture.

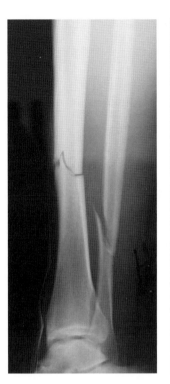

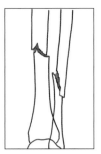

Figure 13.3 X ray of a fractured lower leg with fracture lines through both the tibia and the fibula.

• Symptoms and signs: Symptoms include severe pain of acute onset and possibly malalignment or skin perforation. The fractured area may eventually become swollen.
• Diagnosis: Physical examination confirms the diagnosis if the fracture is grossly unstable. X rays will usually confirm suspected fractures if they are simple fissures in the tibia or fibula. On occasion supplemental skeletal scintigraphy or MRI may be necessary.
• Treatment: Initial on-site treatment consists of rough correction of the axes of the lower leg and stabilization of the fracture as soon as possible (simple splinting, pillows, or the like), to minimize further soft-tissue damage and to reduce pain during transport. Any wounds are covered in as sterile a manner as possible. Immediately after the injury occurs, pain is often less intense, so rapid intervention may make a rough correction of alignment possible without any type of pain-relieving medication. Simple stable fractures are reduced in the hospital, and a cast is applied. By contrast, unstable fractures (particularly open fractures) require surgery with medullary nailing or external fixation. Surgery allows immediate knee and ankle joint mobility and partial loading. If a crus fracture is treated with a cast, the cast must extend from the groin to the toes in order to achieve rotational stability. This cast must be removed as soon as possible, preferably after 2 to 4 weeks, when the fracture has become "set." The patient is then fitted for a lower leg orthosis so that he can begin mobility training and partial loading, which are of great importance to both joint and muscle function.
• Prognosis: Fractures of the tibia shaft tend to heal slowly, because of poor soft-tissue coverage and a poor blood supply to the anterior medial portion of the bone. It usually takes 8 to 12 weeks before healing has progressed sufficiently to permit the patient to gradually and carefully resume sport activity. After a crus fracture, the patient can count on at least 6 months' absence from contact sports or other sports that place a heavy load on the lower leg.

Fibular Fracture

This type of fracture is usually caused by direct trauma (such as a kick), or it may occur when the patient has a sprained ankle with a simultaneous syndesmosis injury. In the latter case, the fracture is usually found in the proximal fibula.

• Symptoms and signs: Severe pain of acute onset following blunt trauma to the fibula is a common clinical scenario. Proximal fibular fractures that occur in connection with ankle injuries are frequently overlooked but may be diagnosed by palpating the proximal leg, provoking pain at the fracture site.

- Diagnosis: X rays usually confirm a suspected fracture. Sometimes supplemental skeletal scintigraphy or MRI may be necessary.
- Treatment: Simple fibular fractures without noteworthy malalignment are usually treated by simply unloading the leg (with crutches) until the patient is pain free. Because of good soft-tissue coverage and an ample blood supply, these fractures usually heal easily. If the ends of the fracture are malaligned or dislocated, then reduction

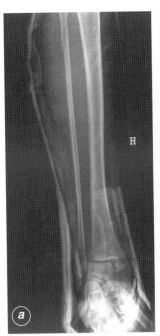
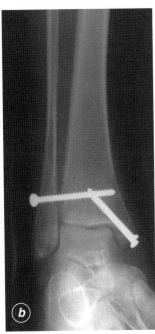

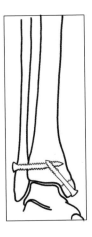

Figure 13.4 Syndesmosis injury. The X ray demonstrates a proximal fibular fracture, syndesmosis rupture, and a fracture of the medial malleolus (a). The patient is initially immobilized in a preliminary plaster cast. Thereafter syndesmosis screws are inserted through the fibula and into the tibia, and screws through the fracture of the medial malleolus are used to surgically stabilize the fracture (b).

and osteosynthesis (fixation) may be necessary to prevent pseudoarthrosis from developing. A combined fracture and syndesmosis injury requires surgical repair of the syndesmosis, with suturing and fixation by means of a syndesmosis screw. This screw is inserted through the fibula into the tibia immediately over the syndesmosis, so that the fibula is pressed in toward the tibia and the position of the ankle mortise is restored (figure 13.4). The syndesmosis screw has to be removed after 8 to 10 weeks to prevent the bone surrounding it from fracturing (fatigue fracture) and to prevent union of the fibula and the tibia (synostosis).

Complete Rupture of the Achilles Tendon

The Achilles tendon is the thickest and strongest tendon in the human body. It plays a very important role in most sport activities and is particularly vulnerable to overloading from repetitive running and jumping. The Achilles tendon forms a joint distal tendon for the gastrocnemius and the soleus muscles. These muscles combine to form the triceps surae muscle (figure 13.5). Athletes who sustain Achilles tendon ruptures most frequently are those who participate in ball sports that demand rapid changes of direction and quick, reactive jumps (e.g., tennis, squash, badminton, and soccer), in addition to runners and jumpers in track and field. Sometimes a patient with a ruptured tendon has a history of long-term pain localized to the tendon, but more often the rupture occurs without warning. Such ruptures are often caused by degenerative changes in the tendon (tendinosis), usually in the segment of the tendon that has the worst blood supply. This segment extends from 2 to 6 cm proximal to the insertion of the tendon onto the calcaneus.

Achilles tendon ruptures may be divided into full thickness ("total") and partial thickness ruptures. Total ruptures usually occur in formerly active athletes (average age 40) who resume sport activity after having been away from it for some time. In these cases, degenerative changes have weakened the tendon so much that sudden, forceful loading of the tendon causes it to tear. To some extent, these changes in the tendon could have been prevented by regular physical activity. In most cases, the injury mechanism is a strong activation of the posterior lower leg musculature, eccentrically overloading the tendon. A typical mechanism of injury involves pushing off hard with the weight-bearing foot while the knee is extended (e.g., running uphill) or sudden, unexpected

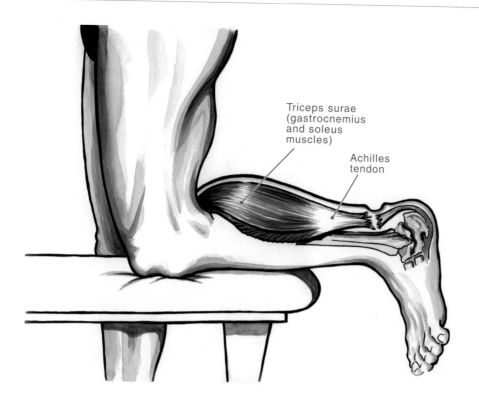

Triceps surae
(gastrocnemius
and soleus
muscles)

Achilles
tendon

Figure 13.5 Full thickness Achilles tendon rupture. If the patient has a total rupture, the Thompson test will be positive (i.e., no plantar flexion will be present in the ankle when the triceps surae is squeezed).

dorsal extension of the ankle with reflex contraction of the calf musculature (e.g., falling down into a hole).

- Symptoms and signs: The athlete experiences acute, intense pain corresponding to the Achilles tendon, often accompanied by an audible "snap." The athlete often spins around to see "who kicked her." She cannot walk on tiptoe, nor can she walk with a normal stride.
- Diagnosis: During the clinical examination, the patient will have significantly reduced ankle plantar flexion strength on the involved side. When the tendon is palpated with one finger on either side, the tendon can be followed from the calcaneus to where it "disappears" in the area of the rupture and to where it then returns 2 to 3 cm proximal to the rupture. If the injury is recent, the patient indicates that her pain is localized at the site of the rupture. The defect eventually fills with blood and edema and the skin over the area becomes ecchymotic. The Thompson test is positive (figure 13.5).
- Supplemental examinations: If the diagnosis is uncertain, ultrasound or MRI can be used to further evaluate the regional anatomy.
- Treatment by physician: All patients who are active in sport at a relatively high level should undergo operative repair of the ruptured tendon as quickly as possible. Postoperatively, the ankle should be immobilized in an orthosis or cast for 2 weeks, with the foot in a slightly equinus position.
- Treatment by physical therapist: After 2 weeks the cast or orthosis is removed. Then the patient's ankle is mobilized in a range-of-motion walking orthosis permitting free plantar flexion and gradually increasing dorsiflexion (beginning from a zero position) over the next 4 weeks. Beginning 6 weeks after surgery, the patient gradually increases the intensity of strength and flexibility training. This treatment plan usually allows the athlete to return to full sport activity after about 3 months. Several studies have shown that early mobilization and loading of a sutured tendon increases collagen formation, remodeling, and strength in the repaired tendon. The risk of recurrent rupture is 1% to 2%, whereas the risk of perioperative infection is between 5% and 10%.

LOWER LEG

Some authors have recommended conservative treatment for total Achilles tendon ruptures. The recommended treatment consists of cast immobilization of the ankle with the foot in a mild equinus position for 4 weeks, after which the ankle is casted in slight plantar flexion for another 4 weeks. When the cast is removed at 8 weeks, the patient uses a buildup (of about 2 cm) under the heel for another 4 weeks, followed by careful strength and flexibility training. This treatment usually results in healing with a lengthened tendon, which reduces jumping ability. In addition, the risk of a recurrent rupture following conservative treatment is between 10% and 30%. Therefore, this method of treatment is not recommended for athletes.

Total Achilles tendon ruptures are frequently overlooked. The patient who sustains this injury will complain of weak calf musculature, and he will not be able to maintain his normal stride. It is impossible for the patient to stand on his toes on the involved side, and plantar flexion is limited. These patients require surgery to resect the scar tissue interposed in the rupture cleft, to mobilize the tendon and muscle proximally, and to suture end to end using either the tendon of the long plantar muscle or a fascia/tendon flap from the proximal part of the Achilles tendon for strength. Rehabilitation is the same as that used after acute repair, except that the progression of activities is somewhat slower and more cautious. The result with respect to strength and jumping ability is often somewhat worse in patients who undergo delayed repair than in those who undergo acute surgical repair.

Partial Rupture of the Achilles Tendon

Partial ruptures of the Achilles tendon (figure 13.6) occur most frequently among participants in the same sports in which total ruptures occur, affecting all age groups. Acute eccentric overload that exceeds the tendon's load capacity usually results in a partial rather than a total rupture. If the symptoms are neglected and loading of the injured area continues, the risk of developing a chronic painful condition increase significantly with the formation of fibrotic granulation tissue in and around the injured area.

- **Symptoms and signs:** Initially, a partial rupture often causes little pain. Loading the affected limb will cause pain, which begins in the area of the rupture and lasts for a while after loading ceases. Eventually, the athlete will experience pain and stiffness corresponding to the injured Achilles tendon from the outset of each training session. The pain may subside somewhat after warm-up, only to worsen again toward the end of the training session. Later in the course, morning stiffness and local pain in the tendon are typical signs of a partial rupture.

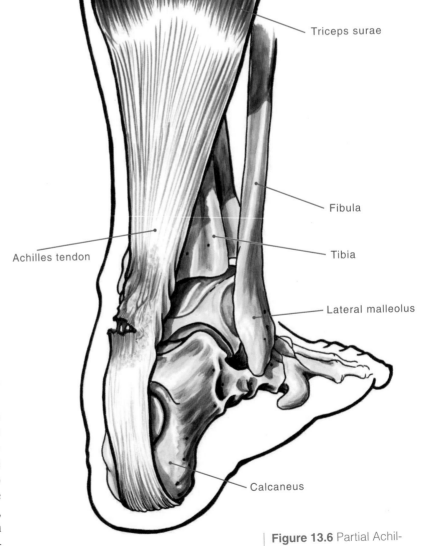

Triceps surae

Achilles tendon

Fibula

Tibia

Lateral malleolus

Calcaneus

Figure 13.6 Partial Achilles tendon rupture.

- Diagnosis: During the acute phase, examination findings include an intensely tender point in the tendon that corresponds to the injured area. Swelling eventually occurs, and the tender areas are easily detected by palpating along the tendon with one finger on each side. Chronic disorders tend to result in some atrophy of the lower leg musculature on the involved side. Ultrasound and MRI will reveal the size and location of the partial rupture, and in chronic cases these modalities will show how much granulation tissue has formed in the area.
- Treatment: Adequate unloading is crucial once the athlete has become symptomatic. Rest is required so that the tendon can heal and a chronic painful condition can be avoided. The patient may need to restrict loading for 2 to 4 weeks or until the tendon pain is gone. Initially, the patient is given NSAIDs for 3 days; after unloading, a heel lift should be used. If the symptoms are neglected and the partial rupture develops into a chronic condition, the athlete may require surgery to remove granulation tissue and separate adherent peritenon from the area of the rupture. Postoperatively, the patient should limit weight bearing with crutches for 4 to 6 weeks but must begin ankle mobility training as soon as pain allows, to stimulate the tendon's revascularization and healing process.
- Prognosis: The prognosis is usually good, if the athlete takes their symptoms seriously and unloads adequately. If the patient develops chronic irritation that requires surgery, he can count on being away from sport activity for at least 4 to 6 months.

Acute Compartment Syndrome

The muscles of the lower leg are divided into four compartments, each of which is surrounded by a relatively non-yielding layer of connective tissue fascia. The four groupings are the anterior, lateral, deep posterior, and superficial posterior compartments (figure 13.7). Acute compartment syndrome occurs when the pressure inside one or

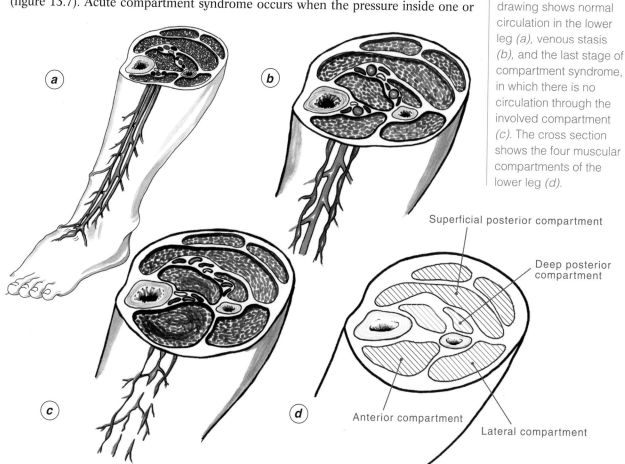

Figure 13.7 Development of acute compartment syndrome. The drawing shows normal circulation in the lower leg *(a)*, venous stasis *(b)*, and the last stage of compartment syndrome, in which there is no circulation through the involved compartment *(c)*. The cross section shows the four muscular compartments of the lower leg *(d)*.

Superficial posterior compartment

Deep posterior compartment

Anterior compartment

Lateral compartment

LOWER LEG

more of the muscle compartments in the lower leg increases. Left untreated, acute compartment syndrome can result in devastating injury to the muscles and nerves within the compartment. This syndrome may occur following a fracture, a significant muscle injury, or even after a single bout of exercise that acutely overloads the muscle groups, such as a long run on hard surfaces by a relatively untrained person.

The mechanism behind the development of acute compartment syndrome can be outlined as follows (figure 13.7): increased pressure inside a compartment (e.g., resulting from bleeding or edema) leads to reduced capillary circulation in the musculature, which in turn precipitates increased production of lactic acid by the muscles, leading to more edema, increased venous stasis (i.e., compression of the vessels through which blood is carried away from the muscles), and ultimately a further increase in pressure. This vicious cycle continues until all circulation in the affected musculature has ceased and the muscles and nerves in the affected compartment become ischemic and necrotic.

- Symptoms and signs: The main symptom of acute compartment syndrome is intense pain that increases when the affected muscles are passively stretched. Muscle function is gradually reduced and ultimately lost. Paresthesias (sensory disturbances) of the cutaneous areas innervated by the affected nerves is a definite, but late, symptom.
- Diagnosis: The history should arouse the suspicion of compartment syndrome. The lower leg musculature will be tense and tender, its function reduced or absent. Paresthesias may occur later in the course of the disorder, although distal circulation in the foot and the dorsalis pedis pulse and that of the posterior tibial artery may be entirely normal.
- Treatment: The patient is referred to a specialist for immediate assistance. Measuring pressure in the affected compartments is an important tool for evaluating the patient, and equipment for this purpose should be available at all hospitals. If increased pressure is suspected on physical examination, or if increased pressure is measured, the patient must undergo immediate surgery to divide the fascia of all four compartments in the lower leg. If the circulation within a compartment is absent for longer than 4 or 5 hours, the muscles will begin to necrose, by which time the damage is irreversible.
- Prognosis: Prognosis is good with early recognition and treatment. It is sometimes difficult to juxtapose the skin edges together after surgery, so skin grafting is occasionally necessary. If the muscle fibers have become necrotic, the injured athlete is at risk for developing fibrosis, shortening, and contracture, as well as chronic neuropathic pain (Volkmann's contracture).

Nerve Contusion

The common peroneal nerve is superficial and relatively unprotected as it passes underneath the head of the fibula (figure 13.8). Direct trauma, such as a kick or persistant pressure over this area, may lead to total or partial paralysis of this nerve (peroneal palsy).

Other nerves in the lower leg that may be subjected to direct trauma or chronic irritation include the superficial cutaneous branch of the peroneal nerve, the sural nerve, and the saphenous nerve (figure 13.9). A slalom ski boot that is strapped too tightly or tight ankle tape may result in a pressure injury to these nerves, with associated sensory disturbance (numbness, or paresthesias), and possibly pain in the corresponding area of cutaneous innervation.

- Symptoms and signs: If the common peroneal nerve is injured proximally, the patient will develop weakness of the ankle dorsiflexors and evertors ("drop foot"),

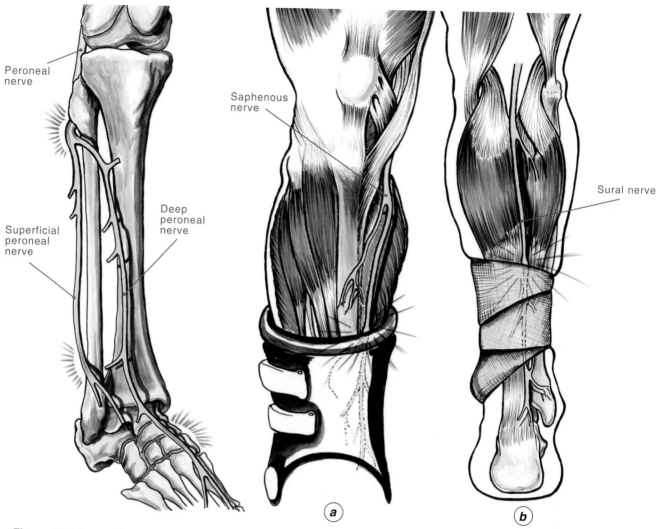

Figure 13.8 Peroneal nerve injury. The peroneal nerve is most vulnerable to injury at the head of the fibula. Less common injury locations are just proximal to the lateral malleolus and on the dorsum of the foot.

Figure 13.9 Saphenous nerve *(a)* and sural nerve *(b)* injuries. Entrapment of these nerves can be caused by a slalom boot or a firm elastic bandage.

in addition to paresthesias on the dorsum of the foot and on the anterior aspect of the ankle.

- Diagnosis: The diagnosis is based on the history and on the physical examination findings. A supplemental electrodiagnostic examination will demonstrate the extent of the nerve damage.
- Treatment: If a contusion injury has occurred and the nerve is intact (neuraproxia), function will gradually return without any type of treatment. If the nerve is torn (axonolysis), it must be surgically repaired.
- Prognosis: The athlete normally recovers completely from neurapraxic injuries in a few days to a few weeks, whereas the prognosis for a surgically repaired transected nerve is much less definite.

Subperiosteal Hematoma

Direct trauma, such as being kicked in the shin, may cause bleeding under the periosteum of the tibia. This type of subperiosteal hematoma is very painful, and the symptoms may persist until the bleeding is resorbed. In some cases, part of the hematoma may be converted to fibrous scar tissue that may subsequently partially or fully calcify.

- Treatment: Treatment is in accordance with the RICE principle during the acute phase. Bleeding must be limited as much as possible. Later, a specially adapted plastic brace can be made to protect against recurrent trauma to the same area. The most important "treatment" is prophylaxis, such as wearing well-adjusted leg padding (shin guards) when playing soccer.

Epiphysiolysis—Slippage of the Growth Plate !

Epiphysiolysis may occur both proximally and distally in the tibia and fibula. In the proximal tibia, avulsions usually occur through the apophysis in the tibial tuberosity or the epiphysis inferior to the knee joint. These injuries usually affect boys during the last stage of their pubertal growth spurt, when the musculature begins to mature and strength increases. If the patient maximally activates his quadriceps (e.g., during jump training for basketball or volleyball), the load on the patellar tendon may be so great that the growth plate is disrupted.

Epiphyseal injuries in the proximal fibula and in the distal tibia and fibula can result from any mechanism of injury that would result in an ankle fracture (with or without associated injury to the syndesmosis) in an adult.

- Symptoms and signs: The principle symptoms include acute pain and possible malalignment (i.e., similar to symptoms caused by a fracture). Because there is less bleeding than results from a fracture, less swelling usually occurs with epiphysiolysis.
- Treatment: Proximal growth plate injuries are usually relatively simple to reduce and to cast. An orthosis should replace the cast after 2 or 3 weeks, after which the patient should begin loading with the knee extended. After 6 weeks, the patient may begin mobility training and gradually progressive strength training. Distal epiphyseolysis is treated according to the same principles but often requires surgical reduction and fixation, because growth zone injuries frequently occur in combination with a fracture. Syndesmotic injuries always require surgical fixation with a syndesmosis screw.
- Prognosis: The prognosis is favorable with precise reduction and proper immobilization. In some cases, all or part of the epiphyseal plate may be so damaged that premature closure of the epiphysis (epiphysiodesis) occurs. This results in asymmetrical growth as the athlete matures, which in turn may create the need for corrective osteotomy.

Chronic Lower Leg Pain

Torbjørn Grøntvedt

Occurrence

The lower leg is the most common location for sport-related chronic overuse disorders. These disorders are usually the result of external and internal risk factors, often in combination. The most common modifiable risk factor for overuse injuries is "too much too soon"–that is, too rapid an increase in the amount or intensity of training (e.g., a great deal of running on a hard [asphalt] or icy surface). Muscle imbalance or structural asymmetry or malalignment are the most important internal risk factors, with the most common types being foot malalignment (particularly overpronation [longitudinal flatfoot]), knee malalignment (genu varum [bowlegged] or genu valgum [knock-kneed]), increased femoral anteversion with toeing in, anisomelia (leg length discrepancy), and poorly rehabilitated musculature from a previous injury or surgery. Athletes in all sports in which running is an important part of the activity are affected by chronic overuse disorders of the lower leg.

Differential Diagnosis

The most common overuse disorders of the lower leg are medial tibial stress syndrome, stress fractures, Achilles tendinosis, and chronic compartment syndrome (table 13.2). As is true for acute lower leg injuries, the differential diagnosis for chronic overuse injuries is relatively limited. The most important ones are tumors of bone and the soft tissues. These can cause long-lasting symptoms that resemble the symptoms of overuse disorders. One of the predilection sites for osteogenic sarcoma is the proximal tibia. This is most common in children and adolescents. Osteoid osteoma, a benign bone tumor, is also often found in the lower extremities. Pain due to osteoid osteoma is often confused with pain caused by stress fractures. Because of the serious differential diagnoses, the practitioner must thoroughly evaluate patients who have long-term or somewhat uncharacteristic symptoms, using radiography and possibly skeletal scintigraphy or MRI.

LOWER LEG

Most common	Less common	Must not be overlooked !
Medial tibial stress syndrome (p. 379)	Chronic compartment syndrome (p. 383)	Nerve contusion (p. 372)
Stress fracture (p. 380)	Calcaneal bursitis (p. 384)	Tumors (p. 375)
Tendinosis (p. 382)	Calcaneal apophysitis (p. 385)	Sciatica (p. 376)
Tendinitis/peritendinitis (p. 381)	Haglund's deformity (p. 386)	Intermittent claudication (p. 376)

Table 13.2 Overview of current differential diagnosis of chronic lower leg pain.

Other relatively common diagnostic considerations are sciatica (with pain radiating down into the lower leg) and intermittent claudication (the result of inadequate arterial blood supply to the lower leg musculature). If claudication is present, mere loading will provoke symptoms; more severe stenosis will result in complaints of pain at rest as well.

Diagnostic Thinking

It is as important to document the causes of chronic overuse injuries of the lower leg. In most cases, if the symptoms are treated and the underlying causes are left untreated, the patient will eventually return to the doctor with identical symptoms. A thorough examination will often reveal major or minor malalignment, and the intensity of training may be only a triggering factor. If structural malalignment is minor, it usually takes a major change in the amount of training to trigger overuse injuries, whereas the opposite is true of major congenital or acquired malalignment (figure 13.10).

Clinical History

A thorough history is essential to determine what may have caused the patient's symptoms. The physician must document factors such as the amount and intensity of training, increases in load, the playing or training surface, the footwear the patient wore, and the timing of the symptoms in relation to these factors. It is also necessary to accurately document the exact location of the pain, whether it is well localized or more widespread, whether it began suddenly or gradually, whether it is continuous or only occurs during training, and whether (and how long) it persists following training. In addition, the practitioner should document whether the pain was initially a minor annoyance and gradually increased in connection with activity, or whether the pain remained unchanged during activity. If the patient has medial tibial stress syndrome, the pain will begin gradually during loading and will be localized to the distal two thirds of the medial border of the tibia. The pain often lasts for some time after loading ends and will increase in intensity if the athlete does not reduce the amount of training. However, the pain associated with a stress fracture tends to be of sudden onset, usually occurring while running, and pain is localized to a small area. The pain also rapidly dissipates with rest, only to return when the athlete attempts to resume running.

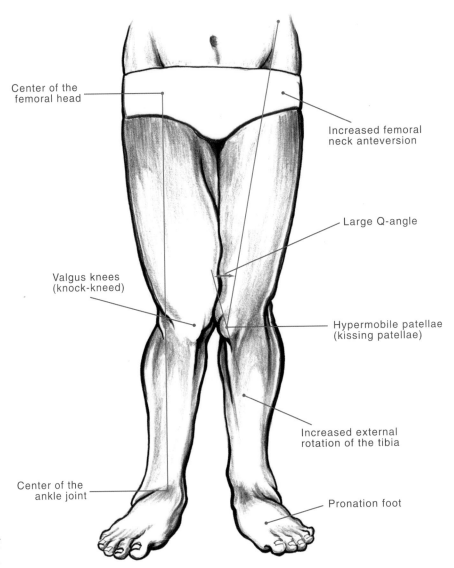

Center of the femoral head

Increased femoral neck anteversion

Large Q-angle

Valgus knees (knock-kneed)

Hypermobile patellae (kissing patellae)

Increased external rotation of the tibia

Center of the ankle joint

Pronation foot

Figure 13.10 Malicious malalignment syndrome. This patient has increased hip anteversion, a large Q-angle, increased external rotation in the tibia, and overpronation of the foot. With increased valgus positioning of the knee, the weight-bearing line goes from the center of the femoral head (hip joint) to the center of the ankle joint, passing lateral to the center of the knee joint.

Clinical Examination

Inspection. If the overuse disorder is chronic, the practitioner must thoroughly examine the patient to detect any malalignment that may have contributed to the onset of symptoms. With the patient standing, the practitioner looks for scoliosis (curvature of the spine), anisomelia, toeing in (as a sign of increased femoral anteversion), varus or valgus malalignment in the knees (figures 13.10 and 13.11), whether the kneecaps point straight ahead or are medially deviated (kissing patella), and whether there is an overpronated, flatfoot or cavus foot (figure 13.12). General postural concerns should also be noted. It is often quite easy to uncover a moderate degree of overpronation if the patient walks back and forth, or walks or runs on a treadmill. The best method is to videotape the athlete from behind while on the treadmill, then analyze the video in slow motion.

Function. Individuals with a stress fracture of the lower leg usually have a positive hop test. For this test, the patient hops on the involved leg. If the patient has a stress fracture, loading the leg in this fashion will trigger well localized pain, in contrast to the more diffuse type of symptoms that occur when the patient has medial tibial stress syndrome. Alignment of lower legs may be assessed with the patient sitting with the hollow of her knee resting against the edge of the examination table. In this position, the toes normally point straight ahead or slightly outward. With the patient lying in a supine position, the practitioner looks for local swelling, redness, or other discoloration in the symptomatic area.

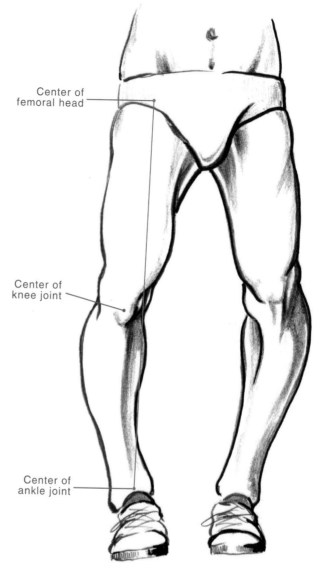

Center of
femoral head

Center of
knee joint

Center of
ankle joint

Figure 13.11 Varus knees (bowlegged). If there is increased varus alignment of the knee, the weight bearing line goes from the center of the femoral head (hip joint) to the center of the ankle joint, passing medially to the center of the knee joint.

LOWER LEG

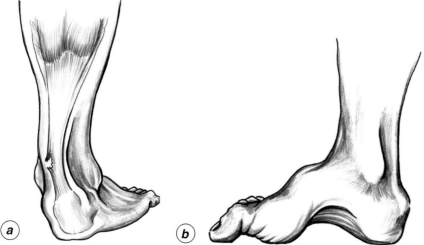

a

b

Figure 13.12 Overpronated, flatfoot (pes planus) *(a)*, and cavus foot (claw foot) *(b)*. Overpronation predisposes the athlete to overuse injuries of the foot, ankle, lower leg, and knee.

Palpation. If the patient has medial tibial stress syndrome, he will indicate that palpation along the distal two thirds of the medial margin of the tibia causes pain. If he has been symptomatic for a long time, the edge of the bone may feel irregular and bumpy. By contrast, a stress fracture causes more localized pain and often some swelling. If the patient has chronic compartment syndrome, the affected compartment will often feel more tense than normal, and the musculature is usually tender to pressure, particularly shortly after training. Chronic Achilles tendinosis often causes all or part of the tendon to become thickened, and it may be intensely tender to palpation from both sides (figure 13.13). If the calcaneal bursa contains a lot of fluid, bursitis is suggested by fluctuation and tenderness to direct pressure over the bursa. Calcaneal apophysitis causes local pain and sometimes mild swelling at the calcaneal insertion of the Achilles tendon to the heel bone.

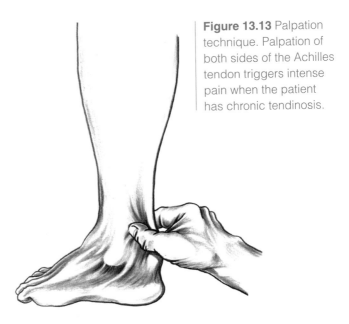

Figure 13.13 Palpation technique. Palpation of both sides of the Achilles tendon triggers intense pain when the patient has chronic tendinosis.

Supplemental Examinations

Radiographic examination. Radiographic examination of the entire lower leg in both the frontal and lateral planes is indicated for most chronic painful conditions of the lower leg. Imaging is particularly useful for excluding possible serious conditions within the differential diagnosis. If the patient has long-term chronic compartment syndrome, X rays will often demonstrate a somewhat thickened and uneven medial cortex in about the distal two thirds of the tibia, whereas a stress fracture may be difficult to visualize before callus forms over the fracture line. On X ray, stress fractures of the anterior margin of the tibia will appear as small rarefactions in the bone cortex (figure 13.14). If the patient has calcaneal apophysitis, the X ray may show sclerosis and possibly fragmentation of the bone at the insertion of the Achilles tendon.

Skeletal scintigraphy. This is an important examination for chronic overuse injuries and is practically diagnostic for stress fractures. One or 2 days after the onset of symptoms, scintigraphy will show strong local uptake corresponding to the fracture site (figure 13.15). More diffuse uptake results from chronic overloading of the osseous substance, such as that caused by medial tibial stress syndrome.

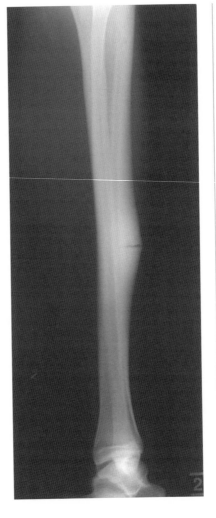

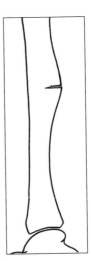

Figure 13.14 Stress fracture of the anterior cortex of the tibia.

Ultrasonography. Scar changes in the musculature after strain injuries as well as changes in the Achilles tendon from chronic tendinosis are easy to demonstrate with ultrasound. If an active ultrasound probe is placed over a stress fracture, it will often trigger significant pain.

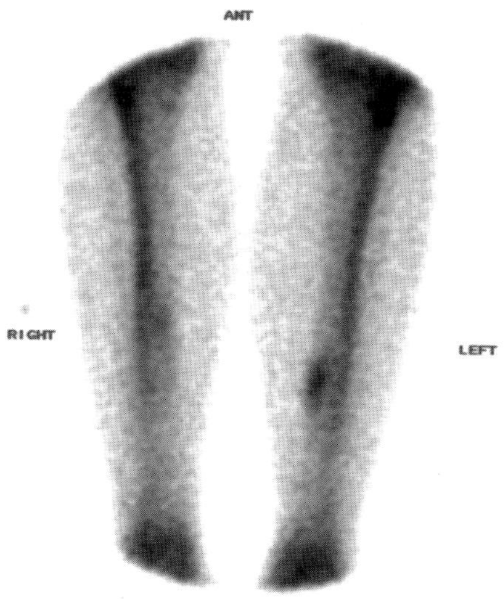

MRI. MRI is used for the same diagnostic purposes as ultrasound. However, MRI can also be used in the evaluation of tumors.

Measuring pressure. Several studies have shown that after loading, increased pressure can be measured in the anterior compartment of the lower leg when clinical symptoms suggest the diagnosis of chronic compartment syndrome. However, measurements in the deep and superficial posterior compartments have not produced analogous results for chronic medial tibial stress syndrome.

Figure 13.15 Skeletal scintigraphy. Stress fracture of the left tibia demonstrated by the focal area of increased uptake.

Common Injuries

Medial Tibial Stress Syndrome

This is the most commonly occurring chronic overuse injury in athletes. It occurs in all sports in which running and jumping constitute a major part of the activity. Muscular hypertrophy and stiffness related to periods of intense training are assumed to be an important underlying cause of medial tibial stress syndrome. The pain is thought to derive from inflammation, fibrosis, and thickening of the fascia in toward the periosteum on the medial margin of the tibia—particularly the distal two thirds. Important predisposing factors include increased external rotation of the lower leg and over pronation. Both of these malalignments cause the athlete to modify the mechanics of weight acceptance during the gait cycle (figure 13.16), placing more load medially, which in turn overloads the deep posterior compartment's fascial insertion to the tibial periosteum.

- Symptoms and signs: During and for a while after training the athlete experiences tenderness and pain along the distal medial tibial margin. Pain gradually increases in proportion to the intensity of training and may become so incapacitating that the affected athlete may have to discontinue running and jumping exercises.
- Diagnosis: The diagnosis can be made on the basis of the case history and a thorough clinical examination. Palpation reveals intense tenderness and possibly swelling over the medial tibial margin (which may feel rough). Most patients with this disorder have either externally rotated lower legs or overpronated feet. A poorly defined thickened medial tibial cortex will be visible on X ray, and diffuse increased uptake along large portions of the tibial margin (known as a stress reaction in the bone) will be visible on skeletal scintigraphy.
- Treatment: During the acute phase, the disorder is treated with rest, alternative training, stretching of the lower leg musculature, and NSAIDs. At the same time, malalignment must be corrected with specially fitted training shoes or insoles, and any training problems (e.g., relating to intensity of exercise or firmness of training surface) should also be corrected. In overpronated feet, orthoses must be used to correct valgus positioning of the heel and to provide good support under the arch of the foot. Some buildup should also be present under the head of the

LOWER LEG

first metatarsal. This will force the foot into a normal gait pattern from heel strike to toe-off, encouraging it to roll from the heel over the lateral arch of the foot and over onto the distal portion of the metatarsals (particularly the first metatarsal and the big toe). It is often difficult to make the proper orthosis on the first attempt, and the pedorthotist may need to make adjustments. In some cases, the results of conservative treatment are not entirely satisfactory. Several studies have shown that a favorable outcome for between 80% to 90% of patients who undergo surgical division of the superficial and deep posterior muscle compartments along the medial edge of the tibia can be expected. This has therefore become a routine intervention for the treatment of long-term disorders. A compression bandage is applied postoperatively and should be worn for 8 to 10 days. The patient usually unloads the operated leg with crutches for about 1 week or until the pain is gone. The athlete can resume running and training after 4 to 6 weeks.

- Prognosis: The prognosis is good if the external and internal causative factors are identified and corrected early. The athlete should plan to be away from high-level sport for up to half a year after surgical intervention.

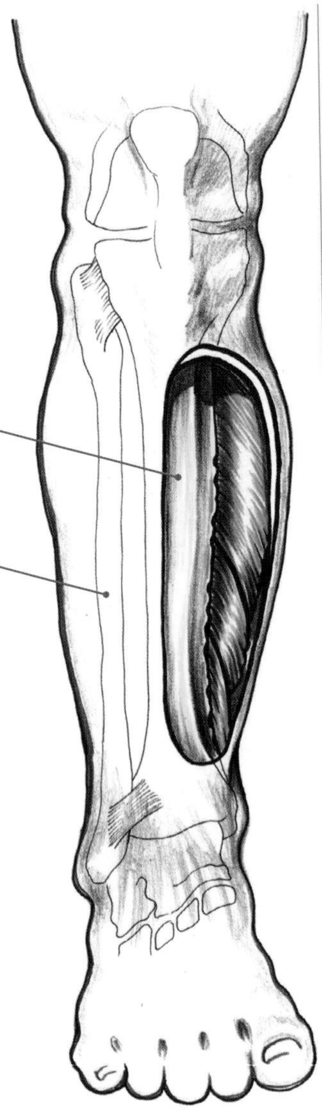

Stress Fracture

Stress fractures of the tibia and fibula occur frequently in athletes for whom running and jumping constitute a major portion of their training and competitive activity. Several studies have shown that up to 50% of all stress fractures in the body occur in the lower leg. The fractures are primarily localized to the distal and proximal portion of the tibia and the distal portion of the fibula (figure 13.17). Stress fractures typically occur between a few weeks and a few months after the athlete begins running training; in athletes who are active at a high level, they occur in connection with increased training intensity, usually when the athlete is preparing for a major competition. Overloading on a hard surface with insufficient shock absorption due to worn out shoes, combined with rapid increases in training intensity, are the most important causative factors. Malalignment may also be a contributing factor, but not to the same extent as in the development of medial tibial stress syndrome.

- Symptoms and signs: Classically, the athlete with a stress fracture complains of significant pain of acute onset, most often during a long training session. The pain is typically well circumscribed and disappears with rest, only to return as soon as the athlete attempts to resume training.
- Diagnosis: A history of pain of typical onset and character should raise the suspicion of a stress fracture. Examination findings include tenderness, possibly some swelling over the fracture site, and a positive hop test. X rays during the early phase are often negative, but callus may be demonstrated over the fracture some weeks later. Skeletal scintigraphy confirms the diagnosis, and bone scan should be positive within 1 or 2 days of symptom onset.

Figure 13.16 Medial tibial stress syndrome. Increased external rotation and overpronation can result in increased loading at the fascial insertion to the medial tibial periosteum. However, the condition may also occur in athletes with normal alignment.

Tibia

Fibula

• Treatment: A period of non-weight bearing of up to 6 to 8 weeks for tibial fractures and of 4 weeks for fibular fractures should normally provide sufficient time for healing. During this period, it is important for the athlete to undertake alternative training–that is, varied activities other than running, jumping, or other activities that directly load the affected lower extremity. Bicycling and aquatic training may be useful to maintain endurance, and strength training that does not include weight bearing is allowed. The practitioner should inform the patient of the necessity of adequate unloading; otherwise, the athlete may want to "test" the effect of treatment too soon, prompting a recurrence of the pain. During the unloading period, it is important to fully investigate why the patient sustained the stress fracture and to correct both the underlying training errors and any malalignment if possible. Stress fractures of the anterior tibial cortex in the midportion of the bone tend to heal slowly (apparently due to poor local blood supply) and may go on to develop pseudoarthrosis. Even unloading the affected limb for a prolonged period may not produce the desired result in these cases. The patient typically remains pain free during normal daily activities but has a recurrence of symptoms as soon as training resumes. Several different treatment methods have been suggested for these fractures. The most-used methods involve surgical fixation of the anterior cortex with a plate and screws, medullary nailing of the tibia, excision of the fracture area, bone transplantation, or excision and drilling of the anterior cortex. Good results have been reported using each of these methods. However, they all involve surgical intervention, with the attendant risk of complications that are related to surgery. Therefore, in recent years we have treated these fractures with extracorporal shock wave therapy. This is an ultrasound based therapy that produces local cortical microfracturing and promotes rapid healing, apparently as the result of the associated inflammatory reaction and increased local blood supply. To date, the results have been encouraging.

• Prognosis: Most stress fractures in the lower leg will heal if they are diagnosed early and adequately unloaded. Prevention is the key to both primary fractures and recurrences, including educating the patient about proper footwear, avoiding excessive training on hard surfaces, and avoiding rapid increases in the intensity of training. Sometimes an athlete (usually a thin, female athlete) will sustain several stress fractures simultaneously. This situation should raise the clinican's suspicion for the female athlete triad: a combination of amenorrhea, anorexia, and predisposition to stress fractures.

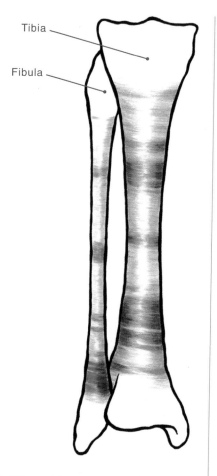

Tibia

Fibula

Figure 13.17 Location of stress fractures in the tibia and fibula. The color intensity reflects the incidence of stress fractures.

LOWER LEG

Tendinitis/Peritendinitis

The following types of tendinitis/peritendinitis may occur in the lower leg: tibialis anterior syndrome, tibialis posterior syndrome, peroneal tendinitis, and Achilles tendinitis. In most cases, acute inflammation in or around tendons is directly triggered by "too much too soon"–that is, the patient increased the amount or intensity of loading too rapidly. External factors (such as running on a hard surface [asphalt], training in a cold climate, or poor footwear) and internal factors (such as foot malalignment–particularly an overpronated foot), are important contributing causes. The physician should attempt to identify both internal and external risk factors when collecting the patient's history and examining the patient. If these factors are not corrected at the same time that training errors are addressed, there is a great likelihood that the athlete will have a recurrence of the symptoms even if initial treatment is successful.

- Symptoms and signs: Patients experience pain of acute onset localized over the involved tendon that is precipitated by movement of the ankle joint.
- Diagnosis: The diagnosis is made on the basis of local swelling, tenderness, and possibly crepitation when the tendon is palpated. If there is severe inflammation, rubor (erythema) of the skin overlying the involved tendon may occur.
- Treatment: The recommended treatment includes unloading until asymptomatic and NSAIDs for up to a week. If the Achilles tendon is involved, patients should follow up the initial treatment with the use of a heel lift for a few more weeks. The athlete must engage in alternative training during the unloading period–that is, she should engage in activities that do not cause pain in the involved area. Practitioners should look for and correct any underlying causes.
- Prognosis: The prognosis is good if unloading and other appropriate treatments are started early. Symptoms usually disappear in 1 or 2 weeks, but the condition can easily become a chronic disorder if the athlete continues loading the leg despite pain.

Tendinosis

Of the tendons in the lower leg, the Achilles tendon is most affected by chronic pathological changes. These changes may occur if the athlete neglects the symptoms of acute tendinitis or other overuse trauma. In such cases, degenerative changes (tendinosis) eventually develops in the tendon. Overpronation is a principle cause of chronic pain in the Achilles tendon. Excessive hindfoot pronation causes the foot to deviate into a valgus position after heel strike, which in turn results in overloading of the medial fibers of the Achilles tendon due to alignment considerations (figure 13.18). Continued overloading may result in microrupture or in chronic irritation of the medial paratenon and in the tendon itself. External factors, such as excessive running on a hard surface, training in a cold climate, footwear that absorbs shock poorly, and shoes with stiff soles, often contribute to the development of chronic Achilles tendinosis.

- Symptoms and signs: The main symptom is pain, which can be graded into four stages. In stage 1, pain occurs only after activity begins and disappears after a

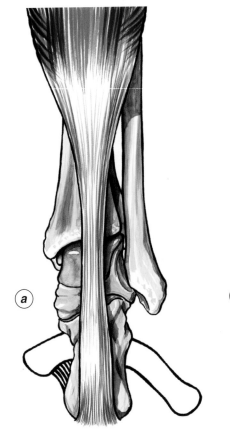
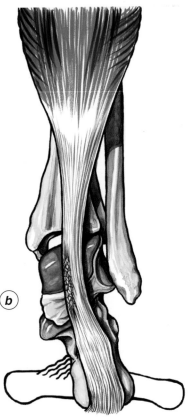

Figure 13.18 Achilles tendinosis—due to excessive hindfoot pronation. If the patient's foot position is normal (a) the Achilles tendon is straight, whereas an overpronated foot (b) causes malalignment of the Achilles tendon and increased loading of the medial fibers of the tendon.

period of rest. In stage 2, pain occurs during activity but does not limit activity. In stage 3, pain is felt during activity and is so intense that it prevents the athlete from participating in normal training. In stage 4, the pain becomes constant—even while the athlete is at rest. Morning stiffness and pain are typical early signs.

- Diagnosis: Findings on palpation may include swelling and tenderness over large portions of the involved tendon, although the musculotendinous junction and the tendon-bone junction are often pain free. Both dorsi- and plantar flexion of the ankle provoke pain, particularly with loading. If the pathological changes include microruptures of the tendon, extra tender "bumps" that correspond to the microruptures can often be palpated. Ultrasound and MRI will demonstrate thickened tendon and paratenon, and in particular will reveal changes corresponding to microruptures and areas with degenerated tendon tissue.

- Treatment by physician: During the early phase of unloading, stretching the leg musculature, alternative training, and NSAIDs often suffice and result in symptom reduction, particularly when combined with correction of the underlying risk factors (such as hindfoot overpronation and training problems). When distance training begins, the athlete often needs to insert a shock-absorbing heel wedge into his shoe, as well as a corrective orthosis. During the early chronic phase, an injection of cortisone around the tendon (in the paratenon) may also have a therapeutic effect. If the desired results are not achieved by a properly placed injection, additional injections are not indicated. Conservative treatment is not successful in all patients. Surgical intervention (designed to divide the paratenon and separate it from the tendon, and to remove granulation tissue from the tendon itself) typically produces good results in cases of chronic, treatment-resistant tendinosis.

- Treatment by therapist: Patients with chronic Achilles tendinosis have achieved good results from eccentric strength training of the triceps surae. The athlete must perform this training routine regularly, twice a day, 7 days a week, for up to 3 months, with gradually increasing loads. After any surgical intervention, subsequent rehabilitation and retraining must be individualized according to the surgical and pathological findings. Generally, however, athletes should not bear weight and must use crutches for 2 weeks, then may gradually increase their loads over the next 2 weeks, eventually progressing up to a normal gait after 4 to 6 weeks. In order to avoid adhesion between the tendon and the skin, mobility training in the ankle joint without loading is started as soon as pain allows. Beginning on the 6th postoperative week, the athlete can gradually increase strength training of the triceps surae, and distance or sprint training may begin after about 3 months.

- Prognosis: The prognosis is good with proper treatment. Most patients become fully or partially asymptomatic and can resume their normal sport activity. However, rehabilitation employing either conservative or surgical treatment may take a long time.

Chronic Compartment Syndrome

Chronic compartment syndrome in the lower leg is a relatively rare disorder that primarily affects the anterior, and (less often) the deep posterior muscle compartments, and only very rarely affects the lateral and superficial posterior compartments. The disorder is most common in athletes who do a lot of running and jumping exercises as part of their training (e.g., team handball and soccer) but may also occur in athletes who engage in strength sports, like weightlifting. Chronic compartment syndrome is usually caused by rapidly increasing muscle volume in connection with intense training, and the fact that the relatively unyielding muscle fascia is not compliant enough to accommodate the enlarging muscle bulk. Muscle volume increases during exercise, due to increased blood volume and retention of fluid, causing intracompartmental pressure to increase, reducing capillary circulation, and (eventually) causing ischemic pain. When loading stops, the pressure decreases, the blood supply normalizes, and the athlete's pain disappears.

- Symptoms and signs: Patients report cramplike pain of gradual onset during loading. The pain usually disappears quickly upon rest. The disorder may become so intense that the athlete develops weakness of ankle dorsiflexion and may also experience paresthesias (numbness), particularly in the area innervated by the peroneal nerve. The pain is usually localized to the affected compartment.
- Diagnosis: The diagnosis is based on tender, tight musculature, particularly upon provocative activity (e.g., running). The diagnosis is confirmed by measuring the pressure of the affected compartment after loading. Pressure in a muscle compartment of the lower leg is normally between 10 and 15 mmHg, both at rest and during training, whereas loading may increase the intracompartmental pressure to over 50 mmHg when a chronic compartment syndrome is present.
- Treatment: During the early stage, the recommended treatments include unloading and stretching of the lower leg musculature, alternative training, and guidelines for training. It is especially important for the athlete to avoid training on a hard surface and to wear well-adjusted footwear with adequate shock absorption. For up to 7 months the athlete should completely avoid loading that provokes symptoms and then gradually should resume training again. If the disorder is chronic, it may be necessary to surgically divide the fascia in the affected muscle compartment. To avoid scar and adhesion formation in the area where surgery was performed, the patient must begin range of motion training and light strength training of the lower leg musculature as soon after surgery as possible.
- Prognosis: The prognosis is good after surgical treatment. The athlete is usually able to resume full training within 6 to 8 weeks after division of the anterior compartment, although return to training may take slightly longer after surgery on the deep posterior compartment.

Calcaneal Bursitis

The calcaneal bursa is found in the area between the calcaneus and the Achilles tendon (figure 13.19). It may become inflamed because of chronic irritation, such as from direct pressure from tight shoes, or indirecly via chronic tendinosis in the distal portion of the tendon.

- Symptoms and signs: Patients with calcaneal bursitis experience pain, possibly swelling, and in rare cases, redness over the Achilles tendon insertion, particularly on the lateral side. Pressure from regular shoes may cause significant discomfort.

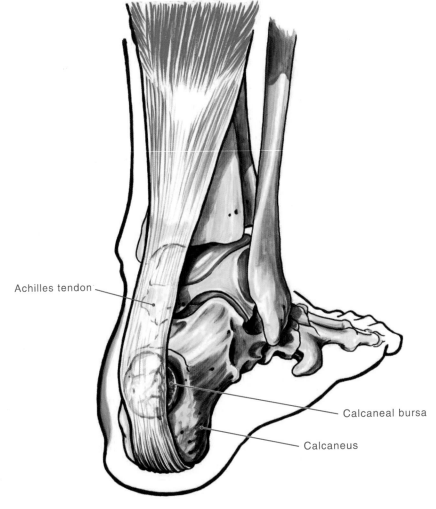

Figure 13.19 Calcaneal bursitis. The bursa is found beneath the Achilles tendon down toward the distal insertion onto the calcaneus.

Achilles tendon

Calcaneal bursa

Calcaneus

- Diagnosis: Pain, swelling, and possibly fluctuation are typical findings upon palpation of the bursa and form the basis of the diagnosis. Ultrasound and MRI show fluid accumulation within the bursa.
- Treatment: The primary intervention is to avoid pressure on the insertion of the tendon. This may be achieved by "blocking out" the athletic shoes in the back, using a piece of foam rubber or felt as padding—with a cutout over the painful area—and a slight heel lift underneath the heel. If symptoms persist, an injection of cortisone into the bursa may be effective. The physician should avoid injecting cortisone into the tendon or the tendon insertion because this may cause the tendon to rupture. If conservative treatment does not bring improvement over time, the bursa must be surgically resected.

Calcaneal Apophysitis (Sever's Disease)

This condition occurs in active adolescents, particularly during the pubertal growth spurt (ages 10-15) when the child's height increases rapidly and muscle strength also develops quickly. The condition is caused by overloading the tendinous insertion onto the calcaneus and the apophyseal growth plate in this area. Additional findings include possible fragmentation and sclerosis of the posterior calcaneus (figure 13.20).

- Symptoms and signs: Pain localized to the posterior aspect of the calcaneus occurs during loading, gradually resolving with rest. The area often feels stiff, and the child may limp.
- Diagnosis: The diagnosis is made on the basis of tenderness to palpation and possibly mild swelling over the site of tendon insertion. An X ray may reveal fragmentation and sclerosis of the posterior portion of the calcaneus if the athlete has been chronically symptomatic.

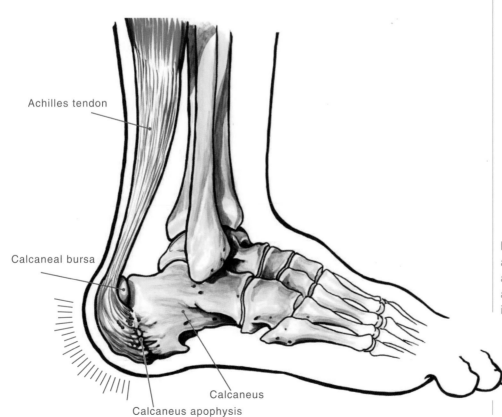

Achilles tendon

Calcaneal bursa

Calcaneus

Calcaneus apophysis

Figure 13.20 Calcaneal apophysitis. This is an overuse injury that affects the growth plate in the calcaneus.

LOWER LEG

• Treatment: The practitioner should inform the patient and the patient's parents that this is not a dangerous disorder and that it will resolve spontaneously as the patient matures (typically between 16 and 18 years of age). Treatment includes unloading the affected leg, alternative training (avoiding running), and use of a heel lift to help unload the tendon. The athlete's activity level should be limited only by pain.

Haglund's Deformity (Bony Prominence at the Insertion of the Achilles Tendon)

Chronic irritation at the insertion of the Achilles tendon onto the calcaneus (e.g., bursitis) may precipitate a periosteal reaction with cartilage and bone formation in the area between the tendon and the calcaneus (figure 13.21), often with overgrowth laterally. Pressure and irritation of this area from tight shoes will worsen the disorder, eventually causing a significant exostosis (Haglund's deformity). Haglund's deformity may be accompanied by an inflammatory subcutaneous bursitis.

• Symptoms and signs: The patient experiences pain and, frequently, erythema over a protruding bump that is located anterior and lateral to the Achilles tendon insertion.

• Diagnosis: The diagnosis is made based on the clinical examination. Oblique X rays may be obtained to demonstrate the exostosis.

• Treatment: In addition to unloading the affected limb, alternative training (avoiding running) and a heel lift to unload the tendon are recommended. The athlete's activity is limited only by pain. If the athlete's symptoms are chronic with a significant exostosis, surgical resection of the exostosis may be indicated.

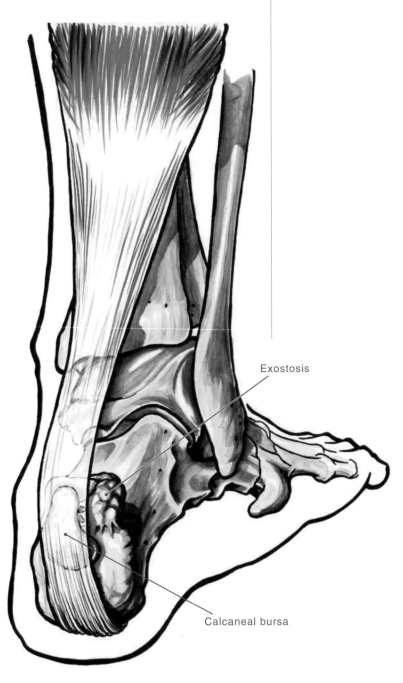

Figure 13.21 Haglund's deformity. The calcaneal exostosis is visible on the lateral aspect of the Achilles tendon.

Exostosis

Calcaneal bursa

Rehabilitation of Lower Leg Injuries

Torbjørn Grøntvedt and Knut Jæger Hansen

Acute Lower Leg Injuries: Goals and Principles

Table 13.3 lists the goals for rehabilitation of acute lower leg injuries.

During the acute phase, tape or an orthosis may be used to provide compression and protection of the affected area(s). During the rehabilitation phase, several of the injuries discussed in this chapter may be treated with an orthotic device instead of a cast, so that the patient is able to train at his normal functional level. One example of this is a total Achilles tendon rupture, where an orthosis will help maintain mobility in the ankle joint while allowing optimal loading of the injured structures. Tape and support devices are rarely used for these injuries during the training phase.

Lower Leg Pain: Goals and Principles

The principles of retraining for chronic lower leg pain are for the most part identical to those for acute injuries. However, the rehabilitation of patients with chronic lower leg injuries almost always focuses on identifying the underlying causes of the injury. This helps patients avoid reinjury. First and foremost, the athlete's training load should be evaluated with respect to both amount and intensity. The practitioner should especially identify the amount of eccentric training that the athlete is performing.

LOWER LEG

	Goals	Measures
Acute phase	Reduce swelling	RICE principle with emphasis on good compression
Rehabilitation phase	Normal mobility and being pain free so as to be able to train with normal function	Exercise, local treatment, and mobilization/stretching
Training phase	Normal strength and neuromuscular function	Sport-specific strength training and neuromuscular training
	Reduce the risk of reinjury	

Table 13.3 Goals and measures for rehabilitation of acute lower leg injuries.

During the rehabilitation and training phases, rehabilitation of chronic conditions is the same as for acute injuries, but the training phase is usually much longer than for acute injuries. A minimum 12-week combination of strengthening, eccentric training, stretching, and ice has proven favorable. Later, the athlete also trains with activities like running and jumping. In addition to strengthening and stretching exercises, the athlete performs balance exercises to guard against the loss of neuromuscular control.

Preventing Reinjury

A training phase that is sufficiently long, combined with the identification of modifiable external and internal risk factors for injury, is the key to preventing reinjury. If the patient has a chronic injury, the training phase should last for up to 12 weeks. It is difficult to specify a time frame for acute injury rehabilitation because injuries and their treatment vary greatly among athletes.

Exercise Program

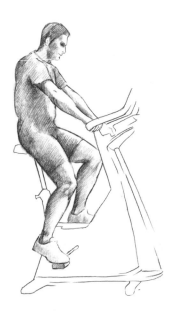

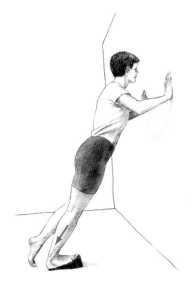

Exercise 13.1 Exercises for circulation

- Use mild resistance.
- Use high frequency.
- Also train for weight transfer and gait so that walking with a normal stride is achieved as quickly as possible.

Exercise 13.2 Stretching the lower leg with the knee extended

- Stretching is often necessary to achieve sufficient dorsal flexion for some lower-leg injuries.
- Stretch without pain.
- Stretch for a long time and with an even pull.

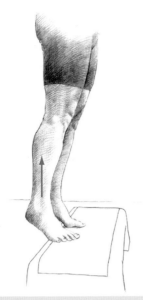

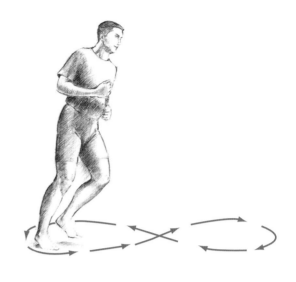

Exercise 13.3 Toe raises on the edge of a step

- Do within pain-free range of motion and, if necessary, without loading.
- Gradually increase range.
- Gradually increase tempo.
- Start with toe raises on both feet. Then transfer loading to the injured leg alone.
- After reaching full range and maximum tempo for one leg, add external resistance. During the training stage, introduce exercises with more emphasis on the eccentric stage (stopping).

Exercise 13.4 Training in function

- Train in exercises that are specific to the sport to which the athlete will return.
- Add turns and distractions.

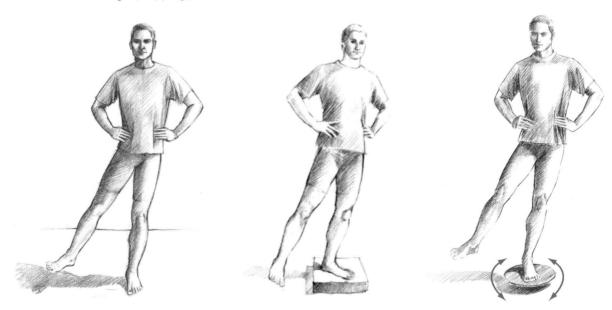

Exercise 13.5 Neuromuscular training: balance exercises while standing

- Do the exercises progressively.
- Use a precise starting position: Keep the knee over the foot, and control the hip.
- Increase difficulty by closing your eyes or by adding distractions, such as a ball and other movements.
- Increase difficulty by switching from a soft to a hard surface.

Acute Ankle Injuries

Roald Bahr

Occurrence

Acute ankle injuries constitute almost 10% of all acute injuries that are treated by physicians. It is estimated that one ankle injury occurs per 10,000 inhabitants every day. Hence, in Norway, with a population of approximately 4.5 million, more than 400 such ankle injuries occur every day, or 150,000 to 200,000 annually. Ankle ligament injuries are clearly the most common injury in sport, accounting for about one-fifth of all sports injuries. In some sports, especially team sports like soccer, basketball, volleyball, and handball, ankle injuries comprise up to half of all acute injuries. A high incidence of ankle injuries also occurs in some individual sports, particularly those sports which involve running over uneven terrain (e.g., orienteering) or require frequent jumping.

Differential Diagnosis

Table 14.1 provides an overview of the differential diagnosis for acute ankle injuries. Young, active patients whose inversion trauma occurred while running, jumping, or falling, usually sustain lateral ligament injuries. Children can sustain epiphyseal plate injuries as a result of this type of trauma, whereas older patients commonly sustain fractures of the lateral malleolus or the base of the fifth metatarsal. Syndesmosis injuries are rare but can occur either in isolation or in combination with other ligament injuries or fractures.

Most common	Less common	Must not be overlooked !
Lateral ligament injuries (p. 398)	Malleolar fractures (p. 401)	Syndesmosis injuries (p. 404)
	Fracture at the base of the fifth metatarsal (p. 400)	Epiphyseal plate injuries (children) (p. 374)
	Talar fracture (p. 405)	
	Calcaneal fracture (p. 428)	
	Medial ligament injuries (p. 399)	
	Ankle dislocation (p. 405)	
	Posterior tibial tendon rupture (p. 417)	
	Peroneal tendon dislocation/rupture (p. 406)	
	Achilles tendon rupture (p. 368)	

Table 14.1 Overview of the differential diagnosis of acute ankle injuries.

Diagnostic Thinking

Most ankle injuries should be treated at the primary-care level. Usually, the main problem is distinguishing between lateral ligament injuries and fractures of the lateral malleolus. Fractures at the base of the fifth metatarsal and syndesmosis injuries are routinely overlooked during the initial examination. This is also true of very rare tendon injuries. A precise clinical examination is necessary to determine whether the patient should be referred for X rays to exclude a fracture. If the patient needs X rays, they should be obtained immediately. If surgery is required for an ankle fracture, it should occur within 6 hours of the injury, before there is excessive swelling.

Thus, the goal of the clinical examination during the acute stage is to determine whether the patient has a lateral ligament injury or some other injury that may require early immobilization or acute surgical treatment. If the most important diagnoses can be excluded by means of the clinical examination, additional examinations are unnecessary during the acute stage.

Clinical History

A precise description of the injury mechanism is essential to establishing the proper diagnosis, particularly for less common injuries.

Inversion trauma (figure 14.1), which causes about 85% of all ankle injuries, usually damages the lateral ligaments in younger patients. Three anatomically and functionally separate units—the anterior talofibular, the calcaneofibular, and the posterior talofibular ligaments—provide ligamentous support on the lateral aspect of the ankle. Normally, the anterior talofibular ligament (ATFL) is injured first (about 50% of acute ankle sprain injuries are isolated ruptures of the ATFL). Once the ATFL fails, the calcaneofibular ligament may then also fail, and only in rare cases (about 1%) are all three of the lateral ligaments injured. The proportion of patients with combined ligamentous damage (i.e., trauma to both the anterior talofibular and the calcaneofibular ligaments) is higher among patients who have been previously injured.

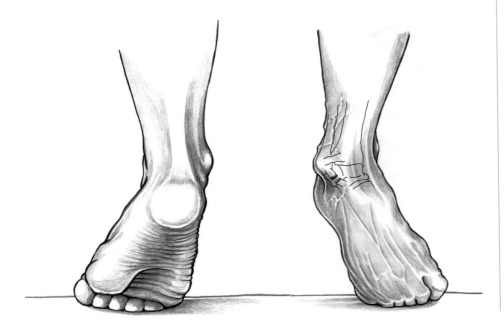

Figure 14.1 Inversion trauma. This is the most common mechanism of injury for ankle sprains. Injuries occur as the ankle is internally rotated and supinated when the athlete lands in plantar flexion. The most common injury is an isolated tear of the anterior talofibular ligament (as shown).

Young patients seldom sustain fractures as a result of moderate trauma (e.g., that typically incurred in an inversion injury while running). If the mechanism of injury involves greater force (e.g., that caused by a jump from a height of 2 m or more), fracture should be suspected, usually in combination with a syndesmosis injury. In older patients, however, moderate inversion trauma commonly causes fractures of either the lateral malleolus or the base of the fifth metatarsal. Avulsion fractures of the fifth metatarsal occur because the most important active stabilizer against inversion trauma, the peroneal musculature, is activated to control the foot so the athlete can make a safe, flat-footed landing and thus avoid ligament injuries.

Eversion trauma usually results in injury to the deltoid ligament (a continuous ligamentous unit that runs along the entire medial malleolus). Medial ligament injuries occur with or without simultaneous syndesmosis injuries and fractures of the lateral malleolus. Isolated ligament injuries on the medial side are rare, totaling only 1% to 2% of all the ligament injuries in the ankle. There are probably several reasons for this, including a natural movement pattern in which landing occurs with the foot in plantar flexion and slight supination. Another important factor, however, may be that the deltoid ligament has greater tensile strength than do the lateral ligaments. For that reason, eversion injuries (when they occur) usually include fractures or syndesmosis trauma, in addition to the medial ligament injury. In rare cases, eversion injuries may result in an isolated syndesmosis injury or peroneal tendon dislocation.

Strict external rotation trauma may cause an isolated anterior syndesmosis injury. If the ankle is locked in an approximately neutral position with limited plantar or dorsiflexion, forceful external rotation of the ankle may cause the tibia and the fibula to be separated so that the anterior syndesmosis tears. This may occur, for example, if the ankle is locked in a downhill ski boot, ski jumping boot, or hockey skate (figure 14.2).

If an athlete lands flatfooted after jumping from a great height (usually more than 2 m) a calcaneal fracture or some other less common fracture must be suspected.

Clinical Examination

Inspection. A lateral ligament injury usually causes swelling anterior to and inferior to the lateral malleolus. Swelling may accumulate quickly and may be quite pronounced. However, athletes, in particular, are likely to have received such good acute treatment (with compression and cooling) that there is minimal or no swelling by the time the patient is examined. If the examiner is unaware of the treatment already received, an injury may be overlooked or underestimated. Ice massage and cold treatment can provide such good pain relief that palpatory tenderness may be significantly reduced as well.

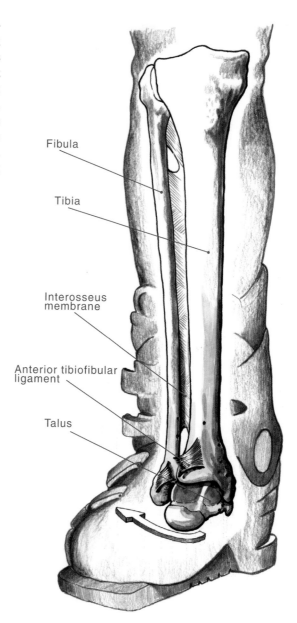

Fibula

Tibia

Interosseus membrane

Anterior tibiofibular ligament

Talus

Figure 14.2 External rotational injury with a syndesmosis rupture. If the foot is locked in neutral or slight dorsiflexion in a downhill ski boot or ice hockey skate, an isolated rupture in the anterior syndesmosis may occur (in addition to injury to the ATFL).

ANKLE

Palpation. Thorough palpation is the most important element of the physical examination. The practitioner should recall that the anterior talofibular ligament is anterior to and just inferior to the tip of the fibula. According to the Ottawa rules, emphasis should be placed on palpation of the following four structures: the lateral malleolus, the medial malleolus, the base of the fifth metatarsal, and the navicular bone (as shown in figure 14.3). Targeted examination of these four structures offers 100% sensitivity for clinically significant fractures, with 59% specificity. Hence, it is necessary to obtain X rays only if the palpatory exam is positive.

Neuromuscular function. It is seldom possible to fully evaluate neuromuscular function during the acute stage of ankle injuries, because the athlete often is limited by significant pain inhibition. Nevertheless, it is usually possible to check peroneal muscle function, to palpate the course of the tendon, and to determine whether an injured retinaculum or a rupture of the peroneus brevis tendon's insertion on the fifth metatarsal is likely. A patient who was able to contract his peroneal muscles in an attempt to dynamically stabilize the ankle and protect himself against an injury will often be tender to palpation over the peroneal musculature itself, because the mechanism of injury may have eccentrically overloaded the peroneal muscle-tendon unit, resulting in a partial muscle tear and significant strain injury. Often, the damage recurs in the tendon down toward the tendon insertion. Frequently, the first indication of such an injury is pronounced stiffness in the musculature after the injury. Neuromuscular function should be monitored during the rehabilitation stage, particularly before the athlete returns to competitive sport. Function can be evaluated by means of a simple test (see page 410).

Syndesmosis tests. One "specific" syndesmosis test is called the squeeze test (figure 14.4), which is performed by squeezing the fibula and the tibia together in the middle of the lower leg. If this compression causes pain distally in the region of the syndesmosis, an injury should be suspected there. Of course, if the test is positive, the patient also needs to be evaluated for alternative diagnoses, such as fracture of the fibula or tibia, compartment syndrome, or contusion injury of the lower leg musculature. An alternative test is the external rotation test (figure 14.4). This test is performed in the same manner as that previously described as the mechanism of syndesmosis injury

Figure 14.3 Ottawa ankle rules. Palpate along the mid-margin of the fibula and tibia, the base of the fifth metatarsal, and above the navicular bone. If the patient does not have palpatory tenderness in these areas and can bear weight on the affected limb, obtaining an X ray is not necessary during the acute stage.

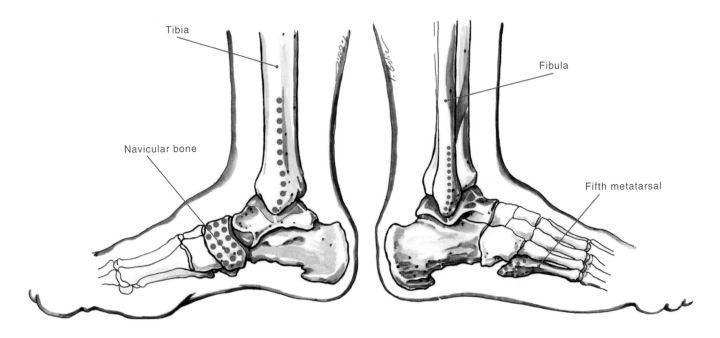

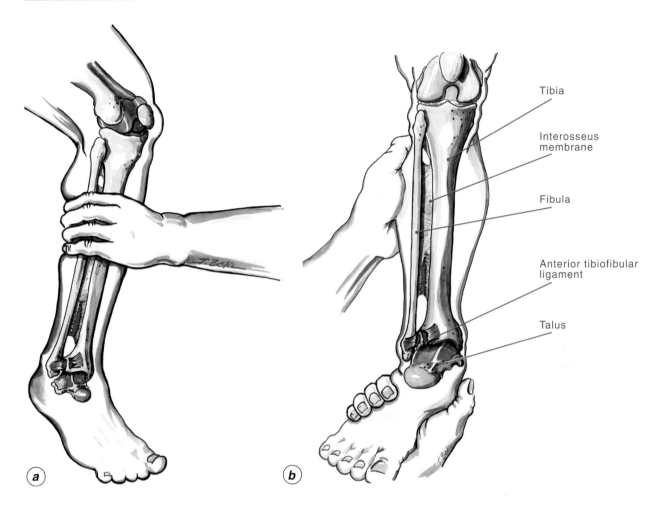

(a)

(b)

Tibia

Interosseus membrane

Fibula

Anterior tibiofibular ligament

Talus

among downhill skiers. Pain in the syndesmosis area caused by external rotation in a neutral position may indicate an injury to the anterior syndesmosis. In addition, a syndesmosis injury usually causes pain when the ankle is placed in forced dorsiflexion. Combined with the findings on palpation, these tests are sensitive indicators of whether or not the patient has suffered a syndesmosis injury.

Stress tests. Two stress tests—the anterior drawer test and the talar tilt test (see page 410)—are used to evaluate the integrity of the lateral ligaments and the mechanical stability of the ankle. The principle behind these tests is that it should be possible to grade lateral ligament injuries. However, in practice, this may be difficult to accomplish during the acute stage. In addition, the choice of treatment is not dependent on an accurate pathoanatomical grading of these injuries; therefore, there is no basis for emphasizing stress tests during the acute stage of an ankle injury.

Supplemental Examinations

Radiographic examination. Unless the clinical examination has created the suspicion of a fracture (see the Ottawa ankle rules) or of a syndesmosis injury, there is no reason to routinely obtain X rays of patients with acute ankle injuries. If X rays are taken, a standard ankle series should include frontal, lateral, and a mortise view (which shows the talus projected in the ankle mortise). The practitioner should look for malleolar fractures and syndesmosis injuries in particular. Syndesmosis injuries may cause lateral displacement of the talus or increased mortise width (figure 14.12). Sometimes eggshell-shaped avulsion fractures from the tip of the fibula are visible

Figure 14.4 Syndesmosis tests. The squeeze test *(a)* is performed by squeezing the fibula and tibia together in the middle of the lower leg, whereas the external rotation test *(b)* is performed by externally rotating the foot with the ankle in neutral (90°). The tests are considered positive if they cause pain in the syndesmosis area; they usually do not result in significant pain if an isolated lateral ligament injury has occurred.

ANKLE

where the anterior talofibular and the calcaneofibular ligaments may have pulled away from their ligamentous insertions.

Other X rays may be indicated in special cases:

- Oblique images may help if a malleolar fracture is suspected and the standard ankle series proves difficult to evaluate.
- If a fracture at the base of the fifth metatarsal is suspected, frontal and lateral images of the fifth metatarsal should be ordered.
- An examination under fluoroscopy may be useful in evaluating syndesmosis injuries but should be administered by an orthopedic surgeon.

Common Injuries

Lateral Ligament Injuries

Injuries to the lateral ankle ligaments are usually classified according to the number of ligaments that were torn (figure 14.5). Grade I is defined as a partial rupture of the anterior talofibular ligament and/or the calcaneofibular ligament; grade II, as a total rupture of the anterior talofibular ligament, but with an intact calcaneofibular ligament; and grade III, as a total rupture of the anterior talofibular ligament and the calcaneofibular ligament. Partial ruptures are uncommon, so the patient almost always has a grade II or grade III injury.

Early functional treatment is always indicated for grade I and II injuries, whereas immobilization in a cast, surgical treatment, and functional treatment have all been used for grade III injuries. However, functional treatment of grade III injuries provides mechanical stability that is nearly equal to that achieved by other methods, and it provides full mobility and full function earlier than the other treatment alternatives. Therefore, most caregivers prefer functional treatment for all lateral ligament injuries. Nevertheless, there are special cases where surgical treatment may be indicated for

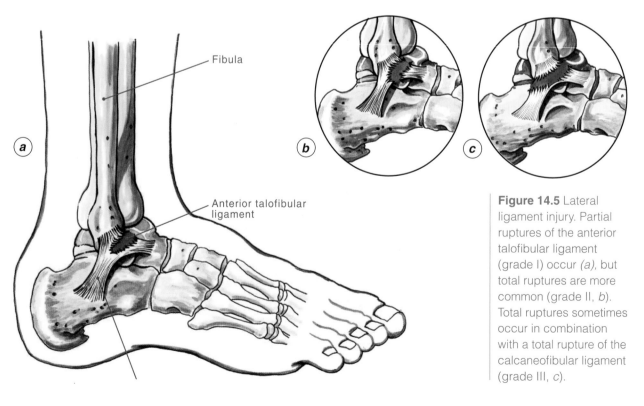

Fibula

Anterior talofibular ligament

Figure 14.5 Lateral ligament injury. Partial ruptures of the anterior talofibular ligament (grade I) occur *(a)*, but total ruptures are more common (grade II, *b*). Total ruptures sometimes occur in combination with a total rupture of the calcaneofibular ligament (grade III, *c*).

an active athlete who sustains a severe grade III injury for the first time. In general, however, it is not necessary to distinguish among grade I, II, and III injuries by means of stress tests or diagnostic imaging during the acute stage.

- Symptoms and signs: Patients experience swelling and tenderness anterior and inferior to the lateral malleolus. Pain and early swelling are usually distinctly localized over the affected ligaments in patients examined immediately after the injury occurs. However, many patients do not seek medical attention until 1 or 2 days after the injury occurs, and they often have significant swelling and ecchymosis diffusely on the lateral aspect of the ankle. In such cases, it may be difficult to distinguish between ligament injuries and fractures.
- Diagnosis: The diagnosis is made clinically, but X rays with a standard ankle series are indicated to exclude fractures or syndesmosis injuries in patients with significant pain on palpatory exam, in accordance with the Ottawa ankle rules or a positive syndesmosis test. The anterior drawer test and the talar tilt test (see page 410) are of little value during the acute stage.
- Treatment by physician: During the acute stage (i.e., the first 48 hours) the goal is to limit bleeding, and this is best achieved through intensive PRICE treatment and inloading the affected limb with crutches. Effective compression is crucial. Treatment with nonsteroidal anti-inflammatory drugs (NSAIDs) should begin as soon as possible. The patient should be given maximum doses, and the treatment should be continued for 4 or 5 days, provided that there are no contraindications. This therapy offers good analgesia and enables more rapid mobilization of the patient. The patient who arrives at the doctor's office more than 24 hours after being injured should be mobilized immediately with an orthosis.
- Treatment by physical therapist: The patient should be referred to a physical therapist after 2 days, for the purpose of obtaining detailed instructions for rehabilitation exercises (see page n) and possibly for instruction on taping the ankle or fitting the orthosis. No definite effects from ultrasound, electrotherapy, electricity, laser, or the like have been documented.
- Prognosis: The prognosis is good. The injured ligament usually heals in 6 to 8 weeks, at least by scarring of the joint capsule, but full function can be achieved earlier with good treatment during the acute stage. However, 10% to 20% of the patients have persisting problems after an acute ankle injury. Therefore, the patient should be told to contact his physician if he has late symptoms.

Other Injuries

Medial Ligament Injuries

Eversion injuries may cause an incomplete tear of the deltoid ligament (figure 14.6). Medial ligament injuries are also seen in combination with malleolar fractures or lateral ligament injuries.

- Symptoms and signs: The main findings are tenderness to palpation and swelling under the medial malleolus. If a total rupture of the deltoid ligament occurs, a defect can often be palpated in the ligament.
- Diagnosis: The diagnosis is made clinically, but X rays (including a standard ankle series) are indicated to exclude fractures or syndesmosis injuries in patients with positive exam findings (in accordance with the Ottawa ankle rules) or if the syndesmosis test is positive.

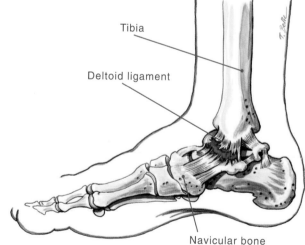

Tibia

Deltoid ligament

Navicular bone

Figure 14.6 Medial ligament injury. Far less common than lateral injuries, medial injuries should be suspected with eversion trauma.

ANKLE

- Treatment: PRICE treatment, orthoses, and functional treatment are all used for isolated medial ligament injuries in the same manner as that for lateral ligament injuries. A medial arch support can also provide some pain relief.
- Prognosis: The prognosis is good, but the progression is generally slower than for lateral ligament injuries.

Fracture at the Base of the Fifth Metatarsal

Inversion injuries may cause a fracture at the base of the fifth metatarsal. These fractures are caused by strong mechanical traction from the lateral bands of the plantar fascia or the peroneus brevis tendon on a weight-bearing inverted foot. There are three types of fractures in the area: avulsion fractures (most common), oblique fractures through the diaphyseal-metaphyseal junction (true Jones fractures), and a fracture through the diaphysis (figures 14.7 and 14.8). The former two are acute fractures, whereas a diaphysis fracture is usually a stress fracture (see page 416).

- Symptoms and signs: The main finding that makes it easy to distinguish this injury from lateral ligament injuries is distinct tenderness to palpation over the base of the fifth metatarsal (figure 14.3). It is palpated as a marked prominence along the lateral edge of the foot. Swelling eventually occurs but is often minimal on the day the injury occurs.
- Diagnosis: The diagnosis is made using X rays of the fifth metatarsal (lateral and frontal views to reveal displacement or angulation and, if necessary, oblique views to look for periosteal reaction). The images must be carefully examined to distinguish between avulsion fractures (figures 14.7 and 14.8) and oblique fractures through the diaphyseal-metaphyseal junction (true Jones fractures) (figure 14.7). In addition, stress fractures often present with acute pain after a lopsided landing, but these fractures usually go through the diaphysis.
- Treatment: Avulsion fractures without significant dislocation will usually heal with functional treatment. Immobilization is necessary only as long as needed to reduce pain. Generally, the patient may bear weight without pain after 1 or 2 weeks, followed by mobilization and rehabilitation as soon as symptoms allow. True Jones fractures go through a zone with a poorer blood supply, and late healing and the development of pseudoarthrosis are more likely to occur. Jones fractures without displacement may be treated by immobilization in a cast for 4 weeks without bearing weight, after which a walking cast is used for 4 weeks. An orthopedic surgeon should evaluate Jones fractures with displacement for possible repositioning and fixation using intermedullary compression screws. Surgical fixation may also be indicated for an athlete who wants to return to sport early, even if there is no malalignment. Stress fractures should also be evaluated to determine if surgical fixation is indicated.
- Prognosis: The prognosis is good for avulsion fractures, and function usually returns to normal in 4 to 6 weeks. However, it is necessary to watch for Jones fractures and acute fractures that are based on stress fractures.

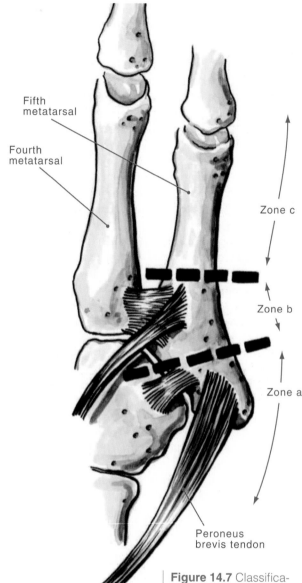

Fifth metatarsal

Fourth metatarsal

Zone c

Zone b

Zone a

Peroneus brevis tendon

Figure 14.7 Classification of fractures of the fifth metatarsal. Acute fractures are usually avulsion fractures (zone a) or oblique fractures through the diaphyseal-metaphyseal junction (so-called Jones fractures, zone b). The third type of fracture, the diaphyseal fracture (zone c), occurs primarily as a stress fracture. Different fracture types have different treatments; therefore, it is important to distinguish between them.

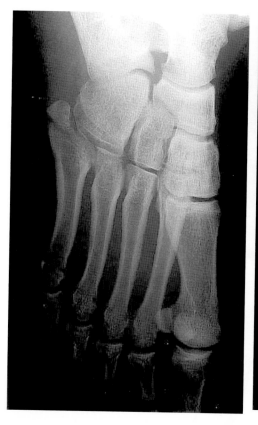

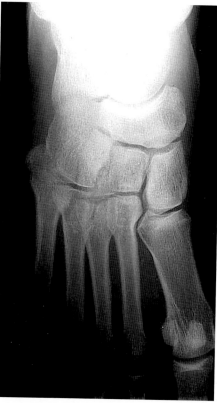

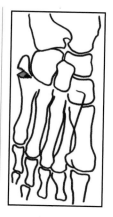

Figure 14.8 Avulsion fracture through the base of the fifth metatarsal.

Malleolar Fractures

Generally, fractures of the lateral malleolus tend to occur in isolation. However, with forceful trauma these fractures often occur in combination with medial malleolar fractures (bimalleolar fractures) or fractures of the posterior malleolus (trimalleolar fractures), especially in older adults. Fractures are usually also accompanied by ligament injuries or syndesmosis injuries. Ankle fractures can be classified according to the location of the fracture line through the lateral malleolus (AO-classification, figure 14.9).

- Symptoms and signs: Symptoms include significant swelling, positive Ottawa ankle rules signs, and obvious malalignment (if the fracture is dislocated). To reduce the risk of skin damage, dislocated ankle fractures must be reduced and stabilized immediately—before sending the patient for X rays or taking other measures.
- Diagnosis: The diagnosis is made with a standard X ray ankle series. Extra oblique images may be helpful if standard images prove difficult to interpret. If a distal fracture has occurred, the entire fibula should be palpated, and if local palpation reveals proximal tenderness, X rays of the entire lower leg, including the proximal fibula, should be obtained. Skin color should be assessed, as should distal capillary filling and the pulse in the dorsalis pedis and the posterior tibial arteries. Distal skin sensitivity should also be evaluated.
- Treatment principles: The main goal of treatment is to maintain (for fractures that are not dislocated) or restore (for dislocated fractures) the normal relationship between the superior articular surface of the talus and the articular surfaces of the tibia and fibula. A malalignment of as little as a couple of millimeters can change the loading pattern of the joints and increase the risk of osteoarthritis. The practitioner should remember to evaluate whether the fracture line through the lateral malleolus is under, in, or above the syndesmosis. Ankle fractures in children often

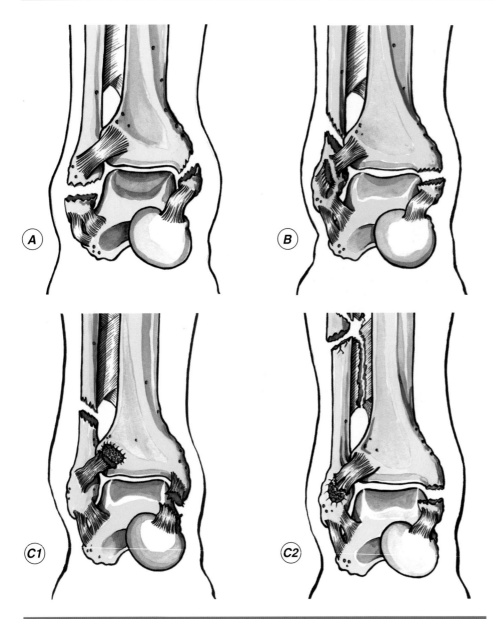

Type	Syndesmosis rupture (%)	Dominant force
A	0	Supination
B	50	External rotation
C1	100	Pronation
C2	100	Pronation

Figure 14.9 Classification of ankle fractures (AO classification).

damage the growth zones in the distal fibula and tibia. This may cause growth disturbance that eventually results in asymmetry in the ankle.

• Treatment of type A fractures (figure 14.9): Eggshell-shaped avulsion fractures from the tip of the lateral malleolus are treated in the same manner as ligament injuries, with early mobilization and functional treatment. Lateral malleolar fractures below the syndesmosis are stable if the medial malleolus is intact. These fractures may also be treated functionally with an orthosis and loading as soon as pain and swelling allow.

- Treatment of type B fractures (figures 14.9 and 14.10): Lateral malleolar fractures (at the syndesmosis level) without significant malalignment are treated with a walking cast for 4 to 6 weeks. Loading is permitted as soon as pain and swelling permit. If malalignment is more than 2 mm and the talus is displaced laterally, the fracture is probably unstable with a simultaneous medial injury (either a rupture of the deltoid ligament or a fracture of the medial malleolus). Patients should be referred immediately to an orthopedic surgeon to evaluate the need for surgery.
- Treatment of type C fractures (figure 14.9): These fractures are characterized by a high fibula fracture, a syndesmosis rupture, and a rupture of the interosseous membrane. These are unstable fractures, and patients who sustain them should

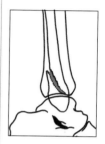

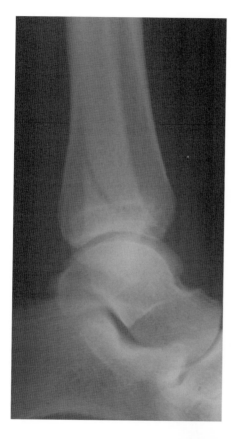

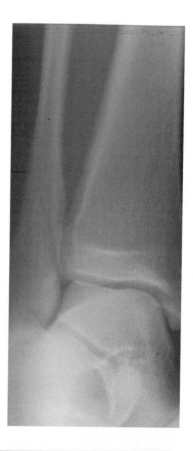

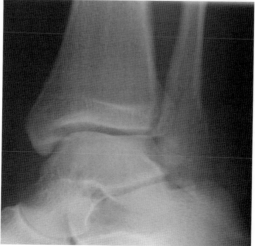

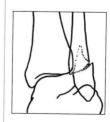

Figure 14.10 Type A lateral malleolar fracture.

be referred immediately to an orthopedic surgeon to evaluate for surgical treatment. The fracture should be roughly reduced and stabilized before the patient is transported to the hospital. Grasp the heel, pull it in the longitudinal direction, and carefully push the tibia posteriorly, if necessary. Apply a mediolateral U-cast before the patient is transported to the hospital.

• Treatment of type epiphysiolysis fractures in children: Often no changes in the epiphyseal line are visible on the X ray. The diagnosis is made clinically if the patient has distinct tenderness to palpation over the epiphyseal line. It may be helpful to compare X rays of both ankles. Growth plate injuries without malalignment should be treated with a short walking cast for 3 to 4 weeks. However, if malalignment is present, the patient should be referred to an orthopedic surgeon for immediate evaluation.

Syndesmosis Injury—Injury to the Ligament Between the Fibula and the Tibia !

A partial or total rupture of the anterior syndesmosis (anterior inferior tibiofibular ligament) (figure 14.11) usually occurs in combination with medial ligament injuries or malleolar fractures. Type A fractures of the lateral malleolus (figure 14.9) rarely involve syndesmosis injuries, type B involve syndesmosis injuries in 50% of the cases, and type C fractures almost always involve syndesmosis injuries. Isolated syndesmosis ruptures can also result from strict external rotating trauma—for example, in a downhill ski boot (figure 14.2).

• Symptoms and signs: Patients experience mild to moderate swelling and maximal tenderness to palpation over the syndesmosis directly proximal to the joint space. A positive squeeze test, a positive external rotation test, and pain from forced dorsiflexion indicate syndesmosis injuries. Patients who are suspected of having a syndesmosis injury must be carefully examined to rule out this type of injury or any other lower limb ligamentous injury or fracture. The proximal fibula should also be examined for possible fracture.

• Diagnosis: The diagnosis is made clinically, but X rays of the ankle are necessary. In such cases, X rays must include the entire fibula. If the patient has a total syndesmosis rupture, widening of the ankle mortise (figure 14.12) will be visible on the X ray. If the practitioner is uncertain about the diagnosis, the patient should be referred to a specialist who can examine him under fluoroscopy or who can request stress X rays, scintigraphy, or magnetic resonance imaging (MRI) as appropriate.

• Treatment by physician: The treatment is the same PRICE treatment that is given for lateral ligament injuries. Partial ruptures are treated functionally, although a period of immobilization (often 2 weeks or longer) in a walking cast may be necessary until the patient can load the affected limb without pain. The patient should be mobilized, and rehabilitation should begin as soon as pain allows. Total ruptures with diastasis are treated surgically with syndesmosis screws, occasionally with concomitant suturing of the ligament, and cast immobilization for 8 weeks. Partial weight bearing, within the limits of pain, is allowed after 3 or 4 weeks. Untreated total syndesmosis ruptures may lead to ankle osteoarthritis.

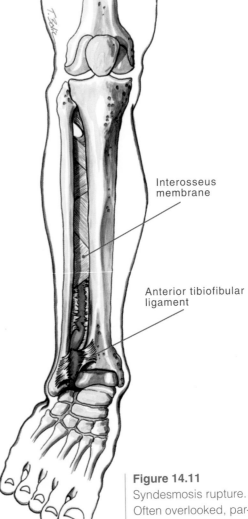

Interosseus membrane

Anterior tibiofibular ligament

Figure 14.11
Syndesmosis rupture. Often overlooked, particularly when isolated and occurring as a result of pure external rotational trauma inside a hockey skate or downhill ski boot.

• Treatment by physical therapist: The training program should emphasize mobility training, strength training, and neuromuscular function. This is particularly true if the patient was surgically treated and subsequently immobilized for a time.

• Prognosis: If the patient has a partial syndesmosis rupture, the rehabilitation period for accompanying ligament injuries or fractures often becomes prolonged. If the patient has an isolated total syndesmosis injury, it will usually take 4 to 6 months before he can return to competitive activity. Ossification of the ligament (synostosis) may occur. This is characterized by increasing stiffness and pain with activity (e.g., kicking) 3 to 12 months after the injury.

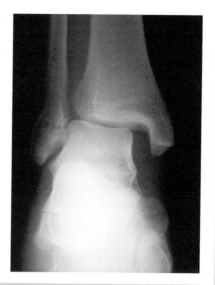

Figure 14.12
Syndesmosis rupture. An X ray of a total syndesmosis injury demonstrates widening of the ankle mortise, resulting in increased space between the fibula and the talus.

Ankle Dislocation

A dislocated ankle is a rare injury (figure 14.13), caused by landing at high speed, falling from a great height in an inverted or everted position, or external trauma to the weight-bearing foot.

• Symptoms and signs: The patient may experience significant swelling, obvious deformity, total ankle dysfunction, and pain. To reduce the risk of skin damage that may complicate further treatment, dislocated ankles should be reduced and stabilized immediately, before the patient is sent to the hospital.

• Diagnosis: The diagnosis is based on the obvious malalignment, but it may be difficult to distinguish a dislocated ankle from fractures (bi- or trimalleolar). The practitioner should check skin color, distal capillary filling, and the pulse in the dorsalis pedis artery and in the posterior tibial artery. Distal sensitivity should also be checked.

• Treatment by physician: The dislocation is reduced by grasping the heel and forefoot and pulling in the longitudinal direction. A splint that resembles a high U-cast should be applied before the patient is transported to the hospital. The patient should be referred immediately to an orthopedic surgeon for evaluation for possible surgery. However, immobilization in a cast is normally the preferred treatment.

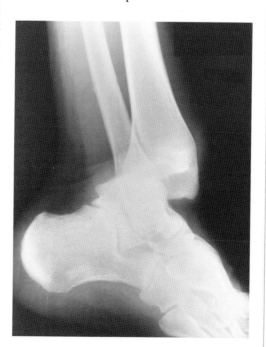

Figure 14.13 Dislocated ankle.

Talar Fractures

A talar fracture is also a rare injury and may result from a fall from a height, from forceful involuntary plantar flexion, or inversion or eversion injuries. The fracture may go through the body or the neck of the talus (figure 14.14). Snowboard ankle is a rare type of fracture through the lateral process of the talus. This type of fracture constitutes about 3% of the ankle injuries sustained by snowboarders. Major portions of the talus are intra-articular, and the talus does not have any muscle insertions. Therefore, the bone has a poor blood supply, and talar fractures tend to heal late with a risk of avascular necrosis.

- Symptoms and signs: Symptoms include swelling and tenderness inferior to the malleoli or in front of the anterior joint space, in addition to pain upon weight bearing.
- Diagnosis: The diagnosis is usually made with a standard ankle series, but a computed tomography (CT) scan may be indicated, to document the fracture in more detail. Snowboard ankle is rarely visible on a standard X ray, so the patient should be imaged with a CT scan if there is continuous lateral ankle pain after an acute ankle injury (particularly if the patient is a snowboarder).
- Treatment by physician: The patient should be referred immediately to an orthopedic surgeon to evaluate the need for surgery.

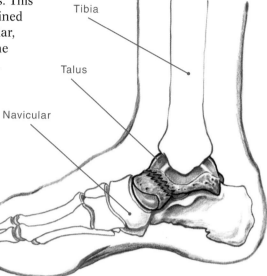

Figure 14.14 Talar fractures. Typical location of a talar fracture, through the neck of the talus. Other types of talar fractures do also occur, with dislocation.

Dislocation/Rupture of the Peroneal Tendons

The peroneal tendons may be injured in the area posterior to the lateral malleolus, particularly as the result of a forceful contraction with the ankle in plantar flexion and eversion. This may result in longitudinal trauma to the tendon in this area, or in tearing of the peroneal retinaculum, so that the tendon may dislocate anteriorly over the lateral malleolus in some positions, particularly in dorsiflexion (figure 14.15). Partial

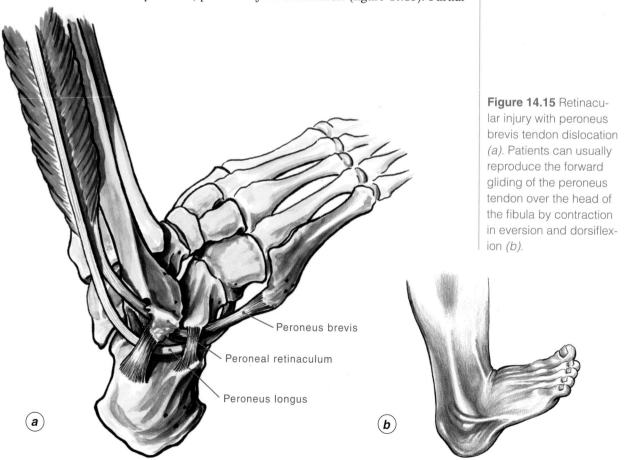

Peroneus brevis

Peroneal retinaculum

Peroneus longus

a

b

Figure 14.15 Retinacular injury with peroneus brevis tendon dislocation *(a)*. Patients can usually reproduce the forward gliding of the peroneus tendon over the head of the fibula by contraction in eversion and dorsiflexion *(b)*.

ruptures of the distal portion of the peroneus brevis tendon down (toward the tendinous insertion on the base of the fifth metatarsal) also occur with inversion trauma.

- Symptoms and signs: The athlete often states that she heard a crack or felt something snapping behind the lateral malleolus. The patient can often reproduce this snapping during the examination if the peroneal tendons are dislocated. The easiest way to do this is to have the patient contract the peroneal musculature with the foot in eversion and dorsiflexion. The entire tendon can be seen and palpated over the lateral malleolus. Some patients have a subluxation condition where the gliding cannot be reproduced. If there is a partial rupture, the tendon is usually tender and thickened in the affected area.
- Diagnosis: The diagnosis is based on symptoms and on the clinical examination, but a standard X ray of the ankle is indicated. In 15% to 50% of the patients, an avulsion fracture of the posterior groove of the lateral malleolus is visible. This type of avulsion fracture is pathognomonic for the diagnosis. Subluxation makes the diagnosis more difficult, and it is usually made late.
- Treatment by physician: If a peroneal tendon injury is suspected, the patient should be referred to an orthopedic surgeon for surgical treatment, which is usually performed acutely. In some cases, a piece of felt can be taped to the ankle behind the lateral malleolus to hold the peroneal tendons in place, so that the athlete can finish the season.

ANKLE

Pain in the Ankle Region

Roald Bahr

Definition

Painful conditions in the ankle area are discussed in this section. Sometimes, over-use injuries occur because of a single hard or unusually difficult training session, but generally, the pain starts gradually, over several days or weeks. This section also describes disorders that may occur in an ankle that was previously sprained, because the main symptom in such situations is usually gradually progressing pain.

Differential Diagnosis

Table 14.2 provides an overview of the diagnosis most relevant to chronic ankle pain. Pain in the heel region, in the midfoot, and in the forefoot are discussed in other chapters. The most common cause of ankle pain is a previous ankle sprain. These sprains can result in osteochondral injuries, synovitis, or recurrent instability. The symptoms may have persisted after an acute injury or may present long after the injury occurred. The patient does not always make the connection between the pain and the previous ankle sprain(s). Stress fractures are also often overlooked. Less common causes of ankle pain (but which are also often related to previous ankle sprain injuries) are sinus tarsi syndrome, syndesmosis injuries, anterior or posterior impingement, ruptures of the tibialis posterior tendon, other injury to the peroneal or the tibialis posterior tendons, and reflex sympathetic dystrophy (also known as complex regional pain syndrome, type I). Other painful conditions are rare, although a few of them may be typical for certain sports.

Most common	Less common	Must not be overlooked
Osteochondral injuries (p. 411)	Sinus tarsi syndrome (p. 413)	Complex regional pain syndrome (p. 418)
Synovitis of the ankle joint (p. 412)	Soccer ankle (anterior impingement) (p. 414)	
Chronic instability (p. 412)	Ballet ankle (posterior impingement) (p. 415)	
	Stress fractures (p. 416)	
	Tibialis posterior syndrome (p. 417)	
	Nerve entrapment (p. 418)	
	Osteoarthritis (p. 418)	

Table 14.2 Overview of the differential diagnosis of ankle pain.

Diagnostic Thinking

If the pain appears to be related to a previous ankle injury (which may have occurred in the remote past), a primary goal of the physical examination is to determine whether there are osteochondral fractures or chronic instability. For athletes who load the ankle in extreme positions, such as soccer players, ballet dancers, and gymnasts, anterior or posterior impingement disorders should be suspected. Athletes who repeatedly load the foot at high intensity must always be evaluated for possible stress fractures. Fortunately, the affected structures within the ankle are superficial and easily palpated. The initial evaluation of patients with ankle injuries should take place at the primary-care level, but a number of conditions require further evaluation by a specialist.

Clinical History

Patients must be thoroughly examined with respect to previous ankle injuries. Patients with a history of ankle trauma usually complain primarily of pain (e.g., from osteochondral fractures, chronic synovitis, sinus tarsi syndrome). They may also experience a feeling of instability or weakness that can be mechanical or functional. In other patients, the history may indicate overuse, particularly from running (e.g., stress fractures, tibialis posterior syndrome), ballet, gymnastics, or soccer dorsiflexion. The practitioner should carefully document the location of pain, instability problems, and any other accompanying symptoms.

Clinical Examination

Inspection. Malalignment is an important predisposing factor to overuse injuries in the ankle area. The patient should be examined while standing and walking, the arch of the foot should be evaluated, and any increased tendency for overpronation or varus/valgus positioning should be assessed. Tibialis posterior dysfunction is indicated if the patient has visible asymmetry with increased unilateral valgus in the hind foot and a positive "too many toes" sign on that side. The practitioner should also evaluate function by having the patient jump and run.

Palpation. All relevant structures—the lateral malleolus, the medial malleolus, the navicular bone, the sinus tarsi, the course of the peroneal tendons, and the course of the tibialis posterior tendon—should be carefully palpated. The ankle and subtalar joints should also be palpated. It may be necessary to have the patient go for a run or do something similar to provoke symptoms before the examination. A positive Tinel sign and radiating pain provoked by lightly tapping over the posterior tibial nerve suggests tarsal tunnel syndrome.

Movement. Active and passive range of motion should be examined. Pain at the end range with forced plantar or dorsiflexion may indicate posterior (ballet ankle) or anterior (soccer ankle) impingement. Pain at maximum inversion or eversion may indicate an osteochondral injury. Normal range of motion in the ankle joint is 20° dorsiflexion, 30° to 50° plantar flexion, 15° to 30° pronation, and 45° to 60° supination. The best way to evaluate range of motion is by comparing the injured ankle with the uninjured one.

Stress tests. The integrity of the ligaments and the mechanical stability of the ankle can be evaluated with the help of two stress tests: the anterior drawer test and the talar tilt test. If the patient has a ruptured anterior talofibular ligament, anterior translation will be increased during the anterior drawer test (figure 14.16). If the

Figure 14.16 Anterior drawer test. The anterior drawer test is performed by holding the calcaneus with the foot resting on the forearm in slight plantar flexion, bringing the foot forward in relation to the tibia. The knee should be flexed to make it easier for the patient to relax completely. Movement occurs around an imaginary medial axis through the intact deltoid ligament.

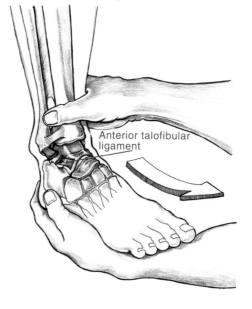

Anterior talofibular ligament

ANKLE

calcaneofibular ligament is also torn, increased supination will be present on the involved side during the talar tilt test (figure 14.17). The practitioner should compare responses to the stability tests on the symptomatic ankle with responses to tests of the ankle on the uninjured side.

Neuromuscular function. The practitioner should assess the integrity of the peroneal and the tibialis posterior tendons and should palpate the course of the tendons.

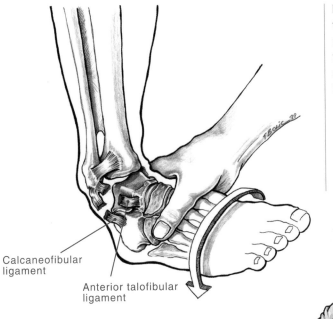

Calcaneofibular ligament

Anterior talofibular ligament

Figure 14.17 Talar tilt test. The talar tilt test is performed by supinating the foot while holding the calcaneus, with the foot in a neutral position.

Neuromuscular function is extremely important to the functional stability of the ankle and is often reduced after a previous ankle injury. Function can be evaluated by means of a simple balance test where the patient stands on one leg with his arms crossed over his chest while looking straight ahead (figure 14.18, basic position). Normally, the patient should be able to accomplish this using only his ankle to correct balance. If the patient is forced to use his hips, knees, or upper body to correct balance, or if he loses his balance, the test result is pathological (table 14.3). The practitioner should evaluate function by comparing it with the opposite side as well.

Supplemental Examinations

If the patient is suspected of having a tendon injury, diagnostic imaging is usually not indicated. X rays of the ankle joint, which often demonstrate ossification or accessory bones in lateral images, are indicated if either anterior or posterior impingement is suspected. However, routine X rays have low sensitivity for detecting suspected osteochondral fractures or stress fractures. Skeletal

Evaluation	Quantitative (time)	Qualitative (movement pattern)
Above normal	Stands on one leg for 1 minute	Uses only the ankle to correct balance the entire time, then manages to stand with his eyes closed for 15 s without losing his balance
Normal	Stands on one leg for 1 minute	Manages >45 s using only the ankle to correct balance
Slightly abnormal	Stands on one leg for 1 minute	Has to correct balance with the knees, hips, and upper body once in a while; otherwise makes corrections using the ankle
Abnormal	Stands on one leg for 1 minute, but sometimes uses the other leg for support	Unable to correct balance with the ankle alone; has to use the knees, hips, and upper body the entire time
Severely abnormal	Manages to stand on one leg, but only for short periods	

Table 14.3 Classification of neuromuscular function in the ankle joint.

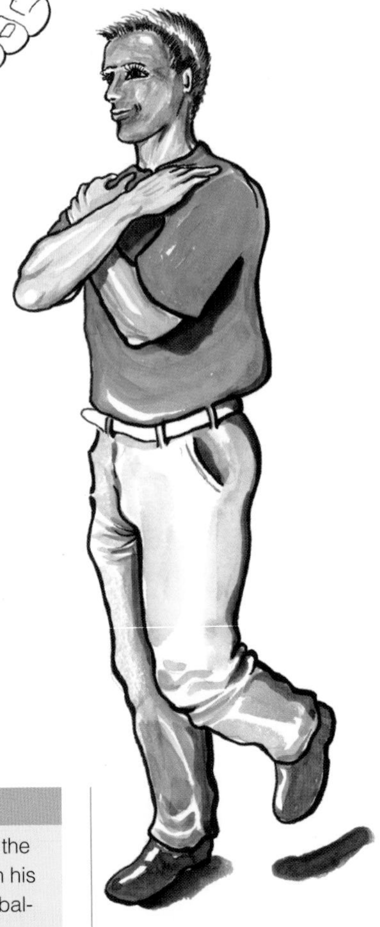

Figure 14.18 Balance test. The patient stands on one leg with the other leg slightly flexed at the knee. He crosses his arms over his chest and looks at a point straight ahead. If he can balance for one minute with his eyes open, he closes his eyes and balances for another 15 seconds.

scintigraphy is required to exclude this type of injury. Positive skeletal scintigraphy generally indicates the need for MRI or a CT scan.

Common Injuries

Osteochondral Injuries

Osteochondral fractures and chondral injuries are common after ankle sprains, particularly when the injury is caused by landing from a jump or by high-speed running. Inversion trauma causes the talus to tilt in the ankle mortise, inflicting a compression injury on the upper medial corner of the talus (figure 14.19). Correspondingly, cartilage or bone on the articular surfaces of the tibia and fibula may be injured. The injury may vary from minor (compression of the bone) to major (a separated piece of bone forming a loose body in the ankle joint). A traumatic osteochondral injury may cause osteochondritis dissecans, but this also often occurs without known antecedent trauma.

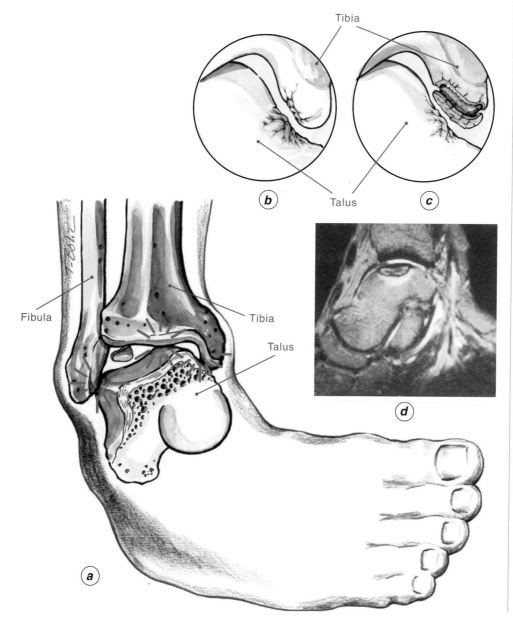

Figure 14.19
Osteochondral injuries. The figure shows the injury mechanism and the typical location of chondral and osteochondral injuries on the talus, tibia, and fibula *(a),* and a superficial (grade I, *b*) and a deep (grade IV, *c*) osteochondral injury. In addition, osteochondritis dissecans may occur without known trauma, as shown on the MRI image *(d).* The fragment is in place and the cartilage above it may be intact. If the bone fragment comes loose, the patient may feel pain and locking in the ankle joint.

ANKLE

411

- Symptoms and signs: Generally, the injury is not recognized when the initial trauma occurs, but eventually the patient seeks medical assistance due to pain that persists or returns some time after the injury occurs. In addition, the patient may be bothered by stiffness and locking. The area is not necessarily tender to palpation.
- Diagnosis: The diagnosis is made using CT or MRI. Scintigraphic evidence of with focally increased uptake also indicates osteochondral damage. CT or MRI makes it possible to distinguish between subchondral fractures (grade I), chondral fractures without detachment (grade II), chondral fractures with detachment but without dislocation (grade III), and chondral fractures with dislocation (grade IV).
- Treatment: An orthopedic surgeon should evaluate patients who have osteochondral injuries. Fractures without detachment (grades I and II) are immobilized in an ankle cast for 6 to 8 weeks without loading, whereas fractures with detachment (grades III and IV) require surgery, either to remove or fix the loose piece of bone. This is often accomplished arthroscopically. After repair, a graded rehabilitation program is necessary before the athlete can return to sport.
- Prognosis: In general, the younger the patient, the less severe the damage, and the better the prognosis. Overall, 70% to 90% of patients with grades III or IV injuries regain normal ankle function.

Synovitis of the Ankle Joint

About 1 to 2 ml of blood often enters the joint immediately upon ankle ligament injury. This blood is usually absorbed quickly, but in a few cases it may contribute to persistent synovitis. Synovitis may also result from increased "play" in the joint due to ligamentous instability. Later in the course, the anterolateral corner of the joint capsule may thicken, making it possible to see on arthroscopy a meniscoid lesion that bulges into the joint (and may cause pain due to impingement).

- Symptoms and signs: Pain upon weight bearing may be localized laterally, medially, anteriorly, and posteriorly. Tenderness to palpation corresponds to the site of greatest discomfort.
- Diagnosis: MRI and arthroscopy may be indicated if anterolateral impingement is suspected.
- Treatment: The treatment of synovitis is primarily NSAIDs and relative rest. A cortisone injection may be helpful. Cortisone is injected intra-articularly through the articular space medial to the tibialis anterior tendon in the posterolateral direction. If the ankle is unstable, the patient should use an orthosis all day until symptoms subside, rather than just during sport activity. Patients who do not respond to conservative treatment should be referred to an orthopedic surgeon for evaluation. Meniscoid lesions can be removed arthroscopically in patients with anterolateral impingement.

Chronic Instability

After an ankle is sprained, some patients experience instability problems from repeated inversion trauma, and they may have the feeling that the ankle will give way in some situations. The disorder may be due to mechanical or functional instability or both. Lengthening of one or more of the ankle stabilizing ligaments (usually as the result of a previous sprain) causes mechanical instability, whereas reduced neuromuscular function causes functional instability.

- Symptoms and signs: The patient reports repeated ankle sprains (usually minor sprains) or a feeling that the ankle simply "gives way" in some positions. Some patients also report associated pain.
- Diagnosis: Positive anterior drawer and talar tilt tests indicate mechanical instability. Balance testing is used to evaluate neuromuscular function. Reduced neuro-

muscular function may cause functional instability, even without signs of mechanical instability.

- Treatment by physician: The patient should tape the ankle or use an orthosis until she has completed an entire rehabilitation program that includes balance and strength exercises. An orthopedic surgeon should evaluate patients with mechanical instability for possible surgical stabilization, if the rehabilitation program does not result in the anticipated gains.
- Treatment by physical therapist: The patient gradually progresses through balance exercises in which he stands on the floor to exercise using balance mats and wobble boards daily for at least 10 weeks. During that time the physical therapist's main job is to instruct the patient in a home exercise program and to evaluate the patient's progress.
- Self-treatment: The patient should use tape or an orthosis in high risk situations to protect the ankle from further trauma at least until he has completed a self-training program in consultation with a physical therapist as described.
- Prognosis: Most patients with instability problems benefit from balance exercises. Surgical stabilization has a good outcome in most cases if there is mechanical instability.

Other Injuries

Sinus Tarsi Syndrome

This encompasses painful conditions that are localized to the tarsal sinus, located on the anterolateral side of the ankle joint (figure 14.20). The syndrome most often occurs among patients who have previously injured their ankle, sustaining damage to the subtalar ligament. The condition may also present as an overuse injury caused by subtalar overpronation.

- Symptoms and signs: The patient usually experiences chronic continuous symptoms after what was considered a "regular" inversion trauma. Pain is localized to the lateral aspect of the ankle, within the tarsal sinus (located in front of the lateral malleolus at the level of the tip of the malleolus). Pain is often described as worse in the morning and usually improves upon warm-up. Worsening pain provoked by running on grass or another soft surface is typical of the syndrome.
- Diagnosis: On physical exam, there is tenderness to palpation over the tarsal sinus. Pain can often be provoked both in full supination and in full pronation. The diagnosis is confirmed if the patient experiences good pain relief after an injection of local anesthetic into the tarsal sinus.
- Treatment by physician: Corrective shoe orthoses should be used if the patient has an increased tendency toward pronation. An injection of cortisone often brings rapid improvement.
- Self-treatment: The patient can treat herself by unloading the affected limb, by applying ice, by modifying her training regimen, and by wearing different shoes.

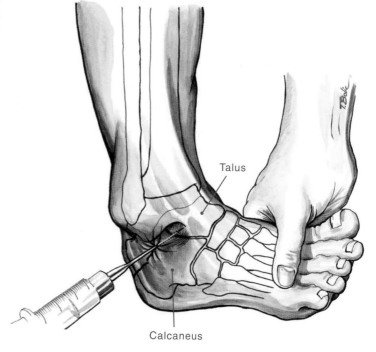

Figure 14.20 Sinus tarsi syndrome. The cortisone injection is given from the lateral side into the tarsal sinus, located a finger's breadth in front and a finger's breadth below the tip of the lateral malleolus. The tip of the needle should be aimed toward the tip of the medial malleolus.

Talus

Calcaneus

ANKLE

413

Anterior Impingement—Soccer Ankle

The anterior impingement syndrome is called "soccer ankle" because it is usually seen in soccer players, but it does also occur among athletes in other sports. Anterior impingement of the ankle joint may cause chronic pain, and it may limit function. Originally, the suggested cause was repeated, forceful plantar flexion from kicking the soccer ball (or the ground) generating a rift in the joint capsule anteriorly (figure 14.21). Another potential cause may be forceful dorsiflexion, resulting in contusion of the anterior tibia against the talus. Over time, this may cause exostoses to develop on the anterior edge of the tibia and eventually on the talus as well. When these osteophytes occur, they cause anterior impingement of the joint capsule. In some cases, osteophyte formation can be seen anteriorly on the tibia, causing a depression ("divot sign") to form in the talus due to repeated "wear."

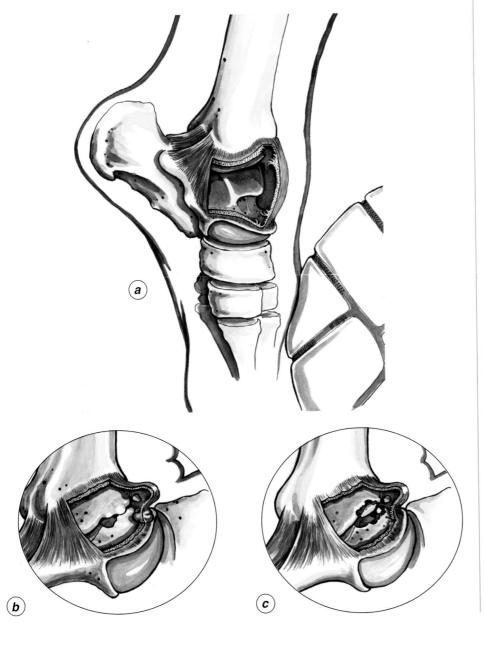

Figure 14.21 Soccer ankle. Possible mechanism of injury resulting in anterior impingement. The injury may be the result of anterior osteophyte formation after bone or capsular injury due to ankle hyperextension in plantar flexion when kicking a ball or the ground (a). Other possible etiologies include repeated contusion of the tibia against the talus in forced dorsiflexion (b, c).

- Symptoms and signs: Pain tends to be activity dependent and is usually triggered in extreme dorsiflexion, often in connection with starting and stopping movements. In subacute cases, the pain may begin after forced dorsiflexion, probably due to bleeding and inflammation in the area. The area is not necessarily immediately tender to palpation anteriorly. Ankle instability after a previous injury may contribute to increased impingement.
- Diagnosis: The athlete's pain may be reproduced by engaging in a starting movement in which the ankle is loaded in forced dorsiflexion. X rays usually demonstrate ossification over the neck of the talus or in the anterior margin of the tibia on a lateral view.
- Treatment by physical therapist: In cases in which instability contributes to the symptoms of impingement, ankle taping or an orthosis may help minimize symptoms.
- Treatment by physician: In subacute cases, antiinflammatory medication may be indicated. If NSAIDs do not work, an injection of cortisone may be attempted. If X rays demonstrate prominent exostoses, the patient should be referred to an orthopedic surgeon for evaluation of possible surgical resection of the exostoses.
- Self-treatment: The patient can self-treat by applying ice, by modifying the loading pattern during training, and by resting.
- Prognosis: The prognosis is good, even in cases that require surgery. Most soccer players return without restrictions after 4 to 6 weeks. The long-term outcome of treatment is unknown, however.

Posterior Impingement—Ballet Ankle

Posterior impingement is caused by a narrowing of the space between the posterior superior talus and the posterior corner of the tibia. The condition is usually called "ballet ankle" because it is common among ballet dancers. Forced plantar flexion (e.g., when assuming demi-pointe and pointe positions) (figure 14.22) is provocative of pain. The condition is also common among gymnasts and soccer players (e.g., after kicks with the ankle extended). In patients with these types of symptoms, ossification usually occurs posteriorly on the talus. The ossicle may become detached, forming an os trigonum (figure 14.22). The practitioner should be aware that an os trigonum (a bone that is not attached to the tibia) is found normally in about 10% of the population. In sports in which forced plantar flexion is preformed repeatedly, this type of ossicle may cause impingement. Posterior contusion injuries are also believed to precipitate ossification in the area.

- Symptoms and signs: The primary symptom of posterior impingement is pain from forced plantar flexion. In subacute cases, pain may begin after one incident of forced plantar flexion (such as a soccer player kicking a ball), probably due to bleeding and inflammation in the area. The patient usually has posterolateral tenderness in the region behind the peroneal tendons, but this does not have to be the case.
- Diagnosis: Pain should be reproduced when the ankle is loaded while in active plantar flexion. X rays (preferably of both ankles) may show osteophytes over the posterior tubercle or an os trigonum. However, osteophytoses (or the lack thereof) does not always correlate with the presence (or absence) of symptoms. Inflammation of the flexor hallucis longus tendon may cause similar symptoms, and the conditions can occur simultaneously. The injection of a small amount of local anesthetic can confirm the diagnosis.
- Treatment by physician: In subacute cases, anti-inflammatory medication may be indicated, and if this does not prove therapeutic, a cortisone injection may be attempted. If neither therapy is effective, the patient should be referred to an orthopedic surgeon to be evaluated for possible surgical removal of the os trigonum or osteophyte.

ANKLE

415

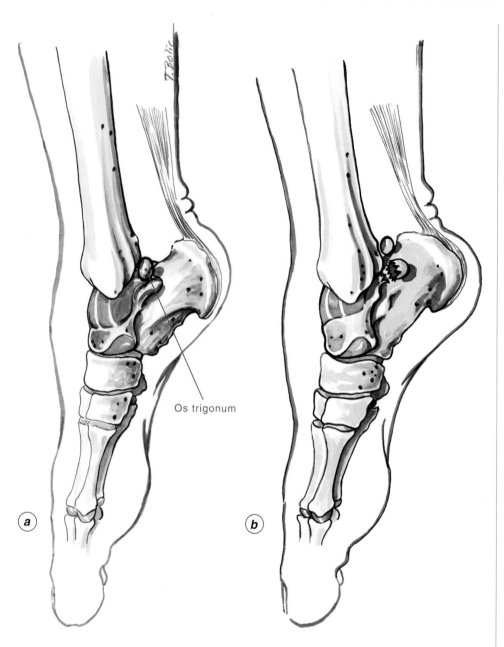

Os trigonum

a

b

Figure 14.22 Ballet ankle. In forced plantar flexion, such as in the pointe and demipointe positions in ballet, the posterior tubercle or an os trigonum *(a)* may become pinched against the posterior aspect of the tibia. Pain may also be caused by the formation of osteophytes, which may subsequently come loose *(b)*.

- Self-treatment: The patient can self-treat by applying ice, by modifying the loading pattern during training, and by resting.
- Prognosis: The prognosis is good, even in cases that require surgery, but rehabilitation may require more than 6 months.

Stress Fractures

Stress fractures may occur both in the talus and the navicular bones, as well as the surrounding bones. Navicular fractures are more common than talar fractures and occur primarily in athletes in flexibility and sprinting sports. Stress fractures of the fifth metatarsal are discussed on page 400.

- Symptoms and signs: Symptoms include exercise-related pain in the affected area. The pain is occasionally described as diffuse and/or radiating. Local tenderness to palpation is a nearly universal finding on physical exam. The navicular bone is palpated by localizing the talonavicular joint first (by moving the forefoot in supination and pronation) and then by palpating the "N-point" (the proximal dorsal portion of the navicular bone). Malalignment, such as overpronation (which presumably predisposes the athlete to the injury), may be found in some patients.

- Diagnosis: The primary radiographic examination for a suspected stress fracture is scintigraphy, because the sensitivity of plain X rays is poor. A positive scintigraphic examination should be followed by an MRI or a CT, to distinguish between stress reaction (negative CT/MRI) and stress fracture (positive CT/MRI).
- Treatment: Stress reactions are treated by unloading without immobilization, but activities that cause pain are not allowed. The athlete's activity level is gradually increased after 2 or 3 weeks. Patients with stress fractures should be referred to an orthopedic surgeon for evaluation. Both the navicular and the talus have poorly vascularized zones where late healing or non-union may occur. Surgery may be indicated in some cases. Normally, the ankle is immobilized in a cast or orthosis for 6 weeks without weight bearing, after which activity can be gradually increased within the limits of pain. To avoid delayed healing, weight bearing should not be allowed during the immobilization stage. Malalignment if present should be corrected with orthoses.

Tibialis Posterior Syndrome—Rupture of the Tibialis Posterior Tendon

Young athletes rarely sustain ruptures of the tibialis posterior tendon (figure 14.23), but older athletes are at relatively greater risk for overuse pathology of the tibialis posterior. In this age group, the distal tendon near the insertion appears to be vulnerable to tearing or overload resulting in pain. The tendon has a broad insertion that includes the navicular bone, all three cuneiform bones, and the second, third, and fourth metatarsals. In rare cases, ruptures of the tibialis posterior may also occur in connection with ankle sprains (usually posterior to the medial malleolus, but trauma may also occur closer to the insertion in the navicular region).

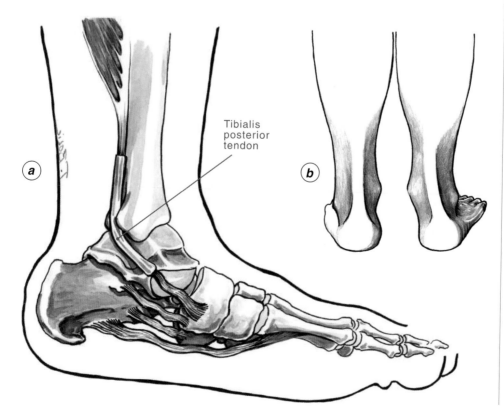

Figure 14.23 Tibialis posterior tendon rupture *(a)*. If a rupture occurs, the patient will develop acute flatfoot. Inspection from behind reveals asymmetry, with several toes visible on the affected side (the "too many toes" sign) *(b)*. In addition, the patient cannot stand on her toes on the affected side.

- Symptoms and signs: If the tendon is not completely torn, the main symptom is continuous activity-related pain along the course of the tendon—either behind the medial malleolus or near the insertion. Patients who sustain a total rupture after an acute episode will occasionally complain of pain medially (e.g., after having stumbled into a hole or having tripped or slipped). In such cases, tenderness will be present above the area of the rupture, and a defect can be palpated if significant swelling has not yet set in. The patient is unable to stand on her toes, the hind foot is in a valgus position, and the "too many toes" sign is present (acute flatfootedness) (figure 14.23). Generally, the patient will state that he has had chronic pain and throbbing in the area. However, many patients will not seek medical assistance in an acute situation. Instead, they wait until after some time has elapsed and their symptoms have increased. These patients may have developed hind foot valgus and overpronation of the forefoot as a consequence of tendon stretching.
- Diagnosis: The best way to confirm the diagnosis is with an MRI, but ultrasound or a CT scan can also be used.
- Treatment: If a rupture of the tibialis posterior tendon is confirmed, the patient should be referred to an orthopedic surgeon for surgical treatment.

Nerve Entrapment—Tarsal Tunnel Syndrome

Nerve entrapment may cause local injury to a peripheral nerve, with inflammation occurring as a result of compression against other anatomical structures. The primary symptom typically is pain or dysesthesia (e.g., numbness, pricking, or a burning sensation). Pain is usually limited if a sensory nerve is involved and is sometimes more diffuse when a motor nerve is affected. In the ankle area, the tibial nerve is affected most commonly, because it passes posterior to the medial malleolus and to the tibialis posterior tendon. Entrapment of the tibial nerve in this region is referred to as "tarsal tunnel syndrome." Entrapment of other nerves in the leg (such as the deep peroneal nerve or the superficial peroneal nerve) is less common. Suspected entrapment disorders should be evaluated and referred to a physiatrist or to a neurologist for confirmatory electrodiagnostic testing.

Osteoarthritis

Arthritis in the ankle joint primarily affects elderly patients who have a history of prior ankle fracture. The main symptoms are pain and stiffness. The diagnosis is confirmed radiographically.

Complex Regional Pain Syndrome !

Complex regional pain syndrome, or reflex sympathetic dystrophy, may occur after ankle injuries (both fractures and ligament injuries alike). The syndrome tends to occur a few weeks or months after initial improvement, with the patient complaining of worsening symptoms. The symptoms consist of increasing pain, swelling, and skin that feels warm or cold. Local sweating and changes in skin color or temperature may occur. Early diagnosis is the key to effective treatment, because the prognosis depends on how soon treatment is started. X rays may eventually show bony demineralization. Patients with reflex dystrophy that do not respond rapidly to conventional pain therapy should be referred to a pain clinic for further evaluation and treatment.

Rehabilitation of Ankle Injuries

Knut Jæger Hansen and Roald Bahr

Acute Ankle Injuries: Rehabilitation Goals and Principles

Table 14.4 lists the goals for rehabilitation of acute ankle injuries.

The injured ankle may be warmed up passively at first, including warm baths, but warm-up should progress to active participation as soon as possible—for example, with the use of a cycle ergometer. Mobilization of the ankle and the joints of the foot may be necessary in rare cases. This can be both active and passive.

The exercise program reflects the goals and uses mobility exercises, strength exercises, functional exercises, and specific exercises to improve neuromuscular function with a gradual progression towards more challenging exercises.

Tape, elastic bandages, or orthoses are used to provide compression during the acute stage. During the rehabilitation stage, tape or an orthosis is used to provide compression and for support, so that training for normal function can begin more quickly. During the training stage, tape or an orthosis is primarily used to prevent reinjury, particularly if the athlete trains on an uneven surface or in other situations that may involve a risk of reinjury.

Ankle Pain and/or Instability: Goals and Principles

The rehabilitation of patients with chronic ankle pain generally focuses on neuromuscular function. The most common cause of ankle pain is a previously sprained

ANKLE

	Goals	Measures
Acute stage	Reduce swelling	The PRICE principle with emphasis on compression
Rehabilitation stage	Normal and pain free range of motion so that the patient can train with normal function	Exercises
Training stage	Normal neuromuscular function; a consequence of ankle injuries may be reduced neuromuscular function with a slow reaction to changes in joint position	Exercises
	Healing of the injured ligament(s) without the loss of mechanical stability or tensile strength	
	Reduce the risk of reinjury	

Table 14.4 Goals and measures for rehabilitation of acute ankle injuries.

ankle that resulted in osteochondral injury and instability. The instability may be mechanical (i.e., the ligaments are permanently overstretched), or functional (i.e., no mechanical instability is present, but neuromuscular function in the ankle is impaired). In almost all cases, a 10-week neuromuscular training program that includes balance exercises should be attempted before the patient is evaluated for possible surgical intervention. The patient should perform 10 minutes of balance training 5 days a week for at least 10 weeks—the 10-5-10 rule.

Preventing Reinjury

Because ankle sprains represent the most common injury in sport, prevention is essential. This is particularly true for athletes with previous ankle injuries, for whom the risk of reinjury is 4 to 10 times greater than for athletes without prior ankle trauma. The risk of reinjury is particularly high during the first 6 to 12 months following a sprain injury for which the athlete has not been adequately rehabilitated.

The following measures have had good results:

Neuromuscular training. Balance training on a wobble board should be performed according to the 10-5-10 rule. The 10-week program may seem excessive, but experience shows that it can easily be completed if the athlete does the exercises daily while doing another activity, such as watching TV. Studies of athletes with instability problems after ankle injuries show that

- neuromuscular function is reduced in patients who complain of instability, including increased reaction time by the peroneal musculature to a sudden inversion stress.
- neuromuscular function may normalize with 10 weeks of training on a balance board.
- training on a balance board substantially reduces the risk of reinjury to the same level as that of ankles that have not been previously injured.

Tape or orthosis. Athletes who do not achieve complete rehabilitation through neuromuscular training should use tape or an orthosis during high risk activities until their rehabilitation is completed. Tests have shown that taping or using an orthotic device prevents reinjury in athletes with a history of ankle sprain, but neither of these methods appear to have any effect on athletes who have not been injured before. This may be due to the manner in which taping and orthotic device apparently work: that is, they improve the ability of the ankle to react quickly to an inversion stress but have a less definite effect as a mechanical support. Recent studies show that the use of an orthosis does not reduce performance with respect to flexibility or speed. If an athlete uses taping or an orthoses, he needs to be well informed about the importance of continuing to use external support until full ankle function is achieved.

Exercise Program

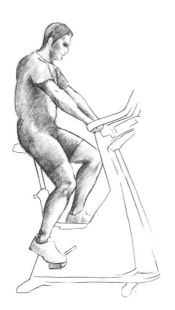

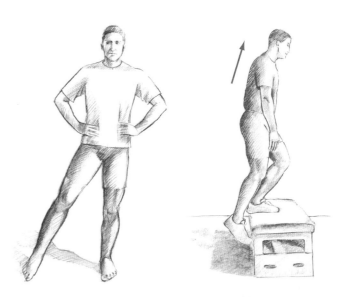

Exercise 14.1 Bicycling

- Use mild resistance.
- Use high frequency.
- Start with your heel on the pedal, then move the loading forward to use your ankle more actively.

Exercise 14.2 Weight transfer and going up a step or stepping on a box

- This is the basis for normal function.
- Train at a controlled pace.
- After long-term injuries, use a treadmill to achieve normal gait.

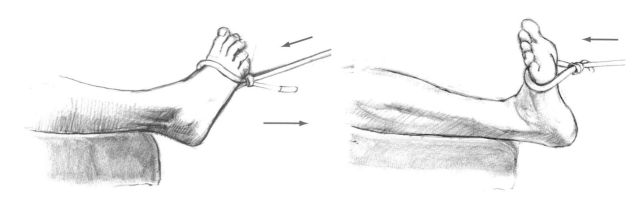

Exercise 14.3 Strength exercise with tension

- Work on endurance strength.
- Consciously use the outer muscle of your lower leg.

ANKLE

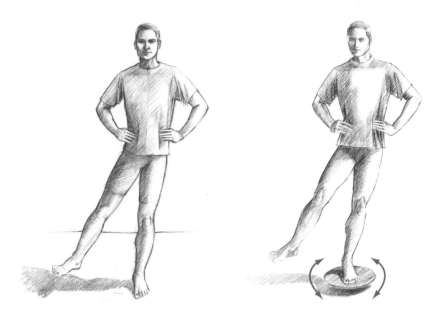

Exercise 14.4 Neuromuscular function: balance exercises while standing

- Be precise about your starting position; keep your knee over your foot and control your hip.
- Increase difficulty by closing your eyes or by adding distractions, such as a ball or other movements.
- Increase difficulty by switching from a soft to a hard surface.

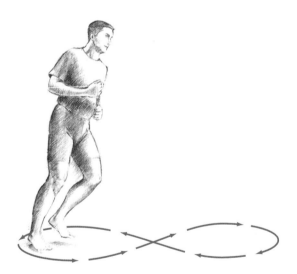

Exercise 14.5 Training in function

- Train in individual exercises for the sport to which the athlete will return.
- Use turns and add distractions.

Acute Foot Injuries

Torbjørn Grøntvedt

Occurrence

The foot serves a complex purpose for athletes, absorbing impact from the ground, carrying body weight, and converting energy from the thigh and lower leg into effective motion for running, jumping, lateral movement, acceleration, and braking. These movements involve significant loading, and a number of factors may contribute to foot injuries. Foot injuries occur most commonly among athletes participating in sports that involve considerable weight bearing activity, such as walking, running, and jumping (table 15.1). In a study of more than 16,000 athletes, 15% of the injuries were localized to the feet. Informing athletes and trainers about routine prophylactic measures, including training conditions, choice of footwear, and the use of insoles, may help to prevent many foot disorders.

Differential Diagnosis

Contusions (injuries caused by impact) and sprains (injuries commonly caused by twisting) are the most common acute foot injuries. Direct trauma, such as having the upper aspect of the foot stepped on by cleats, is common in soccer, whereas orienteering runners usually sprain the ankle because of uneven terrain. More forceful injury mechanisms may result in a fracture or a dislocation in various places in the foot. The foot contains 26 bones that form 30 different joints, and all these bones and joints are vulnerable to injury. Fractures are most common in the toes and metatarsals, less common in the calcaneus and talus, and extremely rare in the

Most common	Less common	Must not be overlooked !
Fractures of the phalanges and metatarsals (p. 427)	Dislocations (p. 428)	Gout (p. 426)
Calcaneal fracture (p. 428)		
Talar fracture (p. 405)		
Fracture at the base of the fifth metatarsal (p. 400)		
Contusions and sprains (p. 429)		
Blisters (p. 429)		

Table 15.1 Overview of the differential diagnosis of acute foot injuries.

tarsal bones (navicular, cuboid, and the three cuneiform bones). Dislocations are most common in the toe joints, less common in the tarsometatarsal joints (together referred to as the Lisfranc joint), and rare in the other foot joints. Foot blisters are common and may be very annoying until the affected area is unloaded. Gout may cause acute severe pain, usually localized to the metatarsophalangeal joint of the big toe, with associated warmth, erythema, and swelling. In young athletes, the symptoms of gout may be misinterpreted as an acute injury.

Diagnostic Thinking

A good clinical history is essential if the patient has an acute injury. Depending on the severity of the trauma, it may be possible to determine whether the patient has a fracture or just a contusion or sprain. If the patient has a mild soft-tissue injury or a sprained joint, it is often possible for the patient to bear weight on the foot; however, if the foot is fractured or dislocated, pain makes weight bearing almost impossible. A thorough clinical assessment that examines, palpates, and tests the structures in the foot will provide good information about injury severity and whether supplemental diagnostic examinations, such as routine X rays or computed tomography (CT), are necessary. Generally, the patient should be referred for X rays anytime there is the slightest suspicion of a fracture.

Clinical History

If the patient has an acute injury, it is usually easy to document the injury mechanism via the clinical history. Fractures or soft tissue contusions are often the sequelae of direct trauma, whereas indirect trauma usually results in a ligament injury (sprain).

Clinical Examination

Inspection. The practitioner should look for malalignment, discoloration of the skin, and swelling, as well as wounds. Dislocated toe joints are easily diagnosed by inspection. In such cases, the differential diagnosis is limited to dislocation with or without concomitant fracture.

Palpation. Thorough palpation of the bones, ligaments, joints, and other soft tissues of the foot provides important information about what is injured, and it can often permit the clinician to determine whether a dislocation or a fracture has occurred. For example, in the case of a metatarsal fracture, direct pressure over the bone, or longitudinal distraction or compression via the corresponding toe will trigger pain (indirect tenderness).

Movement. The various joints in the foot are tested for abnormal laxity and to determine whether movement triggers pain. The best way to determine whether foot motion is normal or not is to compare it with the opposite, healthy side.

Supplemental Examinations

Radiographic examination. X rays must be taken for acute injuries if there is the slightest suspicion of a fracture.

CT. If a tarsal fracture or dislocation has occurred, CT is often indicated to further define the extent of injury. A CT with three-dimensional reconstruction of the injured area can provide useful supplemental information to X rays. This is done routinely prior to surgical treatment of complicated foot injuries.

Common Injuries

Fractures of the Phalanges and Metatarsals—Toe and Midfoot Fractures

The metatarsals and phalanges are frequently fractured in athletes and nonathletes alike. Fractures usually result from direct trauma to the dorsum of the foot or to the toes but may also be caused by strong torsional trauma. Fractures resulting from direct trauma are usually transverse in orientation but may also be comminuted whereas oblique or spiral fractures typically result from indirect trauma (figure 15.1). Intra-articular fractures occur most commonly in the metatarsophalangeal joint of the big toe.

- Symptoms and signs: Symptoms and signs include pain (particularly in response to loading), swelling, possibly discoloration of the skin or skin perforation, and malalignment.
- Diagnosis: Palpation causes significant pain that corresponds to the fracture. Indirect tenderness is typical of metatarsal fractures. The diagnosis is confirmed by X rays.
- Treatment: Fractures of the metatarsals and phalanges that are not dislocated or are only slightly dislocated are treated by unloading, until the patient is pain free. Short-term casting (3 to 4 weeks) is an option if the patient is in considerable pain. Wearing stiff-soled shoes provides sufficient pain relief for most patients. Dislocated fractures, particularly intra-articular ones, must be surgically reduced and fixed. Avulsion fractures at the base of the fifth metatarsal may be somewhat slow to heal, due to persistent distraction by the action of the peroneus brevis (which inserts at the proximal end of the metatarsal). Therefore, open reduction and screw fixation may be necessary to ensure healing.
- Prognosis: Simple fractures of the metatarsals and phalanges heal quickly, and the athlete can usually return to training in 4 to 6 weeks. If surgery is necessary, the patient can count on a somewhat longer rehabilitation period.

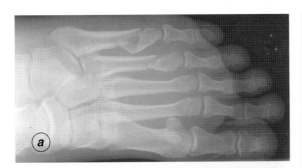

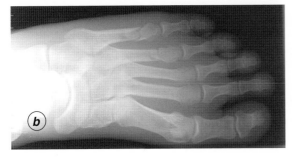

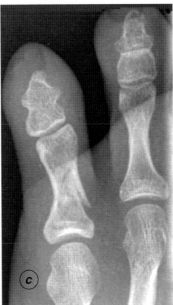

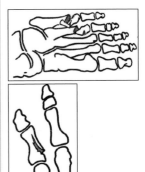

Figure 15.1 Fractures. Oblique fractures through the distal portions of the fourth and fifth metatarsals *(a)* and *(b)*. Fractures of the proximal phalanx of the little toe *(c)*.

Calcaneal Fractures—Heel Bone Fractures

Calcaneal fractures (figure 15.2) result when an individual lands on his heels after usually jumping or falling from a height. Calcaneal fractures often occur bilaterally. Parachute jumpers frequently sustain calcaneal fractures. The force of impact affects injury severity. Minimal force (from low-energy trauma) usually results in a simple fracture without significant malalignment that can be treated conservatively. High-energy trauma is more likely to crush the calcaneus. The most striking radiographic finding in such cases is a decrease in Boehler's angle (the subtalar joint angle). Clinically, this may cause the foot to flatten, and the talar-calcaneal articulation may be more or less dislocated.

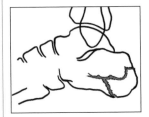

Figure 15.2 Nondisplaced Y-fracture in the calcaneus.

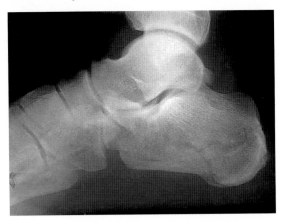

- Symptoms and signs: Calcaneal fractures are typically extremely painful, particularly when weight bearing. Slight swelling occurs during the early phase, while acquired flatfoot, a dislocated Achilles tendon insertion, and a widened heel are visible even before swelling and discoloration of the skin begin. Ankle joint motion is often normal.
- Diagnosis: The diagnosis is based on X rays of the heel in two planes. To demonstrate the extent of injury before surgical intervention, a three-dimensional CT reconstruction of the calcaneus is often obtained.
- Treatment: Non-displaced fractures may be treated with a low boot-shaped cast for 4 weeks. The patient is allowed to bear weight as soon as it can be done painlessly. Displaced fractures should be treated surgically, to restore the subtalar joint angle and to reduce the upper articular surface of the calcaneus.
- Prognosis: Fractures that are not dislocated heal without sequelae, and the patient regains normal foot function. In case of a comminuted calcaneal fracture, particularly with concomitant depression of the subtalar articular surface, the outcome depends on how well the calcaneus is surgically reconstructed. Many of these patients end up with a somewhat flatter and wider foot, and some eventually develop osteoarthritis of the subtalar joint.

Dislocations

Dislocations involving the toes and the tarsometatarsal joint (Lisfranc joint) are relatively common. Dislocations of the talonavicular-calcaneocuboid joint (Chopart joint) are less common, and dislocations of the talus and the calcaneus are even rarer.

- Symptoms and signs: Pain, malalignment, and swelling are the primary symptoms and signs.
- Diagnosis: The diagnosis is based on the clinical examination, supplemented by frontal, lateral, and (usually) oblique X rays. Three-dimensional CT reconstruction may provide useful additional anatomic detail of the dislocated joint. Dislocation is often combined with fracture in these areas.
- Treatment: If the dislocation is unstable after reposition, the preferred treatment is exact anatomical reduction and pin fixation. Early mobilization is important to prevent the joint from becoming stiff.
- Prognosis: The prognosis is good if exact reduction is achieved and the patient is mobilized rapidly. If the injury results in chronic subluxation, the patient often has chronic pain exacerbated by loading and osteoarthritis will develop in the involved joint(s).

Contusions and Sprains

Contusions and sprains often affect the soft tissues and joints of the foot. Most of the time, if no dislocation has occurred, the articular capsules and ligaments will heal without lasting symptoms.

- Symptoms and signs: Pain, swelling, and bruising over the injured area are the primary symptoms and signs.
- Diagnosis: The history and clinical examination are usually diagnostic. In doubtful cases, an X ray examination should be done to exclude fracture.
- Treatment: PRICE and nonsteroidal anti-inflammatory drugs (NSAIDs) are used during the acute phase. To avoid stiffening of the foot, the athlete must begin weight bearing and mobility training as soon as pain allows. Sometimes taping provides effective pain relief.
- Prognosis: The prognosis is generally good. If a contusion has occurred, the athlete is usually back at full activity after a few days, whereas painful sprains of the tight articular capsules of the foot may take 4 to 6 weeks to heal.

Blisters

Blisters are typically harmless but may sometimes be extremely painful and even disabling. Blisters affect all types of athletes, particularly those for whom running is a major feature of their sport. Blisters are usually caused by new shoes or by switching to an unfamiliar surface, such as from outdoor to indoor training.

- Symptoms and signs: The patient experiences gradually increasing pain over the area that is subjected to friction, most often over the calcaneus or under the big toe. The skin becomes erythematous and a vesicle develops. At first the blister contains a clear fluid, but the contents may become bloody. When the blister bursts, it may cause an open wound to form if friction and irritation continue.
- Diagnosis: The diagnosis is made on the basis of the history and physical inspection.
- Treatment: Blister prevention is undoubtedly the best type of treatment. If friction is anticipated, the skin over the expected area of involvement is treated with ointments (such as salicylic acid ointment) or is protected with special bandages (e.g., Compeed). These simple interventions may also prove effective if applied when symptoms first appear. Clean, dry, soft socks also provide good protection. When the blister first forms, a sterilized needle or hypodermic cannula should be inserted into the edge of the blister to empty it without damaging the skin above it. The layer of skin above the blister should not be removed, as it serves to protect the exposed dermis while new epidermis forms. The dead skin can be cut off after a few days. If an open wound forms, no loading is allowed, and the area must be kept as clean as possible, to minimize the risk of infection. If infection ensues it should be treated with cleansing baths, systemic antibiotics, and sterile bandages changed daily.

FOOT

Foot Pain

Torbjørn Grøntvedt

Occurrence

Running, jumping, and lateral movements all repetitively load the feet, which in turn transfer this load up through the ankle, lower leg, knee, thigh, hips, and pelvis to the spinal column. Running on a flat surface has been shown to load the foot with a force equivalent to roughly three times body weight. Jumping and running downhill increase this load even further. When running, the foot strikes the ground 480 to 1200 times per kilometer. Therefore, a significant cumulative load must be absorbed by the foot and transferred elsewhere. The ability of the foot to tolerate repetitive loading depends on the anatomy and biomechanics of the athlete's foot, which should have an appropriate combination of stiffness and elasticity. A foot that deviates from the norm will have a lower threshold for developing chronic overuse injuries. Although overuse injuries are caused by anatomical deviation (malalignment), they are precipitated by weight bearing. Foot malalignment is relatively common, even among athletes. A foot that was originally normal, with good height on both the longitudinal and the transverse arches, may gradually become overpronated. A runner who has no prior history of overuse disorders may suddenly develop an injury, such as Achilles pain, a stress fracture of the tarsus, or plantar fasciitis, during a period of intense training.

Differential Diagnosis

The most common chronic painful conditions of the foot are stress fractures and plantar fasciitis (table 15.2). Chronic irritation of the soft tissues around a sesamoid bone (sesamoiditis), injuries to the joint capsule of the metatarsophalangeal joint of the big toe, and irritation of the periosteum and soft tissues around the heads of the second to the fourth metatarsals (metatarsalgia) also occur frequently. Morton neuroma and cuboid syndrome may occur in athletes

Most common	Less common	Must not be overlooked !
Stress fractures (p. 433)	Sesamoiditis (p. 436)	Morton's neuroma (p. 438)
Plantar fasciitis (p. 435)	Hallux rigidus (p. 436)	Cuboid syndrome (p. 439)
	Metatarsalgia (p. 438)	Tarsal tunnel syndrome (p. 418)
	Calcaneal apophysitis (p. 385)	Sinus tarsi syndrome (p. 413)
	Hallux valgus (p. 437)	Heel pain (p. 441)
		Osteoarthritis

Table 15.2 Overview of the differential diagnosis of chronic foot pain.

but are relatively rare. Heel pain due to repeated impact to the heel pad with irritation of the underlying periosteum is common in sport and in some cases may be difficult to treat. Rheumatic disorders may affect the joints in the feet, and gout often causes typical pain, rubor, and swelling over the metatarsophalangeal joint of the big toe. Sciatica may cause pain that radiates distally into the foot. Reduced blood supply due to arteriosclerosis can cause ischemic pain with activity, particularly in diabetics. Acute pain, if left undiagnosed and untreated, may become chronic in time.

Diagnostic Thinking

Chronic overuse disorders may be difficult to understand. Training problems and the development of symptoms can be uncovered in the clinical history. The two goals of the physical examination are to make the diagnosis and to identify any anatomical or biomechanical predisposing factors. The patient must be examined while standing, walking, and preferably while running on a treadmill, to determine whether there is any lower limb malalignment. A video taken while the patient is running, which can thereafter be analyzed in slow motion, may be useful. Minor malalignment can be discovered and possibly corrected with simple aids such as sole orthoses. Therefore, the goal of the treatment of chronic overuse disorders is to change the athlete's loading pattern by correcting training problems and malalignment.

Clinical History

If the patient has a chronic overuse disorder, a more detailed history is necessary to determine whether the injury was caused by internal or external factors or by a combination thereof. High volume running on hard surfaces predisposes an athlete to stress fractures and to plantar fasciitis, and if the foot is malaligned, the athlete often will observe that his shoes have become worn on one side. Information about when and where the foot symptoms originated with respect to the loading pattern is critical to making the correct diagnosis. For example, an acute stress fracture of one of the metatarsals might occur during training. Pain associated with stress fractures is usually well-localized, whereas the symptoms of plantar fasciitis typically develop more gradually and are diffusely located on the plantar surface of the foot.

Clinical Examination

It is necessary to be familiar with normal foot motion and mechanics while running. The first stage of the weight bearing portion of the gait cycle is heel strike, which occurs when the heel strikes the ground in a slightly supinated position (i.e., so that the outer side of the heel pad strikes the ground first). The next stage is the support stage. After heel strike, the foot pronates until the foot contacts the ground. As the heel transitions from a supinated to a more neutral position, the foot softens to permit it to adapt to the surface and the lower leg rotates medially. The third stage is "toe-off" stage, during which the forefoot pushes off against the ground, the heel raises up, and the foot supinates. This "locks" the tarsus, stiffening the foot and enhancing toe-off. The final stage of the gait cycle is the swing phase, during which the foot once again prepares for heel-strike.

The two main types of foot malalignment that predispose the athlete to injury are flatfoot (pes planus) and cavus foot. Flatfoot causes overpronation and valgus positioning of the heel with weight bearing. Overpronation also results in increased internal rotation of the tibia, thereby increasing the load on the medial aspect of the lower leg, the knee, and the patellofemoral joint. At toe-off, the amount of supination is insufficient to allow the foot to "lock," and consequently the athlete becomes less efficient in

FOOT

toe-off. In addition to predisposing the athlete to overuse disorders of the lower extremity, a flat foot will tend to impair performance in sports that require good jumping ability (such as the high jump and long jump).

Athletes who run with their foot externally rotated overload the medial arch of the foot and eventually develop longitudinal flatfoot.

A cavus foot is characterized by a high longitudinal arch, and in addition the athlete is frequently found to have a deep-lying anterior portion of the first metatarsal. This causes the anterior medial portion of the foot to contact the ground too early during weight acceptance, making the pronation movement too small and preventing the foot from unlocking. As a result, a cavus foot tends to remain stiff during the entire loading phase, which in turn compromises shock absorbency. Consequently, the plantar fascia, the midfoot bones, and the metatarsal fat pad are prone to overloading. Thus, athletes with cavus feet are susceptible to overuse disorders but tend to do well in sports that require good jumping ability.

An imprint of the foot may provide useful information about the athlete's foot type (figure 15.3).

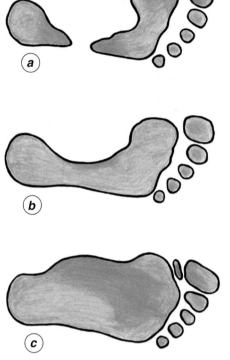

Figure 15.3 Footprints. Cavus foot (clawfoot, pes cavus) *(a)*, normal foot *(b)*, and overpronated foot (flatfoot, pes planus) *(c)*.

Inspection. An athlete with an overuse injury of the foot must be carefully examined when walking, standing, and lying down. The entire lower extremity, the pelvis, and the back must also be systematically examined. The physician must look for scoliosis, anisomelia, toeing in, varus and valgus positioning of the knee(s), malrotation of the lower leg(s), tightness of the Achilles tendon(s), and, last but not least, foot malalignment (particularly cavus foot and overpronation). All these conditions may be important contributing factors to chronic injuries. Well-worn jogging shoes should always be examined and will often reveal wear patterns characteristic of foot malalignment that may be difficult to detect during a clinical examination.

Palpation. If the patient has a metatarsal stress fracture, pain will be triggered by direct palpation over the area of the fracture and by indirect pressure along the bone's longitudinal axis. The plantar fascia should be carefully palpated with the toes in a dorsiflexed position (thereby tightening the fascia) (figure 15.4). Circulation in the foot is examined by palpating the dorsalis pedis and the posterior tibial arterial pulse. Microcirculation can be examined by pressing on the nail bed of the big toe and then

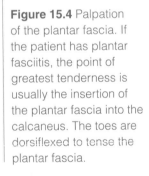

Figure 15.4 Palpation of the plantar fascia. If the patient has plantar fasciitis, the point of greatest tenderness is usually the insertion of the plantar fascia into the calcaneus. The toes are dorsiflexed to tense the plantar fascia.

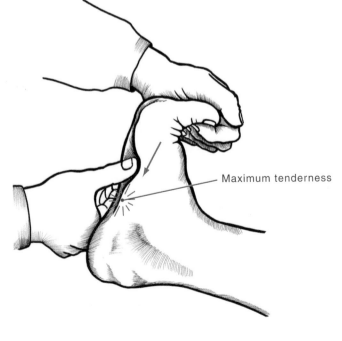

— Maximum tenderness

measuring how long it takes for the natural pink color to return. Cutaneous sensibility may be tested both by palpation and by gentle poking with a sharp object. These tests make it possible to document whether a specific nerve is injured, as might occur in a distal lower-leg pressure injury.

Supplemental Examinations

Radiographic examination. Plain X rays in two planes are often indicated if the patient has a chronic, painful condition of the foot. X rays are useful in demonstrating any malalignment and particularly helpful for excluding other pathology. Stress fractures result in either callus formation (i.e., healing) or the development of pseudoarthrosis (i.e., incomplete healing), whereas chronic plantar fasciitis often causes a beak-shaped calcification (heel spur) to form at the insertion of the fascia on the inferior aspect of the calcaneus.

Scintigraphy should always be ordered if a stress fracture is suspected. It is particularly difficult to demonstrate tarsal stress fractures radiographically: plain films may be negative even if the disorder is chronic, while skeletal scintigraphy is generally positive 1 or 2 days following the onset of symptoms.

Magnetic resonance imaging (MRI) is rarely indicated for foot injuries. If the patient has sinus tarsi syndrome, an MRI may show local changes after subtalar ligament injuries (see chapter 14). A Morton's neuroma, and even a ganglion that may be producing symptoms, can be demonstrated on MRI. An MRI with appropriate detail of the affected bone will also demonstrate the stress fracture shortly after the onset of symptoms.

CT may be indicated for evaluating stress fractures that do not resolve despite adequate treatment. In such cases, CT may demonstrate the development of a pseudoarthrosis.

Stress Fractures

Stress fractures of the foot are relatively common among athletes whose training regimen consists predominantly of running and/or jump training. Several studies have shown that up to 25% of all stress fractures involve the tarsus, particularly the navicular bone. Both overpronation and cavus foot increase loading of the navicular bone, predisposing this tarsal bone to stress fractures. Stress fractures of the foot are almost always directly related to sudden increases in the amount or intensity of training, to exercising on unforgiving hard surfaces, and to footwear that lacks adequate shock absorption. Other bones in the foot that are particularly vulnerable to stress fractures are the metatarsals ("march fractures") and the sesamoid bones beneath the head of the first metatarsal and the base of the fifth metatarsal.

- Symptoms and signs: Patients typically experience pain of acute onset often during a training session. The pain may disappear at rest but rapidly returns in response to loading.
- Diagnosis: A history of acute, localized pain associated with loading should lead the clinician to suspect a stress fracture. Findings on examination include local tenderness and possibly mild swelling over the fracture. The "hop test" (see page 377, in the chapter on the lower leg) is positive if the patient develops localized pain. An X ray may demonstrate a fissure in the shaft of the involved metatarsal, at the base of the fifth metatarsal, or through the affected sesamoid bone, but radiography is usually negative in the case of a tarsal fracture. Skeletal scintigraphy is diagnostic in this situation, with intense radiotracer uptake corresponding to the location of the fracture (figure 15.5). An MRI of the affected bone will also reveal the diagnosis.

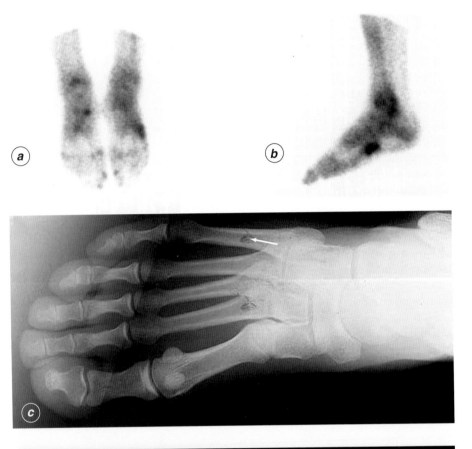

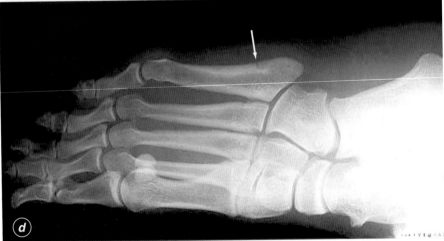

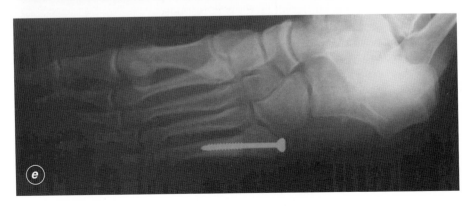

Figure 15.5 Stress fracture at the base of the fifth metatarsal. Skeletal scintigraphy demonstrates strong radiotracer uptake at the base of the fifth metatarsal *(a)* and *(b)*. The X ray view demonstrates a fissure (fracture line) through the base of the fifth metatarsal *(c)* and *(d)*. The X ray view demonstrates the status after surgical fixation of the fracture using a compression screw in the bone marrow canal of the fifth metatarsal *(e)*.

- Treatment: The affected limb should be unloaded, preferably making it non-weight bearing (with crutches) for 4 to 8 weeks, depending on the location of the fracture. For metatarsal fractures, a brief period without weight bearing is often sufficient, whereas fractures of the tarsus in general and of the navicular bone in particular take longer to heal, apparently because of a poorer blood supply. Alternative exercises, such as bicycling, aquatic training, and strength training are important during the non-weight bearing period. Active training with appropriate loading must be resumed gradually and carefully, preferably under the guidance of a physical therapist. When possible, foot malalignment and other intrinsic risk factors should be identified and corrected; otherwise, the injury often recurs. It is difficult to heal stress fractures of the base of the fifth metatarsal and of the sesamoid bone under the head of the first metatarsal due to traction exerted on these bones by the peroneus brevis and the flexor hallucis brevis, respectively. Therefore, these fractures are often treated surgically, with reduction and screw osteosynthesis of the fifth metatarsal (figure 15.5) and extirpation of one fragment of the bifid sesamoid bone. In some cases, pseudoarthrosis may develop in other bones as well, particularly the navicular bone. A CT examination can demonstrate the pseudoarthrosis, for which the recommended treatment is surgical screw fixation of the two fragments to each other.
- Prognosis: Stress fractures of the foot generally heal well if the patient begins an appropriate treatment in a timely manner. Secondary prevention is important, with correction of any malalignment, reduction in the amount and intensity of training, and avoidance of training on hard surfaces.

Plantar Fasciitis—Tendinosis of the Fascia in the Sole of the Foot

The most common cause of heel pain in athletes is plantar fasciitis, a chronic painful condition at the insertion of the plantar fascia onto the calcaneus (figure 15.6). Plantar fasciitis is caused by chronic traction of the fascia, which often results in microruptures of the aponeurosis. Over time, the disorder may cause a heel spur (calcification at the calcaneal insertion) to form. Heel spurs can be easily demonstrated radiographically. Cavus foot, overpronation, and a high volume of running on hard surfaces are the most common predisposing factors associated with plantar fasciitis.

- Symptoms and signs: Patients experience well-localized inferior calcaneal pain with weight bearing in addition to significant morning stiffness. In mild cases, pain may occur only at the onset of training or on the first steps out of bed every morning. In more serious cases, every single step causes pain.
- Diagnosis: The diagnosis is based on an appropriate history, documenting gradually progressive symptoms. On exam, the patient typically identifies his greatest pain on palpation of the inferior-anterior aspect of the calcaneus (figure 15.4). An X ray may demonstrate a calcaneal spur in this region.
- Treatment: Treatment options include a period of restricted weight bearing, alternative exercises, NSAIDs, a heel lift, and shoe inserts with cutouts corresponding to the painful area. Stretching the plantar fascia and the calf musculature may also be useful. An injection of cortisone in the vicinity of the insertion of the fascia may be attempted once, but it should not be repeated if the desired effect is not

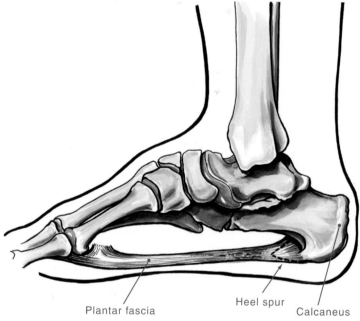

Plantar fascia

Heel spur

Calcaneus

Figure 15.6 Plantar fasciitis. The figure shows the area for maximal histopathological changes and pain in red. Heel spurs (calcification of the insertion of the plantar fascia onto the calcaneus) may form in this area.

FOOT

achieved. Inadvertent injection into the fascia itself may weaken the tissue and lead to rupture. Good results have been achieved by using a night splint for 1 or 2 months (to stretch the plantar fascia). Correction of the external and internal factors that trigger the disorder is critical to prevention of recurrent symptoms. Occasionally, conservative treatment does not produce satisfactory results, in which case the patient may be offered surgery to separate the plantar fascia from its insertion on the calcaneus. Removal of any calcaneal spurs is unnecessary.

• Prognosis: The outcome of surgical treatment in athletes is good; most patients become asymptomatic quickly and may resume their training routines within 4 to 6 weeks. Overpronation may worsen somewhat with time after surgery, and the patient should be fitted with orthoses to help prevent this.

Sesamoiditis—Inflammation Around the Sesamoid Bone

The sesamoid bones found beneath the head of the first metatarsal are surrounded by tendinous tissue. The sesamoid articular surface with the metatarsal is covered with hyaline cartilage. The sesamoid bones are subjected to significant loading, not only from traction exerted by the flexor hallucis brevis, but by direct ground reactive force produced by the gait cycle. Overuse may trigger an inflammatory reaction (sesamoiditis) in the soft tissues surrounding the sesamoid bone. "Toe runners" (i.e., athletes who load only the forefoot when running) are particularly vulnerable to this disorder.

• Symptoms and signs: Pain beneath the metatarsophalangeal joint of the big toe that is associated with weight bearing is the primary symptom.
• Diagnosis: The diagnosis is based on local tenderness and possibly mild swelling over the affected sesamoid bone. Scintigraphy may demonstrate increased radiotracer uptake, whereas plain X rays do not typically show signs of a stress fracture.
• Treatment: Recommended treatment options include a brief period of unloading, NSAIDs, correction of the amount of training, and, when feasible, examination of the athlete's running technique. Footwear with good shock absorption, possibly incorporating extra insoles or padding with a cutout for the painful area, is often the best therapy. Cases that are resistant to treatment for a long time may require surgical extirpation of the sesamoid bone.

Hallux Rigidus (Turf Toe)—Degeneration of the Metatarsophalangeal Joint of the Big Toe

High energy trauma, or repeated minor trauma to the metatarsophalangeal (MTP) joint of the big toe with the joint in dorsiflexion (turf toe syndrome) or plantar flexion (sand toe syndrome), may cause irritation of the MTP. The joint capsule may become inflamed, prompting gradually progressive cartilage formation and calcification in this region, particularly on the head of the first metatarsal. This gradually restricts joint mobility, and dorsal flexion in particular becomes painful. Excessive training on artificial turf with rapid stops and dorsal sprains of the joint are the principle triggering causes for turf toe. Athletes who play beach volleyball may develop sand toe syndrome due to repeated plantar flexion trauma to the joint.

• Symptoms and signs: Patients experience pain in the region of the metatarsophalangeal joint of the big toe from activities such as running and cross-country skiing. This pain is precipitated by movements that involve dorsiflexion of the MTP joint or by running and jumping on a soft surface, like sand.
• Diagnosis: The diagnosis is made on the basis of tenderness, particularly on the dorsal side of the metatarsophalangeal joint of the big toe, possibly with associated swelling. A protruding cartilaginous edge can occasionally be palpated near the joint dorsally and medially. Dorsal flexion is restricted and painful. An X ray

may demonstrate osteophytes, particularly close to the edge of the distal articular surface of the first metatarsal.

- Treatment: For acute injuries, the recommended treatment consists of PRICE and NSAIDs. Taping the joint to avoid excessive dorsiflexion should be attempted; the patient should be advised to wear shoes that have slightly stiff soles for a while. For long-term disorders with manifest osteophytosis, surgery to remove cartilage and new bone formation (cheilectomy) is an option.
- Prognosis: The prognosis is good if degeneration of the cartilage in the joint has not occurred. If there is articular degeneration, the patient will likely have lasting symptoms, and arthrodesis of the big toe's metatarsophalangeal joint may be necessary.

Hallux Valgus

Hallux valgus is defined as excessive lateral displacement of the big toe (figure 15.7). The condition is most common in older women but may even occur in teenage girls. Hallux valgus is caused by one or more anatomical displacements in the foot, and the disorder occurs most in association with transverse flatfoot. In small children the axis goes through the first metatarsal and the big toe together, whereas at the end of the growth period the great toe is normally angulated in 15° to 20° of valgus. This valgus positioning seems to be partially related to wearing shoes, since the condition almost never occurs in people who do not wear shoes. If the valgus position exceeds the upper normal limit of 20°, biomechanical factors (including traction on the metatarsophalangeal joint by the flexor and extensor tendons) will further reinforce the big toe's tendency to assume a valgus position. The head of the first metatarsal is pressed medially, and pressure from the shoe will produce chronic irritation of the bursa on the medial side of the head. Eventually, an exostosis will form in this area, which will aggravate the pressure imbalance. Lateral migration of the big toe will cause the adjacent toes to assume hammertoe deformity.

- Symptoms and signs: Pain gradually increases over a "corn" that develops on the medial aspect of the head of the first metatarsal. Pain also occurs from wearing tight shoes. The skin over the corn becomes red, irritated, and tender. The patient will eventually develop pain in the second and third toes, because of increasing malalignment and pressure.
- Diagnosis: Clinical examination reveals the typical corn that is both red and tender, a broadened forefoot, valgus positioning of the big toe, and possibly hammertoe deformity of the second and third toes. If motion at the metatarsophalangeal joint of the great toe triggers pain, it may indicate that osteoarthritis is developing in the joint. X rays of the foot are always indicated when evaluating the patient for surgical treatment.
- Treatment: For moderate malalignment and only minimal symptoms, initial treatment is conservative. A transverse flatfoot can be corrected by using a transverse pad, which should rest behind the heads of the middle (second to fourth) metatarsals elevating them up off the sole of the shoe. In addition, the patient should wear footwear that has a roomy toebox of sufficient depth and width. Narrow, pointed shoes

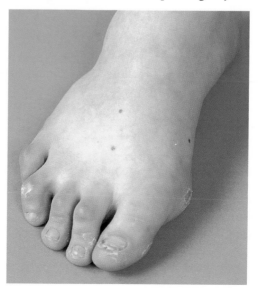

Figure 15.7 Hallux valgus. The patient is flatfooted and has significant valgus alignment of the first metatarsal. Pressure points are visible over the head of the first metatarsal medially and dorsally on the other toes. The patient also has nail fungus on the big toe.

FOOT

will rapidly worsen the patient's symptoms. If the symptoms and malalignment are advanced, the patient should be offered surgical treatment. This is accomplished by removing the exostoses in combination with either corrective osteotomy of the first metatarsal or a soft tissue correction of the tendons and joint capsule to align the toe. Postoperatively, the patient must wear a redressing cast for 6 weeks, after which free mobilization is allowed.

- Prognosis: The prognosis is good if both the associated transverse flatfoot and the patient's shoes are corrected early on. Surgical treatment usually also produces good results, but some patients have a recurrence of the malalignment and symptoms after a while. If the cartilage of the big toe's metatarsophalangeal joint is severely damaged, primary MTP arthrodesis should be performed.

Metatarsalgia

Metatarsalgia (pain under the heads of the second to fourth metatarsal bones) occurs frequently in people with transverse flatfoot where the heads of the second to the fourth metatarsals are deeper than normal. This results in slight hammertoe deformity of the corresponding toes, and the heads of the metatarsals are subject to greater loading than normal. Eventually, the periosteum and soft tissues surrounding the heads of these metatarsals become irritated.

- Symptoms and signs: Pain with weight bearing is the primary symptom.
- Diagnosis: The diagnosis is based on tenderness over the heads of the metatarsals upon palpation of the plantar aspect of the forefoot. Most patients have manifest transverse flatfoot, possibly combined with nascent hallux valgus malalignment.
- Treatment: Recommended treatment includes a brief period of unloading, followed by correction of the transverse arch of the foot by an appropriately fitted shoe insert.
- Prognosis: The prognosis is good with early correction of the transverse arch.

Morton's Syndrome (Interdigital Neuroma)

The nerves to the toes enter the soft tissue between the metatarsals proximally (figure 15.8). Sometimes these nerves become pinched as they pass between the heads of the metatarsals. The nerve between the third and fourth toes is the most vulnerable to injury. Pressure may irritate the nerve, resulting in neuroma formation. As the neuroma enlarges, the pressure further increases and the symptoms worsen. The disorder is most common in patients with transverse flatfoot.

- Symptoms and signs: Typical symptoms include potentially disabling pain in the forefoot upon walking and running.
- Diagnosis: The diagnosis is made on the basis of upon palpation of the space between the heads of the involved metatarsals. The patient's pain may radiate out into the affected toes, and sensation may be reduced in the cutaneous distribution of the involved nerves. Squeezing the forefoot from side to side or a forceful dorsiflexing of the toes will often provoke pain. The neuroma may be sufficiently large that it can be palpated as a fluid-filled sac between the metatarsals. An MRI may show thickening of the involved nerve (figure 15.8c).
- Treatment: Correction of transverse flatfoot with insoles and the use of wide shoes often provides relief from symptoms. If the symptoms are chronic, surgical resection of the neuroma is often necessary. Postoperatively, the patient should unload the affected foot for 2 weeks, after which loading is gradually increased and the athlete may resume training.
- Prognosis: Surgical treatment may have a surprisingly positive effect on patients with long-standing symptoms. Usually, the pain disappears completely, although some patients may experience slight discomfort for a few weeks following the intervention.

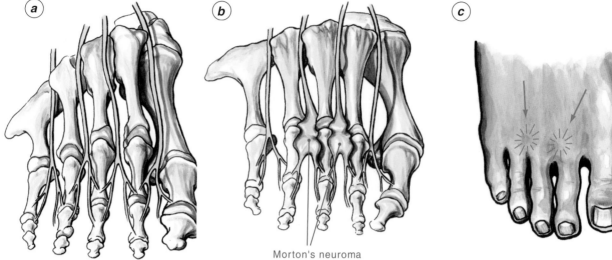

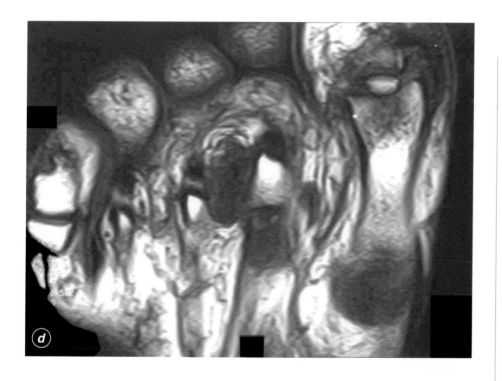

Morton's neuroma

Figure 15.8 Morton's neuroma. Normal toe nerves *(a)*. Morton's neuroma ("nerve tumors") between the heads of the second and third metatarsals, and between the third and fourth metatarsals *(b)*. The areas of maximum tenderness with pressure from either the dorsal or plantar side are located in the space between the metatarsal heads *(c)*. MRI demonstrates a large neuroma between the second and third metatarsals *(d)*.

Cuboid Syndrome—Subluxation of the Cuboid Bone !

The peroneus longus tendon courses beneath the foot, entering laterally from directly in front of the calcaneus and then sloping anteriorly and medially until it inserts onto the base of the first metatarsal (figure 15.9). The tendon is normally located in a small groove on the underside of the cuboid bone. Excessive running (or other training involving repetitive cyclical weight bearing) may precipitate lateral heel pain, radiating along the course of the peroneus longus tendon. Such symptoms may result from plantar subluxation of the cuboid bone. Long-term loading causes the ligaments to be overstretched and the cuboid bone may glide slightly downward.

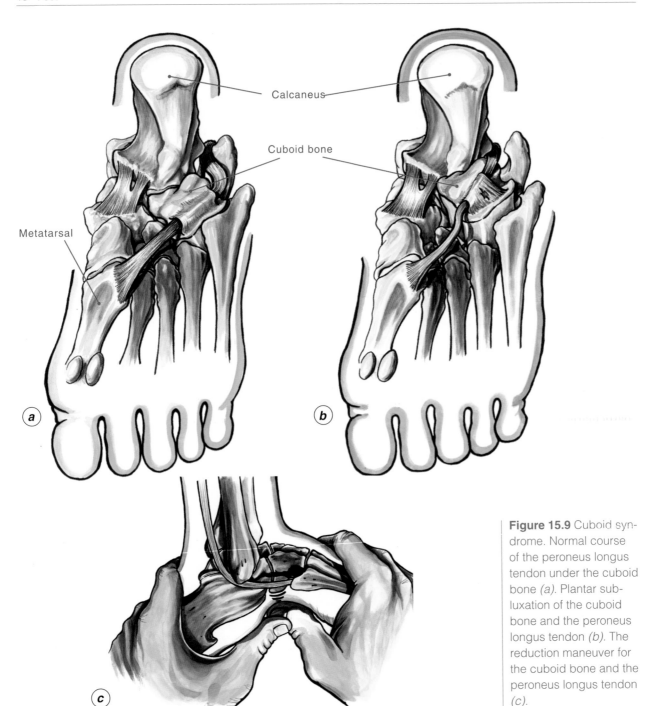

Calcaneus

Cuboid bone

Metatarsal

a

b

c

Figure 15.9 Cuboid syndrome. Normal course of the peroneus longus tendon under the cuboid bone *(a)*. Plantar subluxation of the cuboid bone and the peroneus longus tendon *(b)*. The reduction maneuver for the cuboid bone and the peroneus longus tendon *(c)*.

This in turn could cause the peroneus longus tendon to slide out of its groove, thereby forcing the cuboid out of position.

- Symptoms and signs: Pain is localized to the lateral aspect of the foot, underneath and slightly behind the lateral malleolus. Loading increases pain.
- Diagnosis: The diagnosis is based on tenderness to palpation over the peroneus tendon where it passes to the plantar side of the foot. Tenderness over the inferior surface of the midfoot (corresponding to the underside of the cuboid bone) is also typically present.
- Treatment: Forceful manipulation of the cuboid bone in an attempt to relocate it is recommended (figure 15.9). With the patient in a prone position and the knee

bent to 90°, the physician grasps the foot with both hands so that the thumbs are on the sole of the foot, under the cuboid. The physician then rapidly plantar flexes the foot while pressing firmly against the cuboid. If manipulation succeeds, a click may be audible as the cuboid is reduced. If initially unsuccessful, manipulation can be repeated after an injection of local anesthetic into the painful area. Following manipulation, the cuboid bone should be held in place with a slight buildup of padding adherent to the sole beneath the midfoot. The athlete may gradually resume his training routine.

Heel Pain—Injury to the Heel Pad !

Sudden forceful impact (or repeated impact) to the heel–such as that incurred by jumping onto or running on a hard surface–may traumatize the calcaneal fat pad, resulting in bleeding and crushing the connective tissue septae that hold the fatty tissue in place. This impairs the heel pad's shock-absorbing properties and eventually repetitive loading will irritate the periosteum of the calcaneus. Long jumpers and triple jumpers are particularly vulnerable to this type of injury (figure 15.10).

- Symptoms and signs: Heel pain on loading is the principal symptom.
- Diagnosis: The diagnosis is made on the basis of tenderness to palpation over the injured part of the heel. Often the reduced volume of fatty tissue covering the calcaneus is obvious on inspection.
- Treatment: Recommended treatment includes unloading the injured area with shock-absorbing inserts or heel cups (such as Tulis), and/or fitting special insoles with cutouts to relieve the most painful area. General unloading is recommended, particularly after acute injury. The patient may need to walk with crutches for 2 or 3 weeks to properly unweight the heel.
- Prognosis: Recovery may be somewhat lengthy, depending on the severity of the injury.

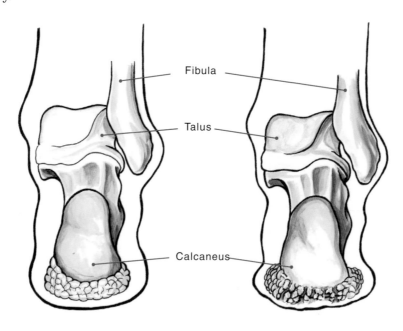

Fibula

Talus

Calcaneus

Figure 15.10 Injury to the heel pad. Normal heel pad with intact connective tissue septae and intact fatty tissue architecture *(a)*. If the fibrous septae are destroyed, the fat of the heel pad will be displaced laterally and medially *(b)*.

FOOT

Index

Note: Page numbers followed by an italicized *f* or *t* refer to the figure or table on that page, respectively.

About the Contributors

Contributing Authors

Arne Kristian Aune, MD, PhD, is a specialist in general and orthopedic surgery and is the head of the orthopedic department at Volvat Medical Center in Oslo. A consulting orthopedic surgeon for the Norwegian national downhill ski team, Dr. Aune has a PhD from the University of Oslo on the biomechanics of knee injuries.

Jens Ivar Brox, MD, PhD, is a staff physician at the department of orthopedics at Rikshospitalet University Hospital, Oslo. Dr. Brox is a specialist in physical medicine and rehabilitation. His PhD thesis was on shoulder problems, and he has published extensively on the treatment for various back disorders. Dr. Brox is the national team physician for the Norwegian track and field team.

Lars Engebretsen, MD, PhD, is a professor at the faculty of medicine at the University of Oslo and at the Norwegian University of Sport and Physical Education. Professor Engebretsen is head of the orthopedic department at Ullevål University Hospital, Oslo, and he is a physician for the Norwegian national soccer team. He has been on the Olympic medical staff since the 1992 Barcelona Games and is the chief medical officer for the 2004 Olympic Games in Athens. Professor Engebretsen is the co-chair of the Oslo Sports Trauma Research Center with professor Roald Bahr. Professor Engebretsen has written numerous publications on sports injuries and their treatment and is involved in several international sports medicine organizations.

Bjørn Fossan, PT, is a certified specialist in manual therapy and sports physical therapy. He is the head of the physical therapy department at the Olympic Training Center in Oslo, has been a member of the Norwegian medical team for six Olympic Games, and will be the head physical therapist for the 2004 Olympic Games. He has also worked with several national teams and elite clubs, specifically in alpine and cross-country skiing, for more than 20 years.

Hilde Fredriksen, PT, is a certified specialist in manual therapy and sports physical therapy, and she works in the physical therapy department at the Norwegian Olympic Training Center in Oslo. She has been a physical therapist for the Norwegian team at two Olympic Games and several international championships, and she has worked with several national teams and elite clubs, specifically in track and field, alpine skiing, and rowing.

Torbjørn Grøntvedt, MD, PhD, is the head of the arthroscopy section at the orthopedic department at St. Olavs Hospital; a senior lecturer at the faculty of medicine at the Norwegian University of Science and Technology; and the head of Rosenborg Sportsklinikk AS, a private sports medicine clinic in Trondheim. His PhD thesis was on the treatment of anterior cruciate ligament injuries, and he is involved in continuing research on this subject. Dr. Grøntvedt is a former president of the Norwegian Society of Sports Medicine and was a physician for the Norwegian women's national team in team handball and for the Norwegian team at the 2000 Olympic Games in Sydney.

Knut Jæger Hansen, PT, is a cofounder and majority owner of the Norwegian Sports Medicine Institute, Norway's largest private sports medicine clinic in Oslo. He is a certified specialist in manual therapy and sports physical therapy. He is president of the Norwegian Society of Sports Physical Therapy and has worked in the emergency room during Norway Cup for 15 years. He has been a physical therapist for the Norwegian teams at several Olympic Games and major international championships, and he has worked with many national teams and elite clubs in various sports.

Jan-Ragnar Haugstvedt, MD, is a senior consultant at the hand and microsurgery section of the department of orthopedics at the Rikshospitalet University Hospital, Oslo. Dr. Haugstvedt's research interests include biomechanics and instability in the carpus and the wrist.

Oddvar Knutsen, PT, is a certified specialist in manual therapy and sports physical therapy. Knutsen was a physical therapist at the Olympic Training Center and was head of the medical team for the Norwegian Skiing Federation, working with the alpine skiing team, for several years. He also worked with the Norwegian team at the 2002 Olympic Games in Salt Lake City and with the Norwegian wrestling and track and field teams during the European Championships and World Championships.

Paul McCrory, MD, PhD, is a neurologist and sports physician and is director of the Head Injury Service at Box Hill Hospital in Melbourne, Australia. He also works at the Centre for Sports Medicine Research & Education and the Brain Research Institute at the University of Melbourne. His PhD thesis was on the clinical manifestations of concussion, and he has published widely on this topic. He was the team physician for a national Australian football team for 15 years. Dr. McCrory is president of the Australian College of Sport Physicians and editor of the British Journal of Sports Medicine.

Grethe Myklebust, PT, MSc, is a certified specialist in sports physical therapy and a research fellow at the Oslo Sports Trauma Research Center at the Norwegian University of Sport and Physical Education. Her research focus is on the prevention of anterior cruciate ligament injuries in sport. She is the team physical therapist for the Norwegian national beach volleyball teams and has been the team physical therapist for the women's handball and soccer teams. She serves on the medical staff of several Norwegian Olympic teams and the Olympic Training Center.

Ingunn R. Rise, MD, PhD, is a staff physician at the department of neurosurgery at Rikshospitalet University Hospital in Oslo. She has a PhD in neurosurgery.

Per Skjelbred, MD, DDS, PhD, is a professor and chair of the department of oral and maxillofacial surgery at Ullevål University Hospital, Oslo. He is chair of the Special Committee for Maxillofacial Surgery and Diseases of the Oral Cavity and an honorary member of the Baltic Organization for Plastic and Maxillofacial Surgery.

Roger Sørensen, MD, is an orthopedic surgeon and head of the spine surgical department at the Rikshospitalet University Hospital in Oslo, a national resource center for deformity surgery.

Stein Tveten, MD, PhD, is the head of a private clinic for facial surgery in Düsseldorf, Germany. He has served as chief physician for the department of oral and facial surgery at Ullevål University Hospital, Oslo, and is trained as both a physician and a dentist, specializing in oral and facial surgery.

Stein Tyrdal, MD, DDS, PhD, is a specialist in general and orthopedic surgery and is the head of the outpatient surgery clinic at Ullevål University Hospital, Oslo. Dr. Tyrdal is the former head of the health department at the Olympic Training Center. His PhD focused on elbow problems among team handball goalies.

Illustrator

Lill-Ann Prøis, illustrator, attended the Bergen Art Academy for four years, training in education and graphic design with an emphasis on illustration. Prøis taught drawing at the upper-secondary school level for 24 years. She has participated in several collective exhibits and is an illustrator of children's books.

About the Editors and Illustrator

Roald Bahr, MD, PhD, is a professor of sports medicine and chair of the Oslo Sports Trauma Research Center and the department of sports medicine at the University of Sport and Physical Education in Oslo, Norway. He also is a consulting physician in the department of sports medicine at the National Sports Center. His primary research area is sports injury prevention. Dr. Bahr is a former national team volleyball player and coach. Dr. Bahr is certified as a sports medicine physician by the Norwegian Society of Sports Medicine and is a fellow of the American College of Sports Medicine. He currently serves as a team physician for the Norway national volleyball and golf teams and is secretary of the Medical Commission of the International Volleyball Federation. He is a former president of the Norwegian Society of Sports Medicine.

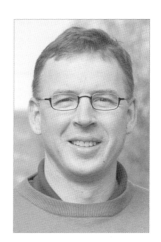

Dr. Bahr lives with his wife, Ingrid, and their three children in Oslo, Norway. He enjoys playing volleyball and golf in his spare time.

Sverre Mæhlum, MD, PhD, is currently the medical director of Pfizer Norway. He has served as chief medical officer for the Norwegian Olympic team at six Olympic Games and worked as a professor of sports medicine at the University of Sport and Physical Education for 10 years. He is a specialist in physical medicine and rehabilitation and an authorized sports medicine physician by the Norwegian Society of Sports Medicine. He is a former president of the Norwegian Society of Sports Medicine. His work is widely published in the field of exercise physiology and sports medicine.

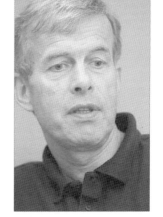

Dr. Mæhlum lives with his wife, Jorunn, in Oslo, Norway, and enjoys running, playing tennis, and hunting in his free time.

Tommy Bolic, medical illustrator, has sport experience as both a top athlete and coach and has more than 10 years of experience teaching on the topic of sports injuries. He has been a medical illustrator for over 30 years, and his work includes *Sports Injuries: Their Prevention and Treatment,* by Peterson and Renström. This work has been translated into 10 languages and is one of the best-selling books on the topic.

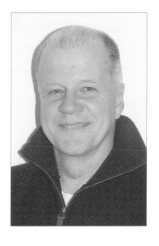

CD-ROM Instructions

The CD-ROM packaged with this text includes the artwork presented in the book. The artwork is organized in folders that correlate to the chapter in which that piece of art can be found. For example, to view figure 5.6 from the book, go to the chapter 5 folder on the CD-ROM and open fig 05.06.

The *Clinical Guide to Sports Injuries CD-ROM* can be viewed on either a Windows®-based PC or a Macintosh® computer.

Microsoft® Windows®

- IBM PC compatible with Pentium® processor, or higher
- Windows® 95/98/2000/ME/XP/NT 4.0
- 1x CD-ROM drive
- Printer (optional)
- Monitor set to display 256 colors
- Mouse

Macintosh®

- System 7.x/8.x/9.x/10.x
- 1x CD-ROM drive
- Printer (optional)
- Monitor set to display 256 colors
- Mouse

Windows® and Microsoft® are registered trademarks of Microsoft Corporation.

Getting Started—Microsoft® Windows®

1. Insert the CD-ROM.
2. Double-click the "My Computer" icon on your desktop
3. Double-click the icon for your CD-ROM drive.
4. Select the folder and artwork you wish to access.

Getting Started—Macintosh®

1. Insert the CD-ROM.
2. Double-click the "Bahr" CD-ROM icon on your desktop.
3. Select the folder and artwork you wish to access.

For technical support contact:

Human Kinetics
P.O. Box 5076, Champaign, IL 61825-5076
217-351-5076 or support@hkusa.com
www.HumanKinetics.com